CONTEMPORARY ENDOCRINOLOGY

Series Editor:
P. Michael Conn, PhD
Oregon Health & Science University
Beaverton, OR, USA

For further volumes:
http://www.springer.com/series/7680

Christian A. Koch · George P. Chrousos
Editors

Endocrine Hypertension

Underlying Mechanisms and Therapy

Humana Press

Editors
Prof. Dr. med. habil. Christian A. Koch
Director, Division of Endocrinology
Head, Endocrine Tumor Program
Cancer Institute
University of Mississippi Medical Center
Jackson, MS, USA

George P. Chrousos, MD, MACP, MACE, FRCP (UK)
Professor and Chairman
First Deparment of Pediatrics
Director, Division of Endocrinology
Metabolism and Diabetes
University of Athens Medical School
Children's Hospital Aghia Sophia
Athens, Greece

ISBN 978-1-60761-547-7 ISBN 978-1-60761-548-4 (eBook)
DOI 10.1007/978-1-60761-548-4
Springer New York Heidelberg Dordrecht London

Library of Congress Control Number: 2012941617

Printed on acid-free paper

Humana Press is a brand of Springer
Springer is part of Springer Science+Business Media (www.springer.com)

Preface

The prevalence of hypertension is almost three times as high as that of diabetes mellitus type 2, with both conditions being major risk factors for stroke, ischemic heart disease, cardiac arrhythmias, and heart failure. The exact prevalence of hypertension related to hormonal derangements, a.k.a. endocrine hypertension, is not known but estimated to affect less than 15% of hypertensive patients. Recent scientific discoveries have increased our understanding of the pathophysiologic mechanisms of hypertension. For instance, there is accumulating evidence on the vitamin D, testosterone, and growth hormone deficiencies as potential risk factors for development of metabolic syndrome, including its constituent hypertension, and cardiovascular disease. In addition to insulin resistance, obesity-associated hypertension may play a role in these conditions, as prevalence rates of obesity have reached up to 34% in several populations. As it is true for many other disorders, better understanding of disease mechanisms may help improve diagnosis and offer affected patients novel targeted therapies.

For many conditions related to endocrine hypertension—for instance, adrenal tumors hypersecreting aldosterone or cortisol—identifying the cause may even lead to curative therapy if undertaken in a timely fashion and in the absence of additional underlying risk factors for hypertension, such as obesity and/or metabolic syndrome. The challenge remains when to assign an endocrine cause in a hypertensive patient and *Endocrine Hypertension* hopefully will assist in this endeavor.

The first part of *Endocrine Hypertension* is dedicated to adrenal hypertension, with the first chapter providing an excellent review on primary aldosteronism, the most frequent cause of hypertension in syndromes of mineralocorticoid excess (Chap. 2). Chapters 3, 4, and 5 discuss rare adrenal disorders linked to glucocorticoid action, such as Cushing's syndrome, primary generalized familial or sporadic glucocorticoid resistance (Chrousos syndrome), and congenital adrenal hyperplasia. Chapter 6 reviews the topic adrenal incidentalomas and hypertension, an important aspect in the era of modern imaging. Catecholamine excess from pheochromocytoma and paraganglioma is discussed in Chap. 7.

The second part of *Endocrine Hypertension* concerns nonadrenal potential causes of hypertension, such as growth hormone excess or deficiency, primary hyperparathyroidism, vitamin D deficiency, testosterone deficiency, insulin resistance, obesity-associated hypertension, and the role of central mineralocorticoid receptors and cardiovascular disease. It should also be mentioned that hypothyroidism can lead to volume-dependent blood pressure elevation with low plasma renin concentrations (Stabouli S, et al., Expert Rev Cardiovasc Ther 2010;8(11):1559–65; Ittermann T, et al., J Clin Endocrinol Metab 2012;97(3):828–34; Cai Y, et al., Hypertens Res 2011;34(10):1098–1105).

The editors of *Endocrine Hypertension* are grateful to the authors for their hard work and the precious time that they spent to produce their outstanding, state-of-the-art chapters. At these hard times, scholarly activity such as this has become difficult, with the ever increasing pressure to publish primary data necessary to generate research grants. *Endocrine Hypertension* will hopefully be a useful resource not only to adrenal investigators and fellow endocrinologists and diabetologists, but to translational scientists and clinicians from cardiology, pediatrics, general internal medicine, family medicine, geriatrics, urology, and reproductive medicine/gynecology.

Jackson, MS, USA — Christian A. Koch
Athens, Greece — George P. Chrousos

Acknowledgement

We are very grateful to Kevin Wright and Richard Lansing from Springer Publisher for their continuous crucial support from the inception, to the execution and finalization of this book project.

Christian A. Koch
George P. Chrousos

Contents

Contributors

Smita B. Abraham, MD The *Eunice Kennedy Shriver* National Institute of Child Health and Human Development, National Institutes of Health, Bethesda, MD, USA

Jacopo Burello, MD Department of Medicine and Experimental Oncology, AOU San Giovanni Battista, Torino, Italy

Angela L. Carrelli, MD Department of Medicine, Division of Endocrinology, College of Physicians and Surgeons, Columbia University, New York, NY, USA

Evangelia Charmandari, MD, PhD Division of Endocrinology and Metabolism, First Department of Pediatrics, University of Athens Medical School, Children's Hospital Aghia Sophia, Athens, Greece

George P. Chrousos, MD, MACP, MACE, FRCP Division of Endocrinology, Metabolism and Diabetes, First Department of Pediatrics, University of Athens Medical School, Children's Hospital Aghia Sophia, Athens, Greece

Valentina Crudo, MD Department of Medicine and Experimental Oncology, AOU San Giovanni Battista, Torino, Italy

Elise P. Gomez-Sanchez, DVM, PhD Research Service, G.V. (Sonny) Montgomery VA Medical Center, Jackson, MS, USA

Division of Endocrinology, Department of Medicine, The University of Mississippi Medical Center, Jackson, MS, USA

Gregory Kaltsas, MD Department of Pathophysiology, Laikon General Hospital, Athens University Medical School, Athens, Greece

Vitaly Kantorovich, MD Division of Endocrinology and Metabolism, Department of Internal Medicine, University of Arkansas for Medical Sciences, Little Rock, AR, USA

Tomoshige Kino, MD, PhD Unit on Molecular Hormone Action, Program in Reproductive and Adult Endocrinology, *Eunice Kennedy Shriver* National Institute of Child Health & Human Development, National Institutes of Health, Bethesda, MD, USA

Christian A. Koch, MD, PhD, FACP, FACE Division of Endocrinology, University of Mississippi Medical Center, Jackson, MS, USA

Eugen Melcescu, MD Division of Endocrinology, University of Mississippi Medical Center, Jackson, MS, USA

Leilani B. Mercado-Asis, MD, PhD Section of Endocrinology and Metabolism, University of Santo Tomas Hospital, Manila, Philippines

Deborah P. Merke, MD The *Eunice Kennedy Shriver* National Institute of Child Health and Human Development and the National Institutes of Health Clinical Center, , Bethesda, MD, USA

George R. Merriam, MD Department of Medicine, Division of Metabolism, Endocrinology and Nutrition, University of Washington School of Medicine, VA Puget Sound Health Care System, Tacoma, WA, USA

Silvia Monticone, MD Department of Medicine and Experimental Oncology, AOU San Giovanni Battista, Torino, Italy

Paolo Mulatero, MD Department of Medicine and Experimental Oncology, AOU San Giovanni Battista, Torino, Italy

Karel Pacak, MD, PhD Program in Reproductive and Adult Endocrinology, Eunice Kennedy Shriver National Institute of Child Health and Human Development, National Institute of Health, Bethesda, MD, USA

Theodora Pappa, MD Endocrinology Department and Diabetes Center, Athens General Hospital "G. Gennimatas", Athens, Greece

George Piaditis, MD Endocrinology Department and Diabetes Center, Athens General Hospital "G. Gennimatas", Athens, Greece

Jeremyjones F. Robles, MD Program in Reproductive and Adult Endocrinology, Eunice Kennedy Shriver National Institute of Child Health and Human Development, National Institute of Health, Bethesda, MD, USA

Sudha S. Shankar, MD Department of Experimental Medicine, Merck Research Laboratories, Rahway, NJ, USA

Shonni J. Silverberg, MD Department of Medicine, Division of Endocrinology, College of Physicians and Surgeons, Columbia University, New York, NY, USA

Helmut O. Steinberg, MD Department of Diabetes and Endocrinology, Merck Research Laboratories, Rahway, NJ, USA

Vin Tangpricha, MD, PhD Section of Endocrinology, Division of Endocrinology, Diabetes & Lipids, Emory University School of Medicine, Atlanta VA Medical Center, Atlanta, GA, USA

Davide Tizzani, MD Department of Medicine and Experimental Oncology, AOU San Giovanni Battista, Torino, Italy

Daniel H.P. Towie, MD Bristol Royal Infirmary, University of Bristol Faculty of Medicine, Bristol, UK

M. Iftekhar Ullah, MD, MPH Division of Internal Medicine and Hypertension, Department of Medicine, University of Mississippi Medical Center, Jackson, MS, USA

Gabriel I. Uwaifo, MD Department of Medicine, Section of Endocrinology, Diabetes and Metabolism, Louisiana State University Health Care System, New Orleans, LA, USA

Franco Veglio, MD Department of Medicine and Experimental Oncology, AOU San Giovanni Battista, Torino, Italy

Andrea Viola, MD Department of Medicine and Experimental Oncology, AOU San Giovanni Battista, Torino, Italy

Tracy Ann Williams, PhD Department of Medicine and Experimental Oncology, AOU San Giovanni Battista, Torino, Italy

Michael Zitzmann, MD Center for Reproductive Medicine and Andrology, Westfaelische Wilhelms University, Muenster, Germany

Part I
Adrenal Hypertension

Chapter 1
Primary Aldosteronism: Progress in Diagnosis, Therapy, and Genetics

Paolo Mulatero, Tracy Ann Williams, Silvia Monticone, Andrea Viola, Davide Tizzani, Valentina Crudo, Jacopo Burello, and Franco Veglio

Abstract Primary aldosteronism (PA) is the most frequent cause of secondary hypertension and its prevalence increases with the severity of hypertension. The importance of PA diagnosis is not just related to offering a targeted treatment, that is, adrenalectomy, for aldosterone-producing adenoma and medical therapy with mineralocorticoid receptor antagonists for bilateral adrenal hyperplasia, but also because it has been demonstrated extensively that patients affected by PA are more susceptible to cardiovascular events and target organ damage compared to essential hypertensives. Herein, we review the pathophysiology of PA and its clinical features and potential complications; the three step approach employed in the diagnosis of PA, established by the Endocrine Society Guidelines, that is, screening, confirmation/exclusion, and subtype diagnosis are discussed; the rarer, familial, and sporadic genetic forms of PA are explained and we conclude with a section on targeted PA therapy.

Keywords Primary aldosteronism • Secondary hypertension • Aldosterone • Vascular and perivascular inflammation • Mineralocorticoid excess • Renin-angiotensin-aldosterone system

Introduction

Primary aldosteronism (PA) was first described by Conn [1] as a frequent cause of secondary hypertension caused primarily by an aldosterone-producing adenoma (APA) associated with hypokalemia and metabolic alkalosis. PA was subsequently considered as a rare and benign condition accounting for less than

P. Mulatero (✉) • T.A. Williams • S. Monticone • A. Viola •
D. Tizzani • V. Crudo • J. Burello • F. Veglio
Department of Medicine and Experimental Oncology, AOU San Giovanni Battista,
Via Genova 3, Torino 10126, Italy
e-mail: paolo.mulatero@libero.it

C.A. Koch and G.P. Chrousos (eds.), *Endocrine Hypertension: Underlying Mechanisms and Therapy*, Contemporary Endocrinology, DOI 10.1007/978-1-60761-548-4_1,

2% of hypertensives [2] and this view persisted for some considerable time; however, over the last 15 years, the ARR (aldosterone/plasma renin activity ratio) screening test has been applied not just to hypokalemics, but also to normokalemic hypertensives, resulting in a 5- to 15-fold increase in PA diagnosis [3]. Recent studies have reported that only a minority—less than a third—of patients are hypokalemic and thus, the presence of hypokalemia should not be considered a prerequisite for pursuing diagnostic tests for PA [4]. PA prevalence increases with the severity of hypertension: from 2% in patients with grade 1 hypertension [5] increasing to 20% in resistant hypertensives [6]. Utilizing new cut-off levels for serum cortisol, aldosterone, and aldosterone/renin ratio, autonomous cortisol and aldosterone secretion from single adrenal adenomas appear to be very common with aldosterone secretion correlating with arterial blood pressure [7]. Nevertheless, the prevalence and the clinical features of PA in the general hypertensive population is still a matter of debate and largely unknown. The reported PA prevalence varies widely, ranging from 1.4 to 32%; this can be explained, at least in part, by differences in either study design (prospective vs. retrospective) and/or diagnostic criteria (including screening and confirmatory strategies). Therefore, the actual prevalence of PA among unselected hypertensives is still unknown, but nonetheless, can be estimated as around 4% [8]. However, it has been hypothesized recently that autonomous aldosterone secretion may be present in more than 30% of hypertensive patients [9].

It should be emphasized that the absence of hypokalemia is often due to the method of blood collection; for example, the use of cuff, tourniquet, and fist clenching can mask the hypokalemia in a significant proportion of PA patients [10].

The importance of PA diagnosis is not just related to offering targeted treatment (surgical, that is, adrenalectomy, for APA and medical with mineralcorticoid receptor antagonists for bilateral adrenal hyperplasia [BAH]), but also because it has been demonstrated extensively that patients affected by PA are more susceptible to cardiovascular events and target organ damage compared to essential hypertensives [11, 12].

Herein, we review the pathophysiology of PA and its clinical features and potential complications; the three step approach employed in the diagnosis of PA, established by the Endocrine Society Guidelines, that is, screening, confirmation/exclusion, and subtype diagnosis are discussed; the rarer, familial, and sporadic genetic forms of PA are explained and we conclude with a section on targeted PA therapy consisting of either surgery (unilateral laparoscopic adrenalectomy) or pharmacological management with a mineralocorticoid receptor antagonist.

Classification

PA comprises a wide spectrum of conditions ranging from a solitary unilateral nodule producing aldosterone to bilateral diffuse or nodular hyperplasia, with several intermediate phenotypes. However, operatively, two major causes of primary aldosteronism are recognized: BAH, accounting for 60–70% of PA patients (Table 1.1), and APAs, accounting for 30–35% of PA [3]. Rarer causes are familial forms of PA,

Table 1.1 Classification of primary aldosteronism subtypes, divided according to therapeutic approach

Unilateral forms of PA (surgically treatable)	
Aldosterone-producing adenoma	30–40%
Unilateral adrenal hyperplasia	<5%
Aldosterone-producing carcinoma	Rare
Bilateral forms of PA (medically treated)	
Bilateral adrenal hyperplasia	60–70%
Familial hyperaldosteronism type I	Very rare

Patients with familial hyperaldosteronism type II should be treated like sporadic forms

unilateral adrenal hyperplasia (UAH), and aldosterone-producing carcinoma, and a few cases of paraneoplastic hyperaldosteronism have also been described [4].

Pathophysiology of Primary Aldosteronism

Adrenal Pathology

Histological analysis of adrenal glands removed from PA patients indicates that the subdivision of APA and BAH, useful from a clinical and operative perspective, oversimplifies the complex alterations that they undergo: in fact, the adrenals of patients with PA exhibit heterogeneous histological alterations. For example, APAs are rarely composed of a single cell type, but rather, exhibit different cell types in varying proportions comprising: *zona fasciculata*-like cells, clear cells with large vacuolated lipid-laden cytoplasm, and round central nuclei; lipid-poor *zona glomerulosa*-like cells; *zona reticularis*-like cells, compact eosinophilic cells; cells with cytological features of both *zona fasciculata* (ZF) and *zona glomerulosa* (ZG) cells showing variable contents of clear lipid micro-vacuoles and granular eosinophilic cytoplasm, also called "hybrid" or "intermediate" cells [13, 14].

Consequently, APA have been classified by some authors according to the prevalent cell type and have attempted to relate the histological findings to some clinical phenotype. For example, the prevalence of ZG-like cells corresponded to responsiveness to angiotensin II infusion and so these APA were denominated, AngII-responsive APA or AR-APA; in contrast to the presence of a prevalence of ZF/reticularis or hybrid cells that correlated to adrenocorticotropic hormone (ACTH) responsiveness (AngII-unresponsive APA, AU-APA) [16]. However, a correlation between cell type and response to posture, and thus to angiotensin II was not observed in another study [17]. Interestingly, most APA patients display either diffuse hyperplasia of the surrounding ZG in the rest of the adrenal or hyperplasia of the ZG with multiple nodules of different sizes, ranging from micro- to macro-nodules [13]. A few reports have studied the contralateral adrenal gland and described similar findings of nodular hyperplasia thereby suggesting that PA may begin, at least in some cases, with one or more unknown stimuli that trigger the development of multiple nodules throughout the adrenal cortex, and a subsequent event stimulates the formation of a single dominant APA that becomes autonomous [14, 15].

In situ hybridization (ISH) studies of *CYP11B2* mRNA have demonstrated that in most cases *CYP11B2* is overexpressed in the APA; however, in some cases the gene is overexpressed not only in the APA, but also in the surrounding adrenal ZG; whilst in others, *CYP11B2* gene expression is not observed in the dominant nodule, but rather, is overexpressed in one or more smaller nodules; in the latter two cases, adrenalectomy did not successfully treat the PA [18, 19].

The recent development of specific antibodies to CYP11B1 (11-beta-hydroxylase) and CYP11B2 (aldosterone synthase) enabled immunohistochemical studies to define the alternative expression patterns of these enzymes from normal adrenals (NA) compared to adrenal glands from PA patients [20].

Normal adrenals display two patterns of expression: (1) a conventional distribution, with CYP11B2 sporadically expressed in the ZG, whereas CYP11B1 is diffusely expressed in the ZF; (2) a variegated pattern with cell clusters strongly expressing CYP11B2 and the remaining areas expressing CYP11B1 [20]. The examination of APA tissues showed that tumors mainly display CYP11B2 positive cells whilst others have a variable proportion of cells expressing the enzyme. APA can consist of three cell types: (a) CYP11B2-positive/CYP11B1-negative cells; (b) CYP11B2-negative/CYP11B1-positive cells; (c) double-negative cells. 3 beta-hydroxysteroid dehydrogenase (3betaHSD) was detected throughout the tumors, irrespective of the expression of CYP11B2 or CYP11B1; whereas CYP17 (17-alpha-hydroxylase) exhibited a similar expression profile to CYP11B1, consistent with its function in cortisol synthesis [20]. In the zone of the adrenal cortex surrounding the APA, two expression patterns have been described: (1) a conventional zonation; and (2) cell clusters expressing CYP11B2 and 3betaHSD, but not CYP11B1, and CYP17, with weak or no expression of CYP11B1 outside the cell clusters [20].

The biochemical and genetic alterations underlying the abnormal cell growth in the *zona glomerulosa* (ZG) cells of the adrenals of PA patients are still largely unknown. A recent study showed that in rats fed with a high salt diet, although the width of the ZG cells was decreased and the expression of *CYP11B2* encoding aldosterone synthase was suppressed, there were nonetheless a number of cells still expressing high levels of CYP11B2 [21]; it is possible to hypothesize that a mutation increased the growth of these cells, thereby resulting in the formation of a nodule of aldosterone-producing cells, not regulated by the increased sodium reabsorption [14].

Genomic Studies in APAs

The molecular basis for the deregulated cell growth and the autonomous hyperproduction of aldosterone observed in PA remains to be fully elucidated. Transcriptosome analysis employing either microarrays or serial analysis of gene expression (SAGE) together with technologies to validate the resultant genetic profiles, such as quantitative real-time PCR (qRT-PCR), have led to several studies attempting to determine the molecular fingerprints of adrenal adenomas. Strict patient selection is of primary importance for such studies and, in fact, insufficiently stringent criteria for APA classification may have caused the discrepancy between the reported differentially expressed genes in APA. Because aldosterone-producing cells are able to store only minimal quantities of the hormone, the synthesis of aldosterone is finely regulated and coupled to its secretion. It is unsurprising therefore, to find aldosterone synthase, up-regulated in APA compared to normal adrenal cortex [22] and all transcriptosome analyses to date have identified the up-regulation of the aldosterone synthase gene (*CYP11B2*) [23–26]; in contrast, one microarray study identified two sub-groups of APA classified on the basis of a paradoxical up- or down-regulation of a set of gene transcripts that included CYP11B2 [27].

Transcripts that code for other steroid metabolizing enzymes, namely *HSD3B2* (encoding 3 beta-hydroxysteroid dehydrogenase type II) and *CYP21* (encoding 21-hydroxylase) have also been identified [24]; the latter gene was also found to be overexpressed in APA in a SAGE analysis and validated by ISH [23].

The *LHR* (luteinizing hormone receptor gene) transcript has been identified as up-regulated by microarray analysis [25, 28] and exogenous expression of the receptor in the aldosterone-secreting adrenocortical carcinoma cell line, NCI H295R [29], and subsequent stimulation with LH resulted in an increased transcription of a luciferase gene reporter construct harboring the *CYP11B2* gene promoter.

A second G protein coupled receptor gene, the serotonin receptor 4 (hydroxytryptamine receptor 4, *HTR4*), that stimulates cAMP release in response to serotonin, has been identified as up-regulated in APA [26, 30, 31]. The aberrant expression of G protein coupled receptors such as LHR and HTR4, among others has been proposed as a putative mechanism for the deregulated steroid production in APA [25, 28].

A recent genomic analysis study by Williams et al. [26] used adenoma tissues from a homogeneously selected group of patients following rigorous diagnostic procedures, including strict criteria for adrenal venous sampling (AVS) interpretation and postadrenalectomy evaluation. Microarray analysis and validation by qRT-PCR identified the epidermal growth factor-like teratocarcinoma-derived growth factor-1 (TDGF1) as the most up-regulated gene in APA compared with NA (21.4-fold). The functional role of TDGF1 was also studied using the H295R cell model: the exogenously expressed growth factor resulted in the activation of phosphatidylinositol 3-kinase (PI3Kinase)/Akt signaling and mediated both an increase in aldosterone secretion (3.8-fold) as well as an inhibition of apoptosis. Both functional effects were blocked by PI3Kinase inhibitors [26].

Interestingly, a sixfold up-regulation of the TDGF1 gene transcript in APA had been identified previously in another study by SAGE [23]. Therefore, two independent methods of transcriptosome analysis have identified TDGF1 as an up-regulated gene transcript in APA compared to normal tissue [23, 26] that, considered together with the functional data, indicate that this gene may represent a key player in the development and pathophysiology of PA.

Role of Aldosterone in Target Organ Damage

Traditionally, aldosterone has been considered the main regulator of water and electrolyte homeostasis due to its effects on epithelial cells, particularly in the collecting ducts of the kidney and distal colon. The physiological actions of aldosterone in non-epithelial tissues are much less evident, but over the last 15 years a wealth of studies both in humans and animal models have allowed new insights on its pathophysiological effects, that are mainly targeted in the heart, blood vessels, kidney, and central nervous system (CNS).

Heart

The main pathological effects of aldosterone excess on the heart are vascular and perivascular inflammation, fibrosis, and myocardial hypertrophy. In a study by Rocha et al. [32] administration of aldosterone and a salt-rich diet to uni-nephrectomized rats resulted in severe arterial hypertension and inflammatory lesions in myocardial vessels, with fibrinoid necrosis in the media and mononuclear leukocyte accumulation in perivascular tissues. These changes were prevented by concomitant administration of the mineralocorticoid receptor antagonist eplerenone, an effect that was independent from blood pressure reduction; similar results have been achieved in other studies [33]. A direct role of aldosterone in myocardial inflammatory damage was further demonstrated in transgenic rats overexpressing the human renin and angiotensinogen genes (dTGR); the hypersecretion of aldosterone promoted hypertrophy, cardiac remodeling and fibrosis, independent of blood pressure. These effects involved an increased expression of NF-kappaB, a key transcription-factor involved in the inflammatory response, and the basic fibroblast growth factor (bFGF) [34]. Therefore, myocardial fibrosis can be determined both as a direct effect of stimulation of cardiac fibroblast proliferation as well as an indirect reparative response to inflammation and cell death [12].

Clinical studies suggested that PA is associated with increased prevalence and severity of left ventricular hypertrophy (LVH) [35]. Napoli et al. [36] demonstrated that PA patients displayed a significantly higher severity of LVH after correction for age, gender, duration, and severity of hypertension compared to essential hypertensives. Myocardial perfusion evaluated by myocardial scintigraphy is significantly more impaired in PA patients compared with matched hypertensive subjects [36]. Rossi et al. [35] demonstrated that, in essential hypertensive and in PA patients, plasma aldosterone levels were directly related to LV wall thickness. Further, myocardial texture was also modified by plasma aldosterone levels [35–37], with an increase in the fibrotic components, resulting in diastolic dysfunction.

In addition to these effects, aldosterone is able to directly affect membrane ionic balance in cardiomyocytes, acting on ionic channels and transporters. Aldosterone reduces Na^+-K^+-pump affinity for sodium and potassium [38], causing a disequilibrium in intra- and extracellular concentrations of these cations, and modifies potassium fluxes during repolarization, especially acting on the rapid component of the delayed rectifier K^+-current. These changes causes a lengthening of the QT-interval at ECG, and can be reversed by spironolactone [39]. Aldosterone also acts on the Na^{2+}/Mg^{2+}-exchanger, with a resultant depletion in intracellular magnesium concentration, and stimulates intracellular calcium influx [40] causing calcium intracellular excess, which can elicit ectopic ventricular beats [41].

Blood Vessels

Vascular and perivascular inflammation elicited by aldosterone excess in myocardium can also be observed in other vascular beds, with similar mechanisms of endothelial activation, leukocyte accumulation, and pro-fibrogenic cytokine production. Aldosterone is in fact able to determine the loss of physiological vasodilating properties of endothelial cells and their imbalance towards a pro-thrombotic and pro-inflammatory phenotype known as "endothelial dysfunction" [42] and also an increased vascular stiffness. Some studies have investigated the mechanisms responsible for these changes, such as overexpression of cyclooxygenase type 2 (COX-2) and overproduction of prostanoids [42], overproduction of endothelin-1 (ET-1) [43] and decrease in expression and activity of NO-synthase [44] with reduced levels of nitric oxide (NO), a well-known vasodilating factor. In agreement with the increased vascular deposition of collagen, a higher level of fibrosis in the walls of subcutaneous small resistance arteries of PA patients has been demonstrated [45].

Kidney

Many studies with animal models of mineralocorticoid excess have shown the involvement of aldosterone in the pathogenesis of renal disease. The first complete demonstration of this causal association was given by the so-called remnant kidney model. In 1996, Greene et al. [46] submitted normotensive rats to sub-total nephrectomy and then compared a group treated with both an ACE-inhibitor (enalapril) and an angiotensin II receptor antagonist (losartan), a group treated with enalapril, losartan, and exogenous aldosterone and a control group without any treatment. Animals in the control group developed arterial hypertension, proteinuria, and glomerulosclerosis associated with overactivity of the renin–angiotensin–aldosterone system (RAAS). The renal lesions that developed in rats treated with RAAS-inhibitors only, were significantly less severe; this protective effect, however, was lost with concomitant administration of exogenous aldosterone. Interestingly, this demonstrate not only a role for aldosterone in renal disease but distinguished its effects from those of angiotensin II. Other animal models were subsequently investigated, for example, spontaneously hypertensive rats—stroke prone (SHRSP), a model of secondary aldosteronism, prematurely develop proteinuria, and malignant nephrosclerosis on a salt-rich diet [47, 48]. Adrenalectomy [33] or mineralocorticoid receptor blocker therapy [33, 48] has proven effective in preventing renal changes in a blood pressure-independent manner [48]. In a model of aldosterone/

salt-treated rats, the animals develop severe hypertension and albuminuria, renal vascular damage, and renal lesions together with myocardial and coronary vascular damage, compared to rats receiving salt alone. Eplerenone significantly reduced blood pressure levels, albuminuria, and renal vascular injury. Renal vascular inflammation after 4 weeks of aldosterone administration was demonstrated by showing elevated expression of osteopontin, monocyte chemoattractant protein, interleukin-1, and interleukin-6. Treatment with eplerenone resulted in renal vascular, glomerular and tubule protection, and attenuated vascular inflammation [49].

Central Nervous System

Mineralocorticoid receptors have been located in several regions of the CNS, especially in peri-ventricular areas, amygdalae, hypothalamus, and cerebellum [50]. The CNS is now considered one of the main targets of aldosterone, as this hormone has been associated with modulation of ACTH secretion, maintenance of arousal and central modulation of salt appetite, water and electrolyte homeostasis, and blood pressure levels [51, 52]. Raised aldosterone levels in CNS can then increase peripheral blood pressure even in the presence of normal plasma aldosterone concentrations [53, 54]. The main mechanisms involved in this effect seem to be the increase in salt appetite, the expansion in extracellular fluid volume, and a marked sympathetic activity [12]; moreover, some studies carried out in dogs have observed a reduction in baroreflex sensitivity following administration of exogenous aldosterone both in acute and in chronic conditions [55].

The main consequence of aldosterone excess on the CNS is the predisposition to acute cerebrovascular events, related to vascular damage that aldosterone may induce in the CNS vascular bed. SHRSP represented a key model to study the causal association between aldosterone and stroke. These animals develop malignant hypertension by 7–10 weeks on salt-rich diet depleted in potassium, with a paradoxical activation of the RAAS and onset of nephroangiosclerosis and premature ischemic stroke which usually results in death within 13–18 weeks [32]. Treatment with mineralocorticoid-receptor blockers can prevent development of severe vascular lesions and decrease mortality in a pressure-independent manner [56].

Clinical Features and Complications of PA

The most relevant feature of primary aldosteronism is an excessive and inappropriate secretion of aldosterone, in relation to blood volume and pressure and to plasma sodium levels. The subsequent rise in blood pressure determines suppression of renin secretion and decrease of angiotensin II production. The excess in aldosterone induces potassium secretion and sodium reabsorption by kidneys, and therefore an electrolyte imbalance; this also determines an increase in magnesium and hydrogen ion excretion, which induces the retention of bicarbonate ions and consequently the onset of metabolic alkalosis. However, even with the powerful effects of aldosterone as kaliuretic and sodium retention agent, plasma concentrations of sodium and potassium can still be within the normal range, due to the activation of compensatory mechanisms.

Sodium retention, in particular, is compensated by escape natriuretic mechanisms, such as an increase in renal perfusion pressure, a rise in natriuretic peptides, and a decrease in sympathetic nervous renal activity and in plasma concentration of angiotensin II [57]; it is because of these mechanisms that patients with primary aldosteronism do not show oedemas.

Hyperaldosteronism induces an increase in blood pressure by sodium retention and the subsequent increase of circulatory volume and cardiac output, which is normalized by reflex vasoconstriction; ultimately, this determines the onset of hypertension. Moreover, recent evidence suggests a direct vasoconstrictory activity of aldosterone itself, in accordance with its rapid secretion after postural changes [58].

Paresthesias and neuromuscular disorders are relatively common in Asian countries [59], but the symptoms are often non specific, in fact, hypokalemia affects only of a relatively small percentage of subjects (less than 30%), who describe muscular weakness and cramps, polydipsia, polyuria, or nycturia.

The two most common features are hypertension and hypokalemia. Hypertension can be moderate or severe, and is often resistant to common antihypertensive therapy; however PA patients with normotension have been nonetheless reported.

A marked hypokalemia can be associated to alterations of electric conduction in myocardium, which manifests as EKG changes, such as T wave flattening, onset of U wave, ST segment sub-elevation, prolongation of PQ, and QT intervals and of QRS; all these conditions can lead to potentially fatal ventricular arrhythmias. It has been shown that PA patients display an increased prevalence of long QT, at least in part independent from potassium levels [60], which is reverted after adrenalectomy or therapy with spironolactone [61].

In the latest decade, many studies have compared patients with PA and essential hypertension, confirming results in animal models that indicate aldosterone per se increases cardiovascular risk, independent of the effect on blood pressure levels.

Patients with PA display a higher incidence of metabolic syndrome compared to essential hypertension [62], and even those without this condition often show a more pronounced insulin-resistance [62, 63]. Metabolic alterations, in turn, can be in part responsible for the increased cardiovascular risk of PA patients [64]. These alterations are ameliorated by PA treatment by spironolactone or adrenalectomy [65]. To date it has not been clarified if metabolic syndrome is secondary to hyperaldosteronism or vice versa. In fact, it has been shown that adipokines such as complement-C1q TNF-related protein 1 (CTRP1), stimulates aldosterone production through an increased expression of CYP11B2 [66]. In the other hand, a longitudinal evaluation of the incidence of metabolic syndrome and changes in metabolic risk factors in the Framingham Offspring Study, showed that higher quartiles of aldosterone were associated to a higher risk of development of metabolic syndrome [67]. However, another study was not able to confirm the association between metabolic syndrome and PA [68]. Finally, a recent retrospective study from the German Conn's Registry, showed that PA patients displayed a higher rate of diabetes compared to a control population of essential hypertensives [69] and others reported a high prevalence of PA in type 2 diabetic patients with resistant hypertension [70, 71].

PA patients also show a significantly higher rate of structural and functional alterations of the heart, kidneys, and blood vessels if compared to patients with essential hypertension. PA patients showed a higher prevalence and degree of LVH compared to essential hypertensives [11, 35, 62] and also a higher prevalence of diastolic dysfunction [72]. At vascular level, PA patients show an increased intima-media thickness [73] and an increased arterial wall stiffness, measured with the pulse wave velocity [74].

PA patients also show a high prevalence of obstructive sleep apnea (OSA) [75]. Calhoun et al. [76] observed that subjects at high risk for OSA were almost two times more likely to have PA diagnosed and had a higher urinary aldosterone excretion. Subsequently, they showed a significant correlation between plasma aldosterone concentration and the severity of OSA [77]. The link between these two conditions is not straightforward: obesity is a common feature in OSA patients and thus, cytokines produced by the adipose tissue may stimulate aldosterone secretion from the adrenals; on the other hand, aldosterone-induced fluid retention may contribute to the upper airway obstruction via an increase of the peripharyngeal oedema.

Few studies have compared renal damage in PA and essential hypertension; the former, though, has higher levels of albuminuria and a higher prevalence of microabuminuria [78–80].

The difference is evident after adrenalectomy or spironolactone therapy; it has been therefore suggested that an increase in albumin urinary excretion could be an indicator of functional damage in early renal disease. Sechi et al. have observed, through the use of Doppler ultrasonography, reduced renal vascular resistances in PA patients when compared to those of essential hypertension; moreover, glomerular filtration rate (GFR) based on creatinine clearance is higher in PA patients [81]. In subjects with higher clearance levels than the population median, the hemodynamic alterations were reversible after adrenalectomy or medical treatment with mineralocorticoid receptor antagonists. Moreover, even though renal excretion of albumin was higher in PA patients than in essential hypertensives, urinary albumin/creatinin ratio (A_U/C_U) did not show a significant difference. These data, as a whole, confirm the presence of glomerular hyperfiltration in PA, as previously reported [78, 80], and correlate these finding to anomalies in intra-renal vascular resistances, which appear responsible for the elevated albumin excretion. However, long-term exposure to high aldosterone levels results in a deterioration of renal function. In the German Conn's Registry, the percentage of patients with a serum creatinine concentration above the normal range was higher in PA patients than in hypertensive controls: age, male sex, low potassium, and high aldosterone concentrations were independent predictors of a lower GFR [82].

Considering the elevated prevalence of multiple cardiovascular risk factors and increased target organ damage in PA patients, an increased prevalence of cardio- and cerebrovascular events is also expected; in fact, PA patients display a fourfold increase in the prevalence of stroke, 6.5-fold of myocardial infarction and 12-fold of atrial fibrillation [11]. These data have been confirmed by further studies [75, 83]. Interestingly, in one of these studies, normokalemic PA patients displayed a higher risk of stroke, highlighting the importance to exclude PA not only in hypokalemic, but also in normokalemic hypertensives [75].

Diagnosis of Primary Aldosteronism

Screening Test

The Guidelines for the diagnosis and treatment of PA recently published the different categories of hypertensive patients that display a relatively high prevalence of PA; it is recommended that patients belonging to these categories undergo a screening test. The screening test should be performed in all patients with: (1) resistant hypertension; (2) hypertension grade 2 or 3; (3) hypertension and spontaneous or diuretic-induced hypokalemia; (4) hypertension with adrenal incidentaloma; (5) hypertension and a family history of early-onset hypertension or cerebrovascular accident at a young age (<40 year); (6) all hypertensive first-degree relatives of patients with PA [4] (Fig. 1.1).

The aldosterone to renin ratio (ARR) is the most reliable, currently available method for PA screening: in fact, many studies have demonstrated that the ARR is superior to measurements of both potassium and aldosterone (which are less sensitive) as well as renin alone (which is less specific) [84–86]. Presently, there is no general consensus on ARR cut-off and therefore, individual centers use different values, ranging from 7.2 to 100 ng dL^{-1} per ng mL^{-1} h^{-1}, with a consequent wide variation in the sensitivity (64–100%) and specificity (87–100%) of the screening test. However, in a recent study published by Rossi et al., the ARR was found to provide a good within-patient reproducibility and an accuracy of 80% for identifying APA patients [87]. The most important confounding factors affecting renin and/or aldosterone measurements thus reducing the sensitivity or specificity of the ARR are antihypertensive drugs [4] (Fig. 1.2). In particular, β-blockers, α-methyldopa and clonidine decrease the beta-adrenoreceptor mediated stimulation of renin production and sympathetic nervous system output thereby causing false-positives. Conversely, other drugs stimulate renin secretion, such as ACE-inhibitors, ATII receptor antagonists, dihydropyridine calcium antagonists, and diuretics. All these drugs (except diuretics that increase aldosterone secretion) may cause a reduction in aldosterone levels and increase in renin levels leading to false-negative results. The recently introduced renin inhibitor Aliskiren reduces plasma aldosterone levels whilst stimulating renin secretion: this results in false-positive ARR levels for renin measured as plasma renin activity (PRA) and false negatives for renin measured as direct renin concentration (DRC) [4]. Antihypertensive medications other than diuretics, that should always be withdrawn for at least 4–6 weeks (6–8 weeks for

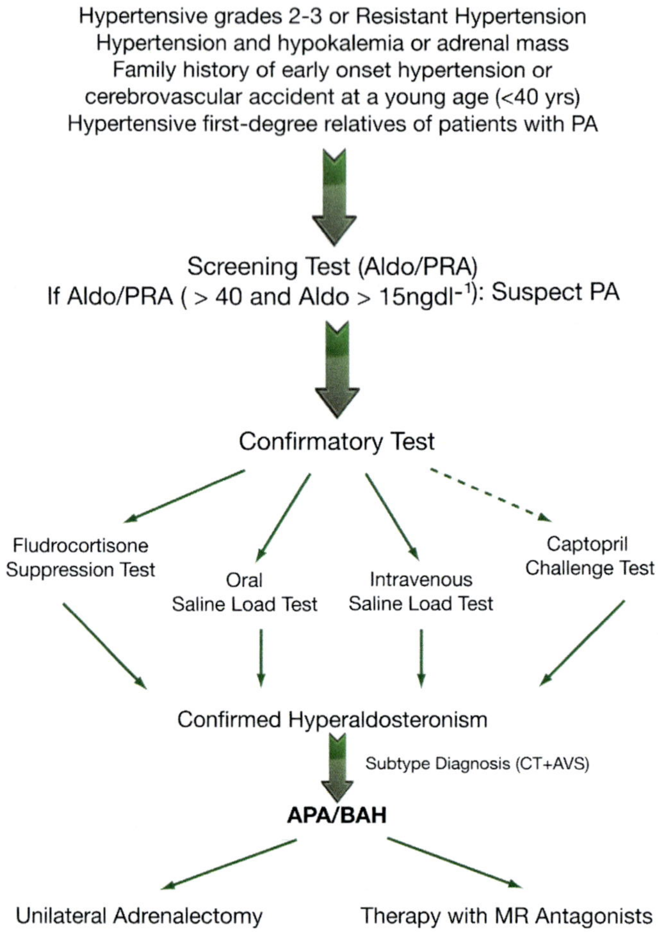

Fig. 1.1 Flow-chart for diagnosis of PA and its subtypes

spironolactone), should be stopped at least 2–3 weeks before ARR testing, but in many patients this is clearly not feasible. Because α-antagonists do not appear to have any significant effect on plasma aldosterone and renin levels, they can be safely used to control hypertension before the screening test is performed. Non dihydropyridine calcium antagonists can cause a modest increase in renin levels and reduce aldosterone secretion, but rarely to an extent that can significantly affect the ARR and confirmatory tests and can be administered to patients whose blood pressure is not adequately controlled by an α-antagonist alone [4, 88].

Further, the effect of oral contraceptive agents has received little attention, but should be considered because estrogen-containing preparations induce angiotensinogen synthesis by the liver. Blood sampling conditions can also have an effect and should be standardized to avoid potential fluctuations in levels of the two hormones and subsequent difficulties in interpreting the ARR [4] (Table 1.2).

Drugs	Aldo	PRA	ARR	Diagnosis
β-Blockers, clonidine, α-methildopa	↓	↓↓	↑	FP
α-Blockers, hydralazine	N	N	N	N
Thiazides and loop duiretics	↑	↑↑	↓	FN
Spironolactone, eplerenone	↑	↑↑	↓	FN
ACE-Is	↓	↑	↓	FN
ARBs	↓	↑	↓	FN
Renin-inhibitors (Aliskiren)	↓	↑	↓↑	FN/FP
Calcium-channel blockers	→↓	→↑	→↓*	N/FN
NSAIDs	↓	↓↓	↑	FP
Advancing age, renal impairment	↓	↓↓	↑	FP

* False positive using PRA, false negative using renin

Fig. 1.2 Effects of drugs on aldosterone, plasma renin activity (PRA), aldosterone to renin ratio (ARR) levels and screening test

Table 1.2 Measurement of aldosterone:renin ratio (ARR)

ARR measurement
Preparation for ARR measurement
Correct hypokalemia
Avoid sodium restriction
Withdraw agents that affect the ARR (see Fig. 1.1)
Conditions for blood collection
Collect blood mid-morning, after the patient has been up for at least 2 h and seated for 5–15 min
Collect blood avoiding stasis and hemolysis
Maintain blood sample at room temperature and not on ice (avoiding activation of renin)
Separate plasma from cells within 30 min of collection
Factors to take into account when interpreting the results
Age
Medications
Method of blood collection
Level of potassium and creatinine

The absolute aldosterone value (>15 ng dL^{-1}) and the lowest detectable level of PRA should also be taken into account. Because the ARR is dependent on PRA, effectively anyone with suppressed PRA will have an increased ARR; this is particularly important in elderly or black populations, who often display PRA values as low as 0.1 ng mL^{-1} h^{-1}, thereby resulting in an increase in the plasma aldosterone concentration: plasma renin activity (PAC:PRA) ratio even with a PAC of 5 ng dL^{-1}. It has been shown that all individuals with aldosterone levels of less than 9 ng dL^{-1} demonstrate normal suppression during a fludrocortisone-suppression test [89].

In the majority of published studies, ARR is reported as a function of renin, measured as PRA, and few data are available for direct active renin (DAR). PRA and DAR are closely correlated (overall correlation coefficient 0.98), but the correlation is weaker for the low compared to the high/normal range of values ($r=0.77$ for samples with PRA <0.65 ng mL^{-1} h^{-1}), i.e., in the range of patients potentially affected by PA [90, 91]. Even newer automated methods for renin measurements have not resolved this issue ($r=0.14$ with PRA<1) [92]. To date, no prospective studies have been performed that have compared the accuracy of the aldosterone to active renin ratio to that of the well-established ARR and therefore, DAR should be considered cautiously as a screening test for PA.

In light of the high prevalence of low renin hypertension [90], it is important to emphasize that an increased ARR is not itself diagnostic of PA and a confirmatory test is always required to avoid patients unnecessarily undergoing costly and potentially harmful lateralization procedures.

Confirmatory Tests

Although the Guidelines clearly recommend that patients with a positive ARR undergo a confirmatory test to definitively confirm or exclude the diagnosis of PA, the choice of test remains a matter of debate and there is currently insufficient direct evidence to recommend one rather than another [4] (Fig. 1.1).

Four testing procedures are approved by the Guidelines: oral sodium loading (OLT), saline infusion (SLT), fludrocortisone suppression (FST), and a captopril challenge (CCT) [4] (Table 1.3).

Briefly, FST consists of fludrocortisone acetate administration for 4 days with KCl and NaCl supplements. If PAC on the fourth day is ≥6 ng dL^{-1}, PA is confirmed (Table 1.3) [4, 16, 93].

In the SLT, PAC is measured after an infusion of 2 L of 0.9% NaCl over 4 h (Table 1.3). If PAC is lower than 5 ng dL^{-1} after the saline infusion, PA is unlikely whereas PAC >10 ng dL^{-1} is diagnostic for PA. PAC between 5 and 10 ng dL^{-1} represents a grey zone, but most clinicians consider such individuals to be affected by PA [4, 93].

OLT is performed with the individual subjected to a high sodium diet for 3 days. Patients should receive adequate potassium chloride supplementation to maintain plasma potassium in the normal range. Normal suppression is usually defined as a 24 h urinary aldosterone concentration <12 μg day^{-1} on the third day (Table 1.3) [4, 93, 94].

In the CC, ARR is measured before and after captopril administration. PA is confirmed when the post-captopril ARR is >30–40 (with aldosterone measured as ng dL^{-1} and PRA as ng mL^{-1} h^{-1}) [95, 96] or post-captopril aldosterone is >8.5–10 ng dL^{-1} [97, 98] (Table 1.3).

Other tests, such as the furosemide upright posture [99] and the losartan test [100, 101], are used in some units, but at present they are not recommended by the Guidelines due to insufficient use and evidence.

The FST is regarded by some investigators as the most reliable means of confirming or excluding the diagnosis of PA because it is the test that more closely

Table 1.3 Confirmatory tests for PA

Primary aldosteronism confirmatory tests		
Test	Procedure	Interpretation
Oral sodium loading test—OLT	Oral NaCl supplementation (>200 mmol Na^+/day for 3 days) and K^+ supplementation to maintain plasma K^+ in normal range Urinary Aldo measured in 24 h urine collection from morning of day 3 to morning of day 4	PA unlikely if urinary Aldo <10 μg/24 h in the absence of renal disease. Elevated urinary Aldo excretion >12 μg/24 h indicates PA highly likely
Intravenous saline loading test—SLT	Intravenous infusion of 2 L 0.9% NaCl solution over 4 h (500 mL h^{-1}) with patient remaining in recumbent position Blood samples for renin and Aldo measurements collected at time zero and after 4 h, with blood pressure and heart rate monitored during the test	Post-infusion plasma Aldo levels <5 ng dL^{-1} indicate no PA; values >10 ng dL^{-1} indicate PA; values between 5 and 10 ng dL^{-1} are inconclusive (57–60); most units consider these patients as PA
Fludrocortisone suppression test—FST	Fludrocortisone acetate (0.1 mg every 6 h), K^+ supplementation (every 6 h at doses sufficient to maintain plasma K^+, measured four times a day, close to 4 mmol L^{-1}) and NaCl (30 mmol every 8 h) and dietary salt to maintain urinary Na^+ excretion rate of at least 3 mmol kg^{-1} body weight for 4 days. On day 4, plasma Aldo and PRA are measured at 10 h with patient seated, and plasma cortisol is measured at 7 and 10 h	Upright plasma Aldo >6 ng dL^{-1} on day 4 at 10 h confirms PA, provided PRA is <1 ng mL^{-1} h^{-1} and plasma cortisol concentration is lower than the value obtained at 7 h (to exclude a confounding ACTH effect)
Captopril challenge test—CCT	25–50 mg captopril orally after sitting or standing for at least 1 h. Blood samples are collected for PRA measurement, plasma Aldo at time zero and at 1 or 2 h after captopril challenge, with patient remaining seated during this period	In patients with PA, aldosterone remains elevated and PRA remain suppressed PA is confirmed when the post-captopril ARR is >30–40 or post-captopril Aldo is >8.5–10 ng dL^{-1}

PA primary aldosteronism; *Aldo* aldosterone; *PRA* plasma renin activity; *ARR* aldosterone:renin ratio

mimics the clinical features of PA, in that both stimulation of the MR and volume expansion due to saline load is determined during the test. However, FST is highly costly since it requires hospitalization in particular for monitoring potassium levels. For this reason, despite the advantages, it is impractical for many centers and it is progressively less used around the world. Furthermore, it is potentially harmful for patients with reduced renal function and previous episodes of heart failure.

The intravenous saline load test (SLT) is widely used; during this test, potassium levels do not change significantly and thus potassium supplementation are usually not necessary [102]. The test requires the patient to remain one morning in the hospital and is performed under controlled conditions. However, the acute expansion of the plasma volume cannot be considered physiological and this test can also be potentially harmful for patients with reduced renal function and previous episodes of heart failure and atrial fibrillation.

The oral saline load (OLT) is the cheapest test but test conditions are not strictly controlled and patient compliance on urine collection is a potential limitation. Furthermore, urinary aldosterone assays usually measure only the 18-oxo-glucuronide fraction that is only a part of the total aldosterone excretion. Again, the test is potentially harmful for patients with reduced renal function and a history of heart failure and atrial fibrillation.

The captopril challenge test (CCT) is the less standardized confirmatory test. The cost of CCT is similar to that of SLT, with the advantage of being less risky for patients with reduced cardiac or renal function; by contrast, the reported substantial number of false-positive and false-negative results [93] has caused many authors to consider this test as a second choice for patients at potential risk for acute saline load requested in the other three tests. A recently published study compared FST and SLT in 100 patients with suspected PA after the screening test. SLT showed a sensitivity of 88% and a specificity of 84% with PAC of 5 ng dL^{-1}. A cut-off of aldosterone post-SLT of 6 ng dL^{-1} resulted in a 100% sensitivity for the diagnosis of APA [102]. Interestingly, a similar level of aldosterone post-SLT was the best cut-off for the diagnosis of APA in the PAPY study [95]. A linear regression analysis of PAC post FST and SLT demonstrated that the two parameters were highly associated. Therefore, SLT is a reasonably reliable alternative to the FST for confirming the diagnosis of PA.

In a small group of eleven patients undergoing both i.v. SLT and FST, the CCT was also performed [103]. Four patients with a negative SLT and FST (i.e., not affected by PA) resulted positive after CCT and thus, would have been incorrectly considered as affected by PA considering the CCT alone. By contrast, one patient with PA, confirmed by both SLT and FST, resulted negative after the CCT. In the PAPY study, the i.v. SLT showed a significantly higher area under the curve compared to the CCT. The performance for the diagnosis of APA, was similar with the CCT compared to the SLT in patients with sodium intake higher than 7.6 g day^{-1}, whereas the SLT was significantly better in sodium depleted patients [104]. Interestingly, even in patients with a high sodium intake, CCT performance was better to exclude rather than confirm PA, with an excess of false-positive diagnoses.

It is important to emphasize that the use of antihypertensive drugs needs to be taken into account not only for the screening test, but also before and during the confirmatory test since they can alter the values of PRA and aldosterone (Fig. 1.2).

In conclusion, it should be noted that the discussion about the optimal cut-off of a confirmatory test (as well as the optimal ARR as screening test) is dependent on the accuracy of the aldosterone assay. It has been demonstrated that different commercially available aldosterone assay kits, although usually reporting good overall correlation coefficients with each other, often display significant differences in the absolute aldosterone concentrations measured for a given sample [105, 106]. Furthermore, the discrepancies are more pronounced in the low-range of aldosterone concentrations (below 10 ng dL^{-1}), that is, the range in which cut-off values for confirmatory tests are found.

Subtype Differentiation

After a positive confirmatory test, further investigation is needed to identify the PA subtype, as some subtypes benefit from surgery and others should be treated pharmacologically with mineralocorticoid receptor (MR) antagonists.

As recommended in the Guidelines, all patients with PA should undergo an adrenal CT scan as the initial study in subtype testing to exclude large masses that may represent adrenocortical carcinomas [4] (Fig. 1.1). High resolution CT scanning with contrast and fine cuts (2.5–3 mm) is the imaging technique that displays the best sensitivity and specificity in identifying adrenal nodules. The CT scan can also provide useful information on the localization of the orifice of the right adrenal vein, thereby facilitating successful cannulation of the vein during the subsequent AVS. However, CT scanning is not sufficiently sensitive to diagnose aldosterone-producing micro-adenomas and also, cannot distinguish between a functional APA and an incidentaloma, that can be found in 2–10% of all adults. Despite these limitations, we recently demonstrated a higher sensitivity, in the detection of adrenal nodules when CT scanning was performed by a motivated, expert radiologist. The use of clinical and biochemical parameters alone cannot be used for the differentiation of PA subtypes because of low sensitivity of detection although they display a high specificity [107]. To reduce the number of patients that undergo AVS, some researchers have attempted to identify other criteria for distinguishing APA from BAH. It has been suggested that patients <40 years old and with an adrenal nodule of >1 cm detected by CT scanning can proceed to unilateral adrenalectomy, and patients >40 years with an adrenal nodule on CT scans >1 cm should undergo AVS [94].

Magnetic resonance has no advantages over CT scanning and should be limited to patients for whom the contrast injected for the CT scan procedure is contraindicated . The adrenal scintiscan with [6β-^{131}I]iodomethyl-19-norcholesterol performed under dexamethasone suppression may potentially correlate morphology with the functional activity of the adrenal nodules, but has demonstrated low sensitivity and specificity for APA [108].

In the past, some hormonal tests have been used to differentiate APA from IHA, including the posture stimulation test and 18-hydroxycorticosterone measurements. The posture test is based on the assumption that APA are angiotensin II unresponsive and that aldosterone secretion follows a circadian rhythm similar to that of cortisol, whereas patients with BAH are sensitive to angiotensin II and posture. The existence of angiotensin II responsive APA as well as patients with BAH in which aldosterone secretion follows a cortisol diurnal rhythm, reduces the accuracy of this test, which therefore cannot have a role in subtype differentiation [3].

For these reasons, The Endocrine Society Guidelines recommend that all patients for whom surgical treatment is practical and desired, should undergo AVS, that is, the gold standard test to differentiate unilateral from bilateral disease [4]. During AVS the adrenal veins are catheterized through the percutaneous femoral vein approach, and the position of the catheter tip is verified by gentle injection of a small amount of contrast. The procedure is technically difficult to perform, the success rate at cannulating adrenal veins increases with experience and dedication of the radiologist and can reach up to 96% [109, 110]. During AVS, because adrenal veins are small, the blood sample is often obtained near the orifice of the vein and may be diluted with other blood, introducing an error in the measurement of aldosterone levels. In particular, the right adrenal vein may be especially difficult to cannulate because it is short, enters the inferior vena cava (IVC) at an acute angle and several anatomical variations may make it difficult to locate and distinguish from other adjacent small vessels.

The simultaneous measurement of cortisol concentrations corrects for this dilution: the cortisol concentration in the blood is thus a measure of the adequacy of cannulation.

Recently, the introduction of a quick and reliable method for real-time rapid cortisol assay in the operation room during AVS, which provides the radiologist with information on the success of the cannulation, offers a new tool to improve AVS performance [111].

Unfortunately, there is no agreement on which criteria should be used for defining both successful cannulation and lateralization, with some centers using more permissive criteria and others using more restrictive criteria [112] (Table 1.4). To define successful cannulation, a ratio between cortisol levels in the adrenal vein and in a peripheral vein should be at least 3, because lower ratios can result in misleading diagnoses [112].

Cosyntropin (infusion of 50 μg h^{-1} initiated 30 min before AVS and continued throughout the procedure or an intravenous bolus of 250 μg) is used in some centers to minimize stress induced fluctuation in aldosterone secretion in non simultaneous AVS, to maximize the gradient in cortisol from the adrenal vein to the IVC and to maximize aldosterone secretion from an APA [94]. However, in some cases ACTH administration may result in the stimulation of the gland contralateral to an APA, thus reducing the gradient of aldosterone production. A recent study showed that the high dose of ACTH can result in incorrect lateralization of aldosterone secretion [113]. The use of continuous ACTH infusion should be considered when AVS is not performed in the early morning and when a patient, at risk for an allergic reaction to the contrast, is pretreated with prednisone [114].

Recently, it was reported that simultaneous secretion of cortisol and aldosterone from adrenal adenomas may not be a rare event, especially when the dimension of the nodule is greater than 20 mm [115]; therefore, it may be advisable to perform a 1 mg-overnight dexamethasone test to exclude subclinical Cushing before performing AVS.

At centers with experienced AVS radiologists, the complication rate is 2.5% or lower. The most frequent complication is a symptomatic groin hematoma; more rare is adrenal hemorrhage and the dissection of an adrenal vein [4].

The diagnosis of APA is considered "proven" when after adrenalectomy the patient displays: (a) normokalemia; (b) cure or significant amelioration of hypertension; (c) normal ARR and normal suppressibility of aldosterone to FST or saline load test; (d) histological confirmation of the diagnosis.

Table 1.4 Criteria for successful cannulation and lateralization after adrenal venous sampling

Criteria	Torino	Brisbane	Cosyntropin infusion (Mayo clinic)
Cannulation criteria	$C_{AV}/C_{IVC} \geq 3$	$C_{AV}/C_{PV} \geq 3$	$C_{AV}/C_{IVC} \geq 5$
Lateralization criteria	$([A/C]_{AV}/[A/C]_{CAV}) \geq 4$ or $([A/C]_{AV}/[A/C]_{CAV}) \geq 3$ and $([A/C]_{CAV}/[A/C]_{IVC}) < 1$	$([A/C]_{AV}/[A/C]_{PV}) \geq 2$ and $([A/C]_{CAV}/[A/C]_{PV}) < 1$	$([A/C]_{AV}/[A/C]_{CAV}) \geq 4$

A aldosterone; *C* cortisol; *AV* adrenal vein; *CAV* contralateral adrenal vein; *IVC* inferior vena cava; *PV* peripheral vein

Genetics of PA

CYP11B1 and CYP11B2 Genes

Aldosterone synthase is a mitochondrial cytochrome P450 enzyme that produces aldosterone from its precursor, deoxycorticosterone (DOC) by three successive reactions comprising 11beta-hydroxylation, 18-hydroxylation, and 18-oxidation [116, 117]. Aldosterone synthase is encoded by the *CYP11B2* gene that is situated on chromosome 8q24.3, adjacent (approximately 40 kb) to the highly homologous *CYP11B1* gene, which encodes 11 beta-hydroxylase [118, 119]. The latter enzyme converts 11-deoxycortisol to cortisol, but is devoid of 18-hydroxylation and 18-oxidation activities. *CYP11B1* and B2 are 95% homologous within their coding regions (comprising nine exons) and approximately 90% homologous in their intronic regions, whilst their aminoacid sequences share 93% identity. Site-directed mutagenesis studies on *CYP11B1* and *CYP11B2* have identified two key amino acid residues (G288 and A320) that confer the additional 18-hydroxylation and 18-oxidation activities to aldosterone synthase [120]. Indeed, substitution of S288 in CYP11B1 by a glycine residue confers efficient 18-hydroxylase activity, and an additional substitution of V320 by an alanine residue confers 18-oxidase activity.

Precise patterns of gene expression underlie the specialized production and secretion of steroid hormones in the different functional areas of the adrenal glands. *CYP11B1* is widely expressed at high levels throughout the adrenal cortex, with ACTH as its main positive regulator. Conversely, *CYP11B2* is selectively expressed in the zona glomerulosa and is primarily regulated by serum potassium and angiotensin II levels. The synthesis of cortisol in the adrenal zona glomerulosa is prevented by the local absence of CYP17. The abnormal presence of a CYP17 activity and the two C18 (18-hydroxylase and 18-oxidase) activities typical of aldosterone synthase, as occurs in glucocorticoid-remediable aldosteronism (GRA), leads to the synthesis of the so-called "hybrid steroids"(18OH- and 18-oxo-cortisol) [121]. In cultured adrenal cells, CYP11B2 mRNA levels have been shown to increase with the administration of angiotensin II and with potassium loading in a time- and concentration-dependent manner [122]. Acute stimulation with ACTH leads to a similar rise in CYP11B2 mRNA levels, but this is reversed by the chronic administration of ACTH [123].

Familial Forms of Primary Aldosteronism

Three forms of familial hyperaldosteronism have been described to date referred to as FH-I, FH-II, and FH-III. FH-I, also known as GRA, is a monogenic form transmitted as an autosomal-dominant disease and responsible for fewer than 1% of PA. FH-I is due to an unequal recombination between *CYP11B1* and *CYP11B2* [124]. GRA is transmitted as an autosomal-dominant disease. Its main clinical features are elevated ACTH-dependent aldosterone secretion, renin suppression, and high levels of the hybrid steroids 18-hydroxycortisol and 18-oxocortisol [125]. Most affected individuals develop severe hypertension early in life [126] and females have an increased risk of pregnancy-aggravated hypertension [127]. Furthermore, GRA patients display higher morbidity and mortality from cerebrovascular events [128]. However, patients with mild hypertension or blood pressure in the normal range are described in many families, some of them displaying a notably milder clinical phenotypes [129]. The most reliable biochemical evidence for GRA is a marked, sustained suppression of plasma aldosterone during several days of dexamethasone administration [130]: the test is considered positive if aldosterone is suppressed below 4 ng dL^{-1} after 4 days of dexamethasone (0.5 mg/6 h) [131]. However, this test may be difficult to perform in very young individuals and is not applicable as a screening test of families; further, a high frequency of false-positive diagnoses has been demonstrated [132]. Nowadays, diagnosis of FH-I is commonly made by a long-polymerase chain reaction (PCR) technique [114]. Genetic testing for FH-I should be considered in patients with onset of PA earlier than 20 year of age and in those who have a family history of PA or of strokes at young age (<40 year) [4]. Others, including our group, suggest to rule out FH-I in all PA patients [114].

A recent study [133], showed that FH-I/GRA is not rare among hypertensive children when obesity and renal causes are excluded. FH-II is a non-glucocorticoid remediable form of PA [134]. This disease is clinically and biochemically indistinguishable from sporadic PA. The molecular basis of FH-II is still unknown, although genetic analyses have shown in families from three different continents, a linkage with chromosomal region 7p22 [135, 136]. However, in other FH-II families the linkage with this region was not observed, indicating a genetic heterogeneity of this disease. Intriguingly, in a linkage analysis that included 1,225 individuals from 328 families, logARR was demonstrated to be in linkage with 7p21-22 with a LOD score of 2.78 [137]. The diagnosis of FH-II requires PA to be confirmed in two or more family members and exclusion of FH-I. The recent PATOGEN study [138] demonstrated that the prevalence of FH-II is much higher than FH-I/GRA, accounting for 6% of PA patients, whereas FH-I/GRA was found in less than 1% of PA patients.

FH-III is a newly described familial form of PA characterized by a particularly severe form of hyperaldosteronism resistant to aggressive pharmacotherapy thus requiring bilateral adrenalectomy [139, 140]. The underlying genetic cause has been recently shown to be due to mutations in the gene encoding the potassium channel KCNJ5 (Kir 3.4, potassium inwardly rectifying channel, subfamily 1, member 5) [141]: the mutation occurs near the selectivity filter for potassium resulting in increased sodium conductance and cell depolarization, which in adrenal glomerulosa cells produces calcium entry and thus increased aldosterone production and cell proliferation.

Genetics of Sporadic PA

In sporadic primary aldosteronism, abnormal adrenal proliferation, development of adrenal tumor/nodularity, and excessive aldosterone secretion may originate from one or more gene variants (mutations or polymorphisms). These variants may have a somatic or germline origin and act alone or in combination with a series of other genetic and/or environmental factors. The somatic mutation hypothesis is especially valid for APA. In most APA patients, aldosterone levels are ACTH-dependent and increased concentrations of hybrid steroids are detectable. Although these findings parallel those in GRA subjects, the presence of the chimeric gene has been ruled out in APA [142].

An *in vitro* site-directed mutagenesis study converted the cortisol producing enzyme, CYP11B1, into an aldosterone-producing enzyme by substituting two amino acids with the corresponding residues from CYP11B2, S288G, and V320A [120].

If these somatic point mutations existed *in vivo* in *CYP11B1*, a gene encoding an enzyme with 18-hydroxylase and 18-oxidase activities and would preserve ACTH responsiveness due to the retained 5′-promoter in the mutated *CYP11B1* gene. However, no point mutations of the *CYP11B1* gene over the two regions examined were found in APA [143]. Furthermore, no mutations have yet been identified in genes coding for p53, RAS, Gsα, renin, angiotensin II type 1 receptor, *CYP21,* and the MEN1 locus [144–147]. In IHA, most studies have focused on germline variants of *CYP11B2* with a possible effect on the enzymatic function or on the level of expression of aldosterone synthase. The most obvious candidate mutation, the chimeric *CYP11B1/B2* gene, was not present in a large population of patients [132, 148]. Interestingly, one study reported that lymphomonocytes from IHA patients overexpress *CYP11B2* compared to normal controls and APA subjects [149]. It is possible that common gene variants may affect the transcription rate of *CYP11B2*, ultimately leading to inappropriate aldosterone levels. Three main polymorphisms of *CYP11B2* have been described: (1) a C-344Tsubstitution; (2) an intron 2 gene conversion; and (3) an R173K (Arg173Lys) substitution.

The first polymorphism, C-344T, is situated in the promoter region of *CYP11B2* and localizes to a putative recognition site for the steroidogenic transcription factor-1 (SF1). The true biological effect of this variant is unclear: in fact, while binding of SF1 is consistently reduced with the -344T allele, there appears to be no clear effect on gene transcription when assessed *in vitro* [150]. The second polymorphism is a conversion of *CYP11B2* whereby part of intron 2 is replaced with the corresponding intronic region of *CYP11B1*. Finally, the R173K polymorphism results from a G/A substitution in the coding region of the gene: this substitution does not affect aldosterone synthesis *in vitro* [151]. Overall, there is considerable data that links the CYP11B2 locus to hypertension and particularly to mineralocorticoid excess-hypertension. In particular, the C-344T polymorphism has been associated by a number of different studies with higher levels of plasmatic and urinary aldosterone, essential salt-sensitive hypertension, and PA itself [152, 153].

Although primary aldosteronism most frequently presents with moderate to severe hypertension, its clinical and biochemical features vary widely. For example, a number of APA patients and several carriers of the GRA mutation have been reported to be normotensive. A significant proportion of this phenotypical heterogeneity may derive from the individual efficiency of the aldosterone-escape mechanisms which counterbalance aldosterone excess, independent of its etiology which may be genetically determined. To test this hypothesis, we focused on genetic variants potentially affecting renal proximal tubule reabsorption (alpha-adducin), vasodilation, and sodium excretion [bradykinin receptor type 2 (B2R), natriuretic peptide receptor type C (NPR-C)], as well as aldosterone production (aldosterone synthase, CYP11B2) [154]. We demonstrated that B2R (C-58T) and alpha-adducin (G460W, Gly460Trp) genotypes appeared to be strong independent predictors of both systolic and diastolic blood pressure levels in PA patients, with PRA and aldosterone as marginal determinants of blood pressure. These data suggest the existence of gene variants affecting the clinical phenotype in patients with PA [154]. Intriguingly, somatic mutations in *KCNJ5*, the same gene responsible for FH-III, have also been shown in APAs from PA patients with severe hypertension and hypokalemia [141].

Therapy of PA

Surgery

Unilateral laparoscopic adrenalectomy should be offered to patients with documented unilateral PA [4]. After adrenalectomy hypertension is cured in around 50% of patients with APA (range 33–70%) [3] whilst the remaining patients display a significant reduction of the blood pressure levels and number of antihypertensive drugs. Factors that have been reported to predict cure after adrenalectomy are: response to spironolactone therapy, young age, short duration of hypertension, family history of hypertension in ≤1 first-degree relative, preoperative use of ≤2 antihypertensive agents, higher ARR and 24-h urinary aldosterone levels [155, 156]. Of note, adrenalectomy in PA patients also improved the quality of life [157]. In a study on APA patients, adrenalectomy was reported to be associated with a significant cost saving (20,472 USD per patient) when compared with the estimated cost of medical treatment over each patient's lifetime [158]. Furthermore, this calculation did not include the potential costs associated with diagnosis and treatment of complications and time off work arising from long-term exposure to increased aldosterone levels and less adequately controlled hypertension in medically treated patients and, of course, did not take into account the improvement in the quality of the life consistently reported by patients who are surgically cured and able to cease antihypertensive medication therapy.

Medical treatment is the first choice for PA patients with bilateral disease; however, a recent study suggests that unilateral adrenalectomy may be beneficial also in carefully selected patients with bilateral PA [159].

Medical Treatment

Medical management with a mineralcorticoid receptor (MR) antagonist is recommended for patients who do not undergo surgery [4]. Spironolactone is a non-selective MR antagonist and displays significant antiandrogenic and progestational activities responsible for its most common side effects (gynecomastia, abnormal menstrual cycles, and impotence). The side effects are more frequent when spironolactone is used at high doses and/or for prolonged periods. Gynecomastia is reversible and dose related: at doses of 50 mg day^{-1} or less the incidence is around 7%, but for doses of 150 mg day^{-1} or higher the incidence increases to 52% [12].

Eplerenone is a selective MR antagonist without anti-androgen and progesterone agonist activity, it displays 60% of the potency of spironolactone and it should be administered twice daily because of its short half-life. A recent study conducted on a small number of patients with BAH, showed similar antihypertensive efficacy of spironolactone and eplerenone [160]. Amiloride is less effective in reducing blood pressure in PA patients: furthermore, due to its specific activity blocking selectively the aldosterone action on sodium reabsorbtion in the kidney, it may not protect non-epithelial tissues from the pro-inflammatory and pro-fibrotic effects mediated by aldosterone. Other drugs such as calcium channel blockers, ACE-inhibitors, and angiotensin II receptor blockers can be used in association with MR antagonists when blood pressure levels are not satisfactorily controlled. In the future, aldosterone synthase inhibitors may provide new options for treatment of PA patients.

At present, it is unknown if there is a prognostic advantage for adrenalectomy compared to therapy with MR antagonists for patients with APA. Furthermore, it is unknown if all MR antagonists confer similar protection in preventing cardiovascular events in PA patients. Finally, it is unknown if PA patients undergoing long-term therapy with MR antagonists should also be treated with angiotensin II receptor blockers to inhibit the potentially detrimental effect of the increased production of angiotensin II due to the chronic activation of the renin–angiotensin system during this therapy.

References

1. Conn J. Presidential address. I. Painting background. II. Primary aldosteronism, a new clinical syndrome. J Lab Clin Med. 1955;45:3–17.
2. Ganguly A. Primary aldosteronism. N Engl J Med. 1998;339:1828–34.
3. Mulatero P, Stowasser M, Loh KC, et al. Increased diagnosis of primary aldosteronism, including surgically correctable forms, in centers from five continents. J Clin Endocrinol Metab. 2004;89:1045–50.

4. Funder JW, Carey RM, Fardella C, et al. Case detection, diagnosis, and treatment of patients with primary aldosteronism: an endocrine society clinical practice guideline. J Clin Endocrinol Metab. 2008;93:3266–81.
5. Mosso L, Carvajal C, Gonzalez A, et al. Primary aldosteronism and hypertensive disease. Hypertension. 2003;42:161–5.
6. Calhoun DA, Nishizaka MK, Zaman MA, Thakkar RB, Weissmann P. Hyperaldosteronism among black and white subjects with resistant hypertension. Hypertension. 2002;40:892–6.
7. Piaditis GP, Kaltsas GA, Androulakis II, Gouli A, Makras P, Papadogias D, et al. High prevalence of autonomous cortisol and aldosterone secretion from adrenal adenomas. Clin Endocrinol. 2009;71:772–8.
8. Mulatero P, Milan A, Rabbia F, Garrone C, Rossato D, Veglio F. Diagnosis of surgically-treatable forms of primary aldosteronism. Curr Hypertens Rev. 2005;1:259–66.
9. Gouli A, Kaltsas G, Tzonou A, et al. High prevalence of autonomous aldosterone secretion among patients with essential hypertension. Eur J Clin Invest. 2011;41:1227–36.
10. Abdelhamid S, Blomer R, Hommel G, et al. Urinary tetrahydroaldosterone as a screening method for primary aldosteronism: a comparative study. Am J Hypertens. 2003;16:522–30.
11. Milliez P, Girerd X, Plouin PF, Blacher J, Safar ME, Mourad JJ. Evidence for an increased rate of cardiovascular events in patients with primary aldosteronism. J Am Coll Cardiol. 2005;45:1243–8.
12. Mulatero P, Milan A, Williams TA, Veglio F. Mineralocorticoid receptor blockade in the protection of target organ damage. Cardiovasc Hematol Agents Med Chem. 2006;4:75–91.
13. Neville AM, O'Hare MJ. Histopathology of the human adrenal cortex. Clin Endocrinol Metab. 1985;14:791–820.
14. Gomez-Sanchez CE, Rossi GP, Fallo F, Mannelli M. Progress in primary aldosteronism: present challenges and perspectives. Horm Metab Res. 2010;42:374–81.
15. Koch CA, Pacak K, Chrousos GP. The molecular pathogenesis of hereditary and sporadic adrenocortical and adrenomedullary tumors. J Clin Endocrinol Metab. 2002;87(12): 5367–84.
16. Stowasser M, Gordon RD, Rutherford JC, Nikwan NZ, Daunt N, Slater GJ. Diagnosis and management of primary aldosteronism. J Renin Angiotensin Aldosterone Syst. 2001;2:156–69.
17. Fallo F, Barzon L, Biasi F, Altavilla G, Boscaro M, Sonino N. Zona fasciculata-like histotype and aldosterone response to upright posture are not related in aldosterone-producing adenomas. Exp Clin Endocrinol Diabetes. 1998;106:74–8.
18. Enberg U, Volpe C, Hoog A, et al. Postoperative differentiation between unilateral adrenal adenoma and bilateral adrenal hyperplasia in primary aldosteronism by mRNA expression of the gene CYP11B2. Eur J Endocrinol. 2004;151:73–85.
19. Shigematsu K, Kawai K, Irie J, et al. Analysis of unilateral adrenal hyperplasia with primary aldosteronism from the aspect of messenger ribonucleic acid expression for steroidogenic enzymes: a comparative study with adrenal cortices adhering to aldosterone-producing adenoma. Endocrinology. 2006;147:999–1006.
20. Nishimoto K, Nakagawa K, Li D, et al. Adrenocortical zonation in humans under normal and pathological conditions. J Clin Endocrinol Metab. 2010;95:2296–305.
21. Romero DG, Yanes LL, de Rodriguez AF, et al. Disabled-2 is expressed in adrenal zona glomerulosa and is involved in aldosterone secretion. Endocrinology. 2007;148:2644–52.
22 Fallo F, Pezzi V, Barzon L, et al. Quantitative assessment of CYP11B1 and CYP11B2 expression in aldosterone-producing adenomas. Eur J Endocrinol. 2002;147:795–802.
23. Assie G, Auzan C, Gasc JM, et al. Steroidogenesis in aldosterone-producing adenoma revisited by transcriptome analysis. J Clin Endocrinol Metab. 2005;90:6638–49.
24. Bassett MH, Mayhew B, Rehman K, et al. Expression profiles for steroidogenic enzymes in adrenocortical disease. J Clin Endocrinol Metab. 2005;90:5446–55.
25. Saner-Amigh K, Mayhew BA, Mantero F, et al. Elevated expression of luteinizing hormone receptor in aldosterone-producing adenomas. J Clin Endocrinol Metab. 2006;91:1136–42.
26. Williams TA, Monticone S, Morello F, et al. Teratocarcinoma-derived growth factor-1 is upregulated in aldosterone-producing adenomas and increases aldosterone secretion and inhibits apoptosis *in vitro*. Hypertension. 2010;55:1468–75.

27. Lenzini L, Seccia TM, Aldighieri E, et al. Heterogeneity of aldosterone-producing adenomas revealed by a whole transcriptome analysis. Hypertension. 2007;50:1106–13.
28. Ye P, Mariniello B, Mantero F, Shibata H, Rainey WE. G-protein-coupled receptors in aldosterone-producing adenomas: a potential cause of hyperaldosteronism. J Endocrinol. 2007;195:39–48.
29. Rainey WE, Saner K, Schimmer BP. Adrenocortical cell lines. Mol Cell Endocrinol. 2004;228:23–38.
30. Cartier D, Jegou S, Parmentier F, et al. Expression profile of serotonin4 (5-HT4) receptors in adrenocortical aldosterone-producing adenomas. Eur J Endocrinol. 2005;153:939–47.
31. Lampron A, Bourdeau I, Oble S, et al. Regulation of aldosterone secretion by several aberrant receptors including for glucose-dependent insulinotropic peptide in a patient with an aldosteronoma. J Clin Endocrinol Metab. 2009;94:750–6.
32. Rocha R, Funder JW. The pathophysiology of aldosterone in the cardiovascular system. Ann N Y Acad Sci. 2002;970:89–100.
33. Rocha R, Stier Jr CT, Kifor I, et al. Aldosterone: a mediator of myocardial necrosis and renal arteriopathy. Endocrinology. 2000;141:3871–8.
34. Fiebeler A, Schmidt F, Muller DN, et al. Mineralocorticoid receptor affects AP-1 and nuclear factor-kappab activation in angiotensin II-induced cardiac injury. Hypertension. 2001; 37:787–93.
35. Rossi GP, Sacchetto A, Visentin P, et al. Changes in left ventricular anatomy and function in hypertension and primary aldosteronism. Hypertension. 1996;27:1039–45.
36. Napoli C, Di Gregorio F, Leccese M, et al. Evidence of exercise-induced myocardial ischemia in patients with primary aldosteronism: the Cross-sectional Primary Aldosteronism and Heart Italian Multicenter Study. J Investig Med. 1999;47:212–21.
37. Kozakova M, Buralli S, Palombo C, et al. Myocardial ultrasonic backscatter in hypertension: relation to aldosterone and endothelin. Hypertension. 2003;41:230–6.
38. Mihailidou AS, Bundgaard H, Mardini M, Hansen PS, Kjeldsen K, Rasmussen HH. Hyperaldosteronemia in rabbits inhibits the cardiac sarcolemmal Na(+)-K(+) pump. Circ Res. 2000;86:37–42.
39. Caballero R, Moreno I, Gonzalez T, et al. Spironolactone and its main metabolite, canrenoic acid, block human ether-a-go-go-related gene channels. Circulation. 2003;107:889–95.
40. Lalevee N, Rebsamen MC, Barrere-Lemaire S, et al. Aldosterone increases T-type calcium channel expression and *in vitro* beating frequency in neonatal rat cardiomyocytes. Cardiovasc Res. 2005;67:216–24.
41. Ouvrard-Pascaud A, Sainte-Marie Y, Benitah JP, et al. Conditional mineralocorticoid receptor expression in the heart leads to life-threatening arrhythmias. Circulation. 2005;111:3025.
42. Blanco-Rivero J, Cachofeiro V, Lahera V, et al. Participation of prostacyclin in endothelial dysfunction induced by aldosterone in normotensive and hypertensive rats. Hypertension. 2005;46:107–12.
43. Pu Q, Neves MF, Virdis A, Touyz RM, Schiffrin EL. Endothelin antagonism on aldosterone-induced oxidative stress and vascular remodeling. Hypertension. 2003;42:49–55.
44. Ikeda U, Kanbe T, Nakayama I, Kawahara Y, Yokoyama M, Shimada K. Aldosterone inhibits nitric oxide synthesis in rat vascular smooth muscle cells induced by interleukin-1 beta. Eur J Pharmacol. 1995;290:69–73.
45. Rizzoni D, Paiardi S, Rodella L, et al. Changes in extracellular matrix in subcutaneous small resistance arteries of patients with primary aldosteronism. J Clin Endocrinol Metab. 2006;91:2638.
46. Greene EL, Kren S, Hostetter TH. Role of aldosterone in the remnant kidney model in the rat. J Clin Invest. 1996;98:1063–8.
47. Rocha R, Chander PN, Khanna K, Zuckerman A, Stier Jr CT. Mineralocorticoid blockade reduces vascular injury in stroke-prone hypertensive rats. Hypertension. 1998;31:451–8.
48. Rocha R, Chander PN, Zuckerman A, Stier Jr CT. Role of aldosterone in renal vascular injury in stroke-prone hypertensive rats. Hypertension. 1999;33:232–7.
49. Blasi ER, Rocha R, Rudolph AE, Blomme EA, Polly ML, McMahon EG. Aldosterone/salt induces renal inflammation and fibrosis in hypertensive rats. Kidney Int. 2003;63:1791–800.

50. Gomez-Sanchez CE, Zhou MY, Cozza EN, Morita H, Foecking MF, Gomez-Sanchez EP. Aldosterone biosynthesis in the rat brain. Endocrinology. 1997;138:3369–73.
51. Brody MJ, Varner KJ, Vasquez EC, Lewis SJ. Central nervous system and the pathogenesis of hypertension. Sites and mechanisms. Hypertension. 1991;18:III7–12.
52. Sakai RR, Ma LY, Zhang DM, McEwen BS, Fluharty SJ. Intracerebral administration of mineralocorticoid receptor antisense oligonucleotides attenuate adrenal steroid-induced salt appetite in rats. Neuroendocrinology. 1996;64:425–9.
53. Janiak P, Brody MJ. Central interactions between aldosterone and vasopressin on cardiovascular system. Am J Physiol. 1988;255:R166–73.
54. Kageyama Y, Bravo EL. Hypertensive mechanisms associated with centrally administered aldosterone in dogs. Hypertension. 1988;11:750–3.
55. Wang W, McClain JM, Zucker IH. Aldosterone reduces baroreceptor discharge in the dog. Hypertension. 1992;19:270–7.
56. Rocha R, Stier Jr CT. Pathophysiological effects of aldosterone in cardiovascular tissues. Trends Endocrinol Metab. 2001;12:308–14.
57. Gonzalez-Campoy JM, Romero JC, Knox FG. Escape from the sodium-retaining effects of mineralocorticoids: role of ANF and intrarenal hormone systems. Kidney Int. 1989;35:767–77.
58. Romagni P, Rossi F, Guerrini L, Quirini C, Santiemma V. Aldosterone induces contraction of the resistance arteries in man. Atherosclerosis. 2003;166:345–9.
59. Huang YY, Hsu BR, Tsai JS. Paralytic myopathy–a leading clinical presentation for primary aldosteronism in Taiwan. J Clin Endocrinol Metab. 1996;81:4038–41.
60. Maule S, Mulatero P, Milan A, et al. QT interval in patients with primary aldosteronism and low-renin essential hypertension. J Hypertens. 2006;24:2459–64.
61. Maule S, Bertello C, Rabbia F, et al. Ventricular repolarization before and after treatment in patients with secondary hypertension due to renal-artery stenosis and primary aldosteronism. Hypertens Res. 2011;34(10):1078–81.
62. Fallo F, Veglio F, Bertello C, et al. Prevalence and characteristics of the metabolic syndrome in primary aldosteronism. J Clin Endocrinol Metab. 2006;91:454–9.
63. Fallo FD, Mea P, Sonino N, et al. Adiponectin and insulin sensitivity in primary aldosteronism. Am J Hypertens. 2007;20:855–61.
64. Sowers JR, Whaley-Connell A, Epstein M. Narrative review: the emerging clinical implications of the role of aldosterone in the metabolic syndrome and resistant hypertension. Ann Intern Med. 2009;150:776–83.
65. Catena C, Lapenna R, Baroselli S, et al. Insulin sensitivity in patients with primary aldosteronism: a follow-up study. J Clin Endocrinol Metab. 2006;91:3457–63.
66. Jeon JH, Kim KY, Kim JH, et al. A novel adipokine CTRP1 stimulates aldosterone production. FASEB J. 2008;22:1502–11.
67. Ingelsson E, Pencina MJ, Tofler GH, et al. Multimarker approach to evaluate the incidence of the metabolic syndrome and longitudinal changes in metabolic risk factors: the Framingham Offspring Study. Circulation. 2007;116:984–92.
68. Matrozova J, Steichen O, Amar L, Zacharieva S, Jeunemaitre X, Plouin PF. Fasting plasma glucose and serum lipids in patients with primary aldosteronism: a controlled cross-sectional study. Hypertension. 2009;53:605–10.
69. Reincke M, Meisinger C, Holle R, et al. Is primary aldosteronism associated with diabetes mellitus? Results of the German Conn's Registry. Horm Metab Res. 2010;42:435–9.
70. Umpierrez GE, Cantey P, Smiley D, Palacio A, Temponi D, Luster K, et al. Primary aldosteronism in diabetic subjects with resistant hypertension. Diabetes Care. 2007;30:1699–703.
71. Mukherjee JJ, Khoo CM, Thai AC, Chionh SB, Pin L, Lee KO. Type 2 diabetic patients with resistant hypertension should be screened for primary aldosteronism. Diab Vasc Dis Res. 2010;7:6–13.
72. Rossi GP, Di Bello V, Ganzaroli C, et al. Excess aldosterone is associated with alterations of myocardial texture in primary aldosteronism. Hypertension. 2002;40:23–7.
73. Holaj R, Zelinka T, Wichterle D, Petrak O, Strauch B, Widimsky Jr J. Increased intima-media thickness of the common carotid artery in primary aldosteronism in comparison with essential hypertension. J Hypertens. 2007;25:1451–7.

74. Strauch B, Zelinka T, Hampf M, Bernhardt R, Widimsky Jr J. Prevalence of primary hyperaldosteronism in moderate to severe hypertension in the Central Europe region. J Hum Hypertens. 2003;17(5):349–52.
75. Born-Frontsberg E, Reincke M, Rump LC, et al. Cardiovascular and cerebrovascular comorbidities of hypokalemic and normokalemic primary aldosteronism: results of the German Conn's Registry. J Clin Endocrinol Metab. 2009;94:1125–30.
76. Calhoun DA, Nishizaka MK, Zaman MA, Harding SM. Aldosterone excretion among subjects with resistant hypertension and symptoms of sleep apnea. Chest. 2004;125:112–7.
77. Pratt-Ubunama MN, Nishizaka MK, Boedefeld RL, Cofield SS, Harding SM, Calhoun DA. Plasma aldosterone is related to severity of obstructive sleep apnea in subjects with resistant hypertension. Chest. 2007;131:453–9.
78. Ribstein J, Du Cailar G, Fesler P, Mimran A. Relative glomerular hyperfiltration in primary aldosteronism. J Am Soc Nephrol. 2005;16:1320–5.
79. Rossi GP, Bernini G, Desideri G, et al. Renal damage in primary aldosteronism: results of the PAPY Study. Hypertension. 2006;48:232–8.
80. Sechi LA, Novello M, Lapenna R, et al. Long-term renal outcomes in patients with primary aldosteronism. JAMA. 2006;295:2638–45.
81. Sechi LA, Di Fabio A, Bazzocchi M, Uzzau A, Catena C. Intrarenal hemodynamics in primary aldosteronism before and after treatment. J Clin Endocrinol Metab. 2009;94:1191–7.
82. Reincke M, Rump LC, Quinkler M, et al. Risk factors associated with a low glomerular filtration rate in primary aldosteronism. J Clin Endocrinol Metab. 2009;94:869–75.
83. Catena C, Colussi G, Lapenna R, et al. Long-term cardiac effects of adrenalectomy or mineralocorticoid antagonists in patients with primary aldosteronism. Hypertension. 2007;50:911–8.
84. Hiramatsu K, Yamada T, Yukimura Y, et al. A screening test to identify aldosterone-producing adenoma by measuring plasma renin activity. Results in hypertensive patients. Arch Intern Med. 1981;141:1589–93.
85. McKenna TJ, Sequeira SJ, Heffernan A, Chambers J, Cunningham S. Diagnosis under random conditions of all disorders of the renin-angiotensin-aldosterone axis, including primary hyperaldosteronism. J Clin Endocrinol Metab. 1991;73:952–7.
86. Stowasser M, Gordon RD, Gunasekera TG, et al. High rate of detection of primary aldosteronism, including surgically treatable forms, after 'non-selective' screening of hypertensive patients. J Hypertens. 2003;21:2149–57.
87. Rossi GP, Seccia TM, Palumbo G, et al. Within-patient reproducibility of the aldosterone: renin ratio in primary aldosteronism. Hypertension. 2010;55:83–9.
88. Mulatero P, Rabbia F, Milan A, et al. Drug effects on aldosterone/plasma renin activity ratio in primary aldosteronism. Hypertension. 2002;40:897–902.
89. Fardella CE, Mosso L, Gomez-Sanchez C, et al. Primary hyperaldosteronism in essential hypertensives: prevalence, biochemical profile, and molecular biology. J Clin Endocrinol Metab. 2000;85:1863–7.
90. Olivieri O, Ciacciarelli A, Signorelli D, et al. Aldosterone to Renin ratio in a primary care setting: the Bussolengo study. J Clin Endocrinol Metab. 2004;89:4221–6.
91. Hartman D, Sagnella GA, Chesters CA, Macgregor GA. Direct renin assay and plasma renin activity assay compared. Clin Chem. 2004;50:2159–61.
92. Dorrian CA, Toole BJ, Alvarez-Madrazo S, Kelly A, Connell JM, Wallace AM. A screening procedure for primary aldosteronism based on the Diasorin Liaison automated chemiluminescent immunoassay for direct renin. Ann Clin Biochem. 2010;47:195–9.
93. Mulatero P, Monticone S, Bertello C, et al. Confirmatory tests in the diagnosis of primary aldosteronism. Horm Metab Res. 2010;42:406–10.
94. Young WF. Primary aldosteronism: renaissance of a syndrome. Clin Endocrinol (Oxf). 2007;66:607–18.
95. Rossi GP, Bernini G, Caliumi C, et al. A prospective study of the prevalence of primary aldosteronism in 1,125 hypertensive patients. J Am Coll Cardiol. 2006;48:2293–300.
96. Lyons DF, Kem DC, Brown RD, Hanson CS, Carollo ML. Single dose captopril as a diagnostic test for primary aldosteronism. J Clin Endocrinol Metab. 1983;57:892–6.

97. Agharazii M, Douville P, Grose JH, Lebel M. Captopril suppression versus salt loading in confirming primary aldosteronism. Hypertension. 2001;37:1440–3.
98. Castro OL, Yu X, Kem DC. Diagnostic value of the post-captopril test in primary aldosteronism. Hypertension. 2002;39:935–8.
99. Omura M, Saito J, Yamaguchi K, Kakuta Y, Nishikawa T. Prospective study on the prevalence of secondary hypertension among hypertensive patients visiting a general outpatient clinic in Japan. Hypertens Res. 2004;27:193–202.
100. Giacchetti G, Ronconi V, Lucarelli G, Boscaro M, Mantero F. Analysis of screening and confirmatory tests in the diagnosis of primary aldosteronism: need for a standardized protocol. J Hypertens. 2006;24:737–45.
101. Wu VC, Chang HW, Liu KL, et al. Primary aldosteronism: diagnostic accuracy of the losartan and captopril tests. Am J Hypertens. 2009;22:821–7.
102. Mulatero P, Milan A, Fallo F, et al. Comparison of confirmatory tests for the diagnosis of primary aldosteronism. J Clin Endocrinol Metab. 2006;91:2618–23.
103. Mulatero P, Bertello C, Garrone C, et al. Captopril test can give misleading results in patients with suspect primary aldosteronism. Hypertension. 2007;50:e26–7.
104. Rossi GP, Belfiore A, Bernini G, et al. Comparison of the captopril and the saline infusion test for excluding aldosterone-producing adenoma. Hypertension. 2007;50:424–31.
105. Pizzolo F, Corgnati A, Guarini P, et al. Plasma aldosterone assays: comparison between chemiluminescence-based and RIA methods. Clin Chem. 2006;52:1431–2.
106. Schirpenbach C, Seiler L, Maser-Gluth C, Beuschlein F, Reincke M, Bidlingmaier M. Automated chemiluminescence-immunoassay for aldosterone during dynamic testing: comparison to radioimmunoassays with and without extraction steps. Clin Chem. 2006;52:1749–55.
107. Mulatero P, Bertello C, Rossato D, et al. Roles of clinical criteria, computed tomography scan, and adrenal vein sampling in differential diagnosis of primary aldosteronism subtypes. J Clin Endocrinol Metab. 2008;93:1366–71.
108. Mansoor GA, Malchoff CD, Arici MH, Karimeddini MK, Whalen GF. Unilateral adrenal hyperplasia causing primary aldosteronism: limitations of I-131 norcholesterol scanning. Am J Hypertens. 2002;15:459–64.
109. Nwariaku FE, Miller BS, Auchus R, et al. Primary hyperaldosteronism: effect of adrenal vein sampling on surgical outcome. Arch Surg. 2006;141:497–502; discussion 502–3.
110. Young WF, Stanson AW, Thompson GB, Grant CS, Farley DR, van Heerden JA. Role for adrenal venous sampling in primary aldosteronism. Surgery. 2004;136:1227–35.
111. Mengozzi G, Rossato D, Bertello C, et al. Rapid cortisol assay during adrenal vein sampling in patients with primary aldosteronism. Clin Chem. 2007;53:1968–71.
112. Mulatero P, Bertello C, Sukor N, et al. Impact of different diagnostic criteria during adrenal vein sampling on reproducibility of subtype diagnosis in patients with primary aldosteronism. Hypertension. 2010;55:667–73.
113. Seccia TM, Miotto D, De Toni R, et al. Adrenocorticotropic hormone stimulation during adrenal vein sampling for identifying surgically curable subtypes of primary aldosteronism: comparison of 3 different protocols. Hypertension. 2009;53:761–6.
114. Mulatero P, Bertello C, Verhovez A, et al. Differential diagnosis of primary aldosteronism subtypes. Curr Hypertens Rep. 2009;11:217–23.
115. Fallo F, Bertello C, Tizzani D, Fassina A, Boulkroun S, Sonino N, et al. Concurrent primary aldosteronism and subclinical cortisol hypersecretion: a prospective study. J Hypertens. 2011;29(9):1773–7.
116. Curnow KM, Tusie-Luna MT, Pascoe L, et al. The product of the CYP11B2 gene is required for aldosterone biosynthesis in the human adrenal cortex. Mol Endocrinol. 1991;5:1513–22.
117. Kawamoto T, Mitsuuchi Y, Toda K, et al. Role of steroid 11 beta-hydroxylase and steroid 18-hydroxylase in the biosynthesis of glucocorticoids and mineralocorticoids in humans. Proc Natl Acad Sci U S A. 1992;89:1458–62.
118. Brand E, Chatelain N, Mulatero P, et al. Structural analysis and evaluation of the aldosterone synthase gene in hypertension. Hypertension. 1998;32:198–204.
119. Taymans SE, Pack S, Pak E, Torpy DJ, Zhuang Z, Stratakis CA. Human CYP11B2 (aldosterone synthase) maps to chromosome 8q24.3. J Clin Endocrinol Metab. 1998;83:1033–6.

120. Curnow KM, Mulatero P, Emeric-Blanchouin N, Aupetit-Faisant B, Corvol P, Pascoe L. The amino acid substitutions Ser288Gly and Val320Ala convert the cortisol producing enzyme, CYP11B1, into an aldosterone producing enzyme. Nat Struct Biol. 1997;4:32–5.
121. Ulick S, Chu MD. Hypersecretion of a new corticosteroid, 18-hydroxycortisol in two types of adrenocortical hypertension. Clin Exp Hypertens A. 1982;4:1771–7.
122. Shibata H, Ogishima T, Mitani F, et al. Regulation of aldosterone synthase cytochrome P-450 in rat adrenals by angiotensin II and potassium. Endocrinology. 1991;128:2534–9.
123. Lehoux JG, Fleury A, Ducharme L. The acute and chronic effects of adrenocorticotropin on the levels of messenger ribonucleic acid and protein of steroidogenic enzymes in rat adrenal *in vivo*. Endocrinology. 1998;139:3913–22.
124. Lifton RP, Dluhy RG, Powers M, et al. A chimaeric 11 beta-hydroxylase/aldosterone synthase gene causes glucocorticoid-remediable aldosteronism and human hypertension. Nature. 1992;355:262–5.
125. Mulatero P, Morello F, Veglio F. Genetics of primary aldosteronism. J Hypertens. 2004;22(4):663–70.
126. Dluhy RG, Anderson B, Harlin B, Ingelfinger J, Lifton R. Glucocorticoid-remediable aldosteronism is associated with severe hypertension in early childhood. J Pediatr. 2001;138:715–20.
127. Wyckoff JA, Seely EW, Hurwitz S, Anderson BF, Lifton RP, Dluhy RG. Glucocorticoid-remediable aldosteronism and pregnancy. Hypertension. 2000;35:668–72.
128. Litchfield WR, Anderson BF, Weiss RJ, Lifton RP, Dluhy RG. Intracranial aneurysm and hemorrhagic stroke in glucocorticoid-remediable aldosteronism. Hypertension. 1998;31:445–50.
129. Mulatero P, di Cella SM, Williams TA, et al. Glucocorticoid remediable aldosteronism: low morbidity and mortality in a four-generation italian pedigree. J Clin Endocrinol Metab. 2002;87:3187–91.
130. Sutherland DJ, Ruse JL, Laidlaw JC. Hypertension, increased aldosterone secretion and low plasma renin activity relieved by dexamethasone. Can Med Assoc J. 1966;95:1109–19.
131. Halperin F, Dluhy RG. Glucocorticoid-remediable aldosteronism. Endocrinol Metab Clin North Am. 2011;40(2):333–41.
132. Mulatero P, Veglio F, Pilon C, et al. Diagnosis of glucocorticoid-remediable aldosteronism in primary aldosteronism: aldosterone response to dexamethasone and long polymerase chain reaction for chimeric gene. J Clin Endocrinol Metab. 1998;83:2573–5.
133. Aglony M, Martínez-Aguayo A, Carvajal CA, Campino C, García H, Bancalari R, et al. Frequency of familial hyperaldosteronism type 1 in a hypertensive pediatric population: clinical and biochemical presentation. Hypertension. 2011;57:1117–21.
134. Mulatero P, Williams TA, Monticone S, Veglio F. Is familial hyperaldosteronism underdiagnosed in hypertensive children? Hypertension. 2011;57:1053–5.
135. Lafferty AR, Torpy DJ, Stowasser M, et al. A novel genetic locus for low renin hypertension: familial hyperaldosteronism type II maps to chromosome 7 (7p22). J Med Genet. 2000;37:831–5.
136. Sukor N, Mulatero P, Gordon RD, et al. Further evidence for linkage of familial hyperaldosteronism type II at chromosome 7p22 in Italian as well as Australian and South American families. J Hypertens. 2008;26:1577–82.
137. Newton-Cheh C, Guo CY, Gona P, et al. Clinical and genetic correlates of aldosterone-to-renin ratio and relations to blood pressure in a community sample. Hypertension. 2007;49:846–56.
138. Mulatero P, Tizzani D, Viola A, Bertello C, Monticone S, Mengozzi G, et al. Prevalence and Characteristics of Familial Hyperaldosteronism: the PATOGEN study (Primary Aldosteronism in TOrino—GENetic forms). Hypertension. 2011;58(5):797–803.
139. Geller DS, Zhang J, Wisgerhof MV, Shackleton C, Kashgarian M, Lifton RP. A novel form of human mendelian hypertension featuring nonglucocorticoid-remediable aldosteronism. J Clin Endocrinol Metab. 2008;93:3117–23.
140. Mulatero P. A new form of hereditary primary aldosteronism: familial hyperaldosteronism type III. J Clin Endocrinol Metab. 2008;93:2972–4.
141. Choi M, Scholl UI, Yue P, Björklund P, Zhao B, Nelson-Williams C, et al. K+ channel mutations in adrenal aldosterone-producing adenomas and hereditary hypertension. Science. 2011;331:768–72.

142. Carroll J, Dluhy R, Fallo F, et al. Aldosterone-producing adenomas do not contain glucocorticoid-remediable aldosteronism chimeric gene duplications. J Clin Endocrinol Metab. 1996;81:4310–2.
143. Pilon C, Mulatero P, Barzon L, et al. Mutations in CYP11B1 gene converting 11beta-hydroxylase into an aldosterone-producing enzyme are not present in aldosterone-producing adenomas. J Clin Endocrinol Metab. 1999;84:4228–31.
144. Higaki J, Miya A, Miki T, et al. Contribution of the activation of the ras oncogene to the evolution of aldosterone- and renin-secreting tumors. J Hypertens. 1991;9:135–7.
145. Gordon RD. Primary aldosteronism: a new understanding. Clin Exp Hypertens. 1997;19:857–70.
146. Zwermann O, Beuschlein F, Mora P, Weber G, Allolio B, Reincke M. Multiple endocrine neoplasia type 1 gene expression is normal in sporadic adrenocortical tumors. Eur J Endocrinol. 2000;142:689–95.
147. Beuschlein F, Schulze E, Mora P, et al. Steroid 21-hydroxylase mutations and 21-hydroxylase messenger ribonucleic acid expression in human adrenocortical tumors. J Clin Endocrinol Metab. 1998;83:2585–8.
148. Mulatero P, Curnow KM, Aupetit-Faisant B, et al. Recombinant CYP11B genes encode enzymes that can catalyze conversion of 11-deoxycortisol to cortisol, 18-hydroxycortisol, and 18-oxocortisol. J Clin Endocrinol Metab. 1998;83:3996–4001.
149. Miyamori I, Inaba S, Hatakeyama H, Taniguchi N, Takeda Y. Idiopathic hyperaldosteronism: analysis of aldosterone synthase gene. Biomed Pharmacother. 2000;54 Suppl 1:77s–9.
150. Bassett MH, Zhang Y, Clyne C, White PC, Rainey WE. Differential regulation of aldosterone synthase and 11beta-hydroxylase transcription by steroidogenic factor-1. J Mol Endocrinol. 2002;28:125–35.
151. Portrat-Doyen S, Tourniaire J, Richard O, et al. Isolated aldosterone synthase deficiency caused by simultaneous E198D and V386A mutations in the CYP11B2 gene. J Clin Endocrinol Metab. 1998;83:4156–61.
152. Mulatero P, Schiavone D, Fallo F, et al. CYP11B2 gene polymorphisms in idiopathic hyperaldosteronism. Hypertension. 2000;35:694–8.
153. Davies E, Kenyon CJ. CYP11B2 polymorphisms and cardiovascular risk factors. J Hypertens. 2003;21:1249–53.
154. Mulatero P, Williams TA, Milan A, et al. Blood pressure in patients with primary aldosteronism is influenced by bradykinin B(2) receptor and alpha-adducin gene polymorphisms. J Clin Endocrinol Metab. 2002;87:3337–43.
155. Sawka AM, Young WF, Thompson GB, et al. Primary aldosteronism: factors associated with normalization of blood pressure after surgery. Ann Intern Med. 2001;135:258–61.
156. Celen O, O'Brien MJ, Melby JC, Beazley RM. Factors influencing outcome of surgery for primary aldosteronism. Arch Surg. 1996;131:646–50.
157. Sukor N, Kogovsek C, Gordon RD, Robson D, Stowasser M. Improved quality of life, blood pressure, and biochemical status following laparoscopic adrenalectomy for unilateral primary aldosteronism. J Clin Endocrinol Metab. 2010;95:1360–4.
158. Sywak M, Pasieka JL. Long-term follow-up and cost benefit of adrenalectomy in patients with primary hyperaldosteronism. Br J Surg. 2002;89:1587–93.
159. Sukor N, Gordon RD, Ku YK, Jones M, Stowasser M. Role of unilateral adrenalectomy in bilateral primary aldosteronism: a 22-year single center experience. J Clin Endocrinol Metab. 2009;94:2437–45.
160. Karagiannis A, Tziomalos K, Papageorgiou A, et al. Spironolactone versus eplerenone for the treatment of idiopathic hyperaldosteronism. Expert Opin Pharmacother. 2008;9:509–15.

Chapter 2
Syndromes of Mineralocorticoid Excess

Eugen Melcescu and Christian A. Koch

Abstract In addition to obesity, diabetes type 2, and the metabolic syndrome, hypertension represents a major public and global health problem, most of which can be improved by lifestyle changes, including changing dietary habits with less consumption of processed and preserved foods, which generally contain higher amounts of salt than freshly prepared food items. Amongst causes for endocrine hypertension are syndromes of mineralocorticoid excess typically resulting from overactive amiloride-sensitive sodium channels located in the distal convoluted tubules and collecting ducts of the kidney, as well as other tissues, including vascular smooth muscle. The net effect of such an overactivation, which occurs mostly in primary aldosteronism is sodium and water retention with volume expansion and hypertension that is exacerbated by a diet high in salt. Biochemically, plasma renin activity is suppressed and hypokalemia may be present. Aldosterone mediates its action through the mineralocortoid receptor (MR), which regulates salt homeostasis in the kidneys and plays a range of other roles in the vasculature, heart, brain, and adipose tissue.

Excessive MR activation can promote inflammation, fibrosis, and heart disease as well as psychiatric illness, including anxiety and depression, through key modulators, including the glucocorticoid receptor and the 11β-hydroxysteroid dehydrogenases.

Apart from aldosterone, the MR is also activated by products of abnormal adrenal steroid biosynthesis, dysregulated metabolism of cortisol in cells that are targets of mineralocorticoids, and activating mutations of the MR or of ion channels that are inducible by the MR. We provide here an overview of mineralocorticoid excess caused by congenital adrenal hyperplasia due to mutations of the 11beta-hydroxylase and 17alpha-hydroxylase genes, by mutations of the 11beta-hydroxysteroid dehydrogenase type 2 gene (apparent mineralocorticoid excess (AME)), mutations of the epithelial sodium channel genes (Liddle syndrome), mutations of the

E. Melcescu • C.A. Koch (✉)
Division of Endocrinology, University of Mississippi Medical Center,
2500 N State Street Clin Sci Building, Room 512, Jackson, MS 39216, USA
e-mail: ckoch@umc.edu

C.A. Koch and G.P. Chrousos (eds.), *Endocrine Hypertension: Underlying Mechanisms and Therapy*, Contemporary Endocrinology, DOI 10.1007/978-1-60761-548-4_2,

mineralocorticoid receptor gene (Geller syndrome), and pseudohypoaldosteronism type 2 or Gordon syndrome.

Most of these conditions are treated by restricted dietary salt intake. However, some require special therapies, including hydrocortisone (CAH), spironolactone/eplerenone, thiazide diuretics (Liddle and Gordon syndrome), while in others spironolactone and other MR antagonists may be contraindicated (Geller syndrome). Understanding the pathophysiology of these rare conditions may help designing future molecular-targeted therapies. Naturally, the mainstay of antihypertensive therapy continues to be reducing the overconsumption of salt in addition to increasing compliance and adherence of patients to currently available indicated therapies.

Keywords Mineralocorticoid excess • SME • Aldosterone • Endocrine hypertension • Congenital adrenal hyperplasia • Licorice-induced hypertension • Liddle syndrome • Pseudohypoaldosteronism type 2 • Geller syndrome

Introduction

Syndromes of mineralocorticoid excess (SME) typically result from overactive amiloride-sensitive sodium channels located in the distal convoluted tubule and collecting ducts of the kidney, as well as of other tissues, including vascular smooth muscle [1]. The effect of such an overactivation is sodium and water retention with volume expansion and hypertension (without hypernatremia) that is aggravated by a diet high in salt, as it is presently the case for many Americans, but also for people in other parts of the world where processed and preserved foods instead of freshly prepared meals are consumed. Biochemically, plasma renin activity is suppressed and hypokalemia may be present (Table 2.1).

Most frequently, the underlying condition for syndromes of mineralocorticoid excess is autonomous secretion of aldosterone or primary aldosteronism (see Chap. 1 in this book and ref. [2]). Aldosterone mediates its action through the mineralocortoid receptor (MR) which regulates salt homeostasis in the kidneys and plays a range of other roles in the vasculature, heart, brain, and adipose tissue. To mediate transcription of target genes, the MR interacts with both mineralocorticoids and glucocorticoids (reviewed in [3]). The MR is able to exert tissue- and ligand-specific effects via its interactions with a range of binding partners. The MR also plays a major role in inducing glomerular podocyte injury and progression of chronic kidney disease which can be reduced by MR antagonists or selective MR inhibition [4].

Excessive MR activation can promote inflammation, fibrosis, and heart disease as well as psychiatric illness including anxiety and depression through key modulators including the glucocorticoid receptor (GR) and 11β-hydroxysteroid dehydrogenases (11βHSDs), which determine the amount of intracellular concentrations of active glucocorticoids [5, 6].

Table 2.1 Conditions with low renin concentrations

Common conditions with low renin concentrations
Mineralocorticoid excess
Primary aldosteronism (see Chap. 1)
Cushing's Syndrome (see Chap. 3)
Glucocorticoid/cortisol resistance (see Chap. 4)
Apparent mineralocorticoid excess syndrome
Licorice or carbenoxolone in excess
Congenital adrenal hyperplasia (11beta- and 17alpha-hydroxylase deficiencies)
11-Deoxycorticosterone (DOC), 18-hydroxy-DOC excess
Salt retention (Gordon and Liddle syndrome)
Geller syndrome
Salt loading (oral or intravenous)
Rare conditions leading to low renin levels
Increasing age
Low renin essential hypertension
Hyporeninemic hypoaldosteronism
Hyperkalemia
Therapy with beta-adrenergic blockers
Autonomic dysfunction
Decrease of renal tissue or being anephric

Koch CA, Wofford MR, Ayala AR, Pacak K. Overview of endocrine hypertension (from Chapter 26) http://www.endotext.org/adrenal/adrenal26/adrenalframe26.htm In: Adrenal physiology and diseases (George Chrousos, section editor), In: Endotext.org (Leslie De Groot, editor)

Aldosterone secretion is stimulated by angiotensin II, high potassium, vasopressin, and ACTH (transient), and inhibited by high levels of natriuretic peptides. Apart from aldosterone the MR is also activated by products of abnormal adrenal steroid biosynthesis (Fig. 2.1), dysregulated metabolism of cortisol in cells that are targets of mineralocorticoids, and activating mutations of the MR or of ion channels that are inducible by the MR to mediate its action.

SME and its inherited forms of mineralocorticoid hypertension have helped our understanding of normal physiology and of the pathogenesis of hypertension called "essential" which represents a major public health problem [8].

Hypertension is defined as a blood pressure exceeding 139/89 mmHg for adults aged 18 years or older based on the mean of two or more properly measured seated BP readings on each of two or more office visits. Hypertension affects approximately 31% of Americans; blood pressure control is suboptimal and is achieved in less than 1 in 3 [9, 10]. The prevalence of resistant hypertension varies from 34 to 53% in different large studies: ALLHAT (34%), NHANES (53%), or Framingham Heart Study (48%) [11]. The Joint National Committee (JNC VII) [12] classified hypertension for adults 18 years and older as follows:

Normal	<120 mmHg (systolic)	<80 mmHg (diastolic)
Pre-HTN	120–139	80–89
Stage 1 HTN	140–159	90–99
Stage 2 HTN	≥160	≥100

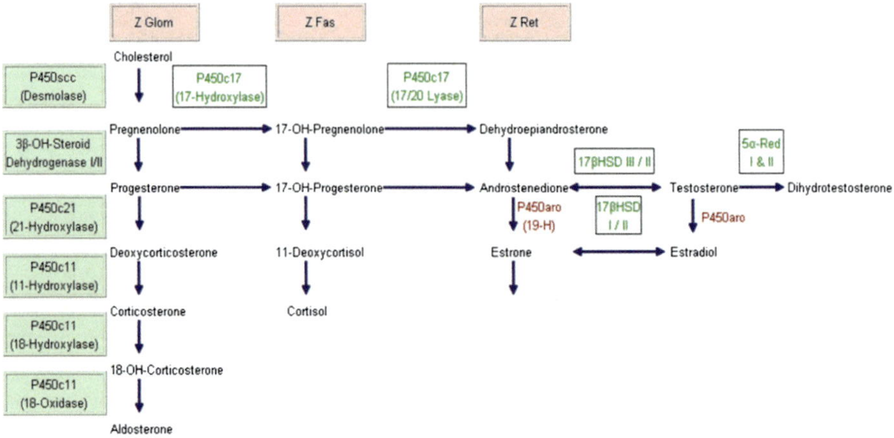

Fig. 2.1 Adrenal steroid synthesis. Modified from ref. [7]. *Z Glom* zona glomerulosa; *Z Fas* zona fasciculata; *Z Ret* zona reticularis; *19-H* 19-Hydroxylase; *HSD* Hydroxysteroid dehydrogenase; *P450aro* aromatase; *5alpha-Red* 5alpha-Reductase. The three adrenal cortex zones Z Glom, Z Fas, and Z Ret stand above the "column" of hormones that are produced in the respective zone. The steroidogenic enzymes on the *left* starting with P450scc (Desmolase) are listed in order for "vertical and horizontal reading," i.e., Desmolase converts cholesterol to pregnenolone, 3beta-OH-Steroid Dehydrogenase I/II convert pregnenolone to progesterone, 17-OH-Pregnenolone to 17-OH-Progesterone, and P450c11 converts deoxycorticosterone to 18-OH-Corticosterone and 11-Deoxycortisol to cortisol, etc

Clinical Findings and Clues to Identify Patients with Endocrine Hypertension Caused by Mineralocorticoid Excess

Individuals homozygous for an inherited condition of SME may develop hypertension very early in life and become refractory to antihypertensive therapy (failing triple-drug treatment). However, the clinical phenotype varies and some patients may not be found to have SME before they reach adulthood (Table 2.2).

Pathogenesis

The pathophysiological mechanisms of mineralocorticoid excess syndromes are better understood at present with the advent of new techniques in molecular biology and genetics. The increasing availability of affordable genetic/molecular testing may elucidate further the pathogenesis of these rather rare genetic conditions and their implication in hypertension seen in the general public. Excessive production of aldosterone (primary: familial hypoaldosteronism, aldosterone-producing adenoma/ carcinoma/hyperplasia [13–16] or secondary: reninoma [17–20]) and sometimes of

Table 2.2 Clinical findings in patients with mineralocorticoid excess

Condition	Clinical presentation
CAH: 11beta-hydroxylase deficiency	Early growth spurt initially, then short adult stature, advanced bone age, premature adrenarche, acne, precocious puberty in males, amenorrhea/hirsutism/virilism in females
CAH: 17alpha-hydroxylase deficiency	Pseudohermaphroditism (male), sexual infantilism (female)
Apparent mineralocorticoid excess	Growth retardation/short stature, nephrocalcinosis
Liddle syndrome	Severe hypertension, hypokalemia, and metabolic alkalosis, muscle weakness
Geller syndrome	Early onset hypertension (before age 20 year), exacerbated in pregnancy
Glucocorticoid remediable aldosteronism (GRA)	Early onset of hypertension, presence of family history of mortality or morbidity from early hemorrhagic stroke
Pseudohypoaldosteronism type 2	Short stature, hyperkalemic and hyperchloremic metabolic acidosis, borderline blood pressure
Glucocorticoid resistance (children) (Chrousos syndrome)	Ambiguous genitalia, precocious puberty. Women may have acne, excessive hair, oligo/anovulation, infertility

deoxycorticosterone (DOC) (primary: DOC-secreting adrenocortical adenoma/carcinoma [21–24] or secondary: 11beta-hydroxylase deficiency [25–27], 17alpha-hydroxylase deficiency [28–30], substances with high mineralocorticoid activity can lead to salt and water retention and consequently hypertension without causing hypernatremia.

11Beta-hydroxylase is responsible for the conversion of DOC to corticosterone (precursor of aldosterone) and 11-deoxycortisol to cortisol. In approximately 2/3 of individuals affected by a deficiency of this enzyme, monogenic low renin hypertension with low aldosterone levels ensues caused by accumulation of 11-deoxycortisol and DOC. Also, adrenal androgens are produced in excess in individuals with 11beta-hydroxylase deficiency compared with 17alpha-hydroxylase deficiency where they are deficient [25–30]. In patients with 17alpha-hydroxylase deficiency a persistent elevation of ACTH increases DOC and corticosterone levels and as a consequence affected patients will develop hypertension, hypokalemia, low aldosterone, and suppressed renin [28–30].

AME is caused by deficiency of the enzyme 11βHSD2) [31–33]. This enzyme is responsible for the conversion of cortisol to the inactive cortisone in renal tubular cells. Cortisol and aldosterone have equal affinity for the mineralocorticoid receptor but normal circulating concentrations of cortisol are 100–1,000-fold higher than those of aldosterone [34]. If 11βHSD2 is oversaturated or defective, more cortisol will be available to bind to the mineralocorticoid receptor [35]. Diminished

11βHSD2 activity may be hereditary or acquired. Acquired deficiency of this enzyme may result from its inhibition by glycyrrhetinic acid, the active metabolite generated when using licorice, certain brands of chewing tobacco, and carbenoloxone. The mutations in the 11βHSD2 gene are responsible for the reduced activity of the enzyme, which causes Na retention, low K, renin, and aldosterone.

In Liddle syndrome, "gain of function" mutations in the genes coding for the beta- or gamma-subunit of the renal epithelial sodium channel, located on chromosome 16p13, lead to constitutive activation of renal sodium and water resorption, hypertension, low renin, and aldosterone [36].

Pseudohypoaldosteronism type 2 or Gordon syndrome is an autosomal dominantly inherited disorder with genes mapping to chromosomes 1, 12, and 17 [37, 38]. Mutations have been identified in WNK kinases WNK1 and WNK4 on chromosomes 12 and 17, respectively. More recently, mutations in the KLHL3, CUL3, and SPAK genes have been linked to Gordon syndrome. Published families with this condition (hypertension, hyperkalemia, metabolic acidosis, normal renal function, low/normal aldosterone levels) are predominantly from Australia [38] or the United States (Lifton and coworkers at Yale University, CT). Hypertension in these patients may develop as a consequence of increased renal salt reabsorption; and hyperkalemia ensues as a result of reduced renal K excretion despite normal glomerular filtration and aldosterone secretion [39–41]. The reduced renal secretion of potassium makes this condition look like an aldosterone-deficient state, thus the term "pseudohypoaldosteronism."

Activating mutations in the amiloride-sensitive sodium channel of the distal renal tubule may explain the pathogenesis of this condition. Overactivation of the NaCl cotransporter results in Na and water retention and increased blood pressure.

Glucocorticoid resistance or Chrousos syndrome (see Chap. 4 in this book) is caused by inactivating mutations of the glucocorticoid receptor gene [42–44]. Chronic elevation of ACTH can lead to stimulation of adrenal compounds with mineralocorticoid activity (corticosterone, DOC), and elevation of cortisol may lead to stimulation of the mineralocorticoid receptor, resulting in hypertension and increasing androgenic activity (androstenedione, DHEA, DHEAS) in women.

Constitutive activation of the MR is an autosomal-dominant condition determined by "gain of function" mutations in the MC gene on chromosome 4q31 [45].

Figure 2.2 provides an overview of these pathogenic mechanisms involved in mineralocorticoid excess syndromes Fig. 2.2.

Diagnosis

As is true for measuring any hormone, when analyzing steroids, it is important to obtain accurate information. The most sensitive and specific method to detect a defect in adrenal steroid biosynthesis is urinary steroid profiling [47]. Particularly robust appears to be measuring steroid precursor/product ratios which are independent of 24-h excretion and usually not determined by commercial laboratories.

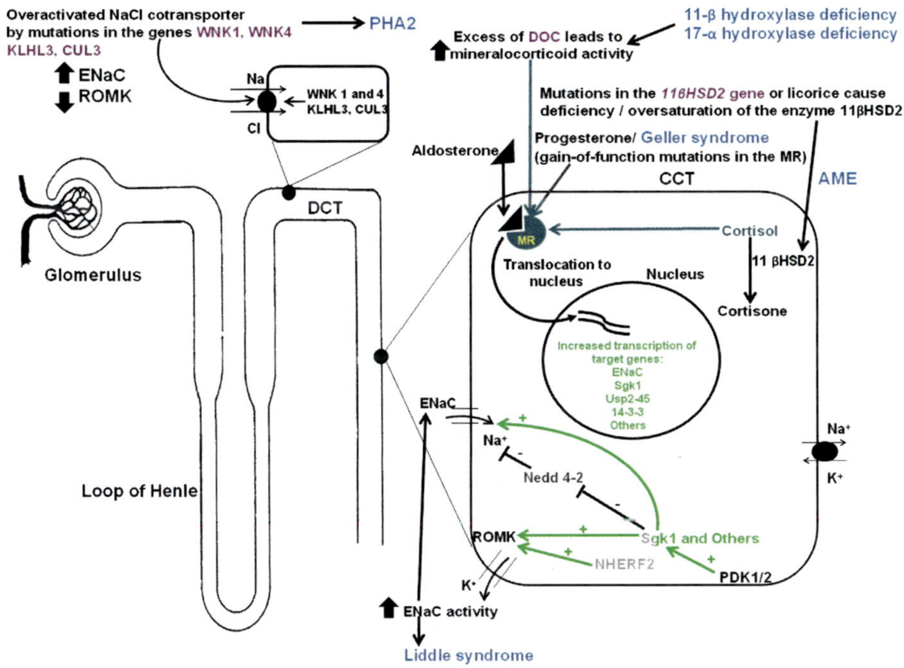

Fig. 2.2 Inherited endocrine conditions related to mineralocorticoid excess (modified after ref. [46, 47], and http://home.comcast.net/~llpellegrini/urinarysystem.htm). Shown are the molecular pathways involved in dysregulation of NaCl homeostasis located in the distal renal tubules. AME - Apparent mineralocorticoid excess, GRA - Glucocorticoid-remediable aldosteronism, PHA2 - Pseudohypoaldosteronism type 2; MR - mineralocorticoid receptor; WNK - with-nolysine (K) kinase 1, 4; ROMK- renal outer medullary potassium channel; ENaC - epithelial sodium channel; KLHL3 - kelch-like 3; CUL 3 - cullin 3; Sgk1 - serum glucocorticoid kinase 1; Nedd4-2, ubiquitin-protein ligase; deubiquitylating enzyme Usp2-45; 14-3-3 proteins; NHERF2 - Na+/H+ exchange regulating factor 2; PDK1,2 - 3-phosphoinositide-dependent kinases 1 and 2; + activation; - inhibition

The diagnostic approach to syndromes of mineralocorticoid excess is based on the clinical presentation, laboratory, and genetic testing. The most important laboratory and genetic tests are described in Table 2.3.

Congenital Adrenal Hyperplasia: 17Alpha-Hydroxylase Deficiency

- This enzyme deficiency is rare and affects both adrenal and gonadal steroid production.
- Cytochrome P450c17 enzyme complex catalyzes both 17-hydroxylase and 17,20 lyase activity [25, 28–30].
- Clinical findings: pseudohermaphroditism (46, XY male), sexual infantilism (46, XX female), varying degrees of hypertension and hypokalemic alkalosis.

Table 2.3 Laboratory testing protocols for some causes of mineralocorticoid excess syndromes

Disease	Laboratory testing	Genetic testing
CAH: 17α-OH deficiency	↑DOC, ↓ 11-deoxycortisol ↓↓ Aldosterone, ↓renin, ↓K ↓Plasma 17-hydroxyprogesterone ↓testosterone ↑Urinary100*THDOC/(THE+THF+5αTHF) and (THA+THB+5αTHB)/(THE+THF+5αTF)	*CYP17* gene
CAH: 11β-OH deficiency	Potassium depletion (variable), ↓renin (The degree of hyporeninemia may vary widely) ↓↓Aldosterone ↓Cortisol, ↑ACTH ↑11-Deoxycortisol, ↑DOC, ↑17-OHP ↑19-nor-DOC ↑↑Urinary 100*THS/(THE+THF+5αTHF) and 100*THDOC/(THE+THF+5αTHF)	*CYP11B1* gene
Apparent mineralocorticoid excess	Check the level of tritiated water in plasma samples when 11-tritiated cortisol is injected ↑24 h Urinary free cortisol/cortisone and ↑urinary (THF+5αTHF)/THE	*11βHSD2* gene
Liddle syndrome	↓Plasma K, ↑urinary K, ↓PRA and suppressed aldosterone secretion, metabolic alkalosis ↓Urinary THALDO (<2 μg/24 h) Normal steroid profile (24-h urine cortisone/cortisol and other ratios)	*ENaC* gene
Pseudohypoaldosteronism type 2	↑↑K, hyperchloremic metabolic acidosis ↓aldosterone, ↓renin ↓Serum HCO_3 (variable in children) Hypercalciuria (occasionally) ↓Urinary THALDO	*WNK1 and 4* gene *KLHL3, CUL3, SPAK* gene
Geller syndrome	K, ↓aldosterone, ↓renin ↓Urinary THALDO	*MCR* gene

DOC - deoxycorticosterone; TH - tetrahydro; A - 11-dehydro-corticosterone; B - corticosterone; E - cortisone; F - cortisol; S - 11-deoxycortisol; ALDO - aldosterone, see also ref. [47, 48]

- Biochemical features: ↑DOC, ↓11-deoxycortisol, ↓↓ aldosterone, ↓renin, ↓K.,

  ↓ Plasma 17alpha-hydroxyprogesterone, ↓testosterone, ↑urinary 100*THDOC/(THE+THF+5αTHF), and (THA+THB+5αTHB)/(THE+THF+5αTHF) ratios [47, 48].
- Diagnosis of this autosomal recessive condition is suggested by delayed puberty, absent secondary sexual characteristics or amenorrhea combined with typical biochemical findings described above.
- Genetic testing for mutations in the *CYP17*.
- Cortisol is the first-line therapy and sometimes mineralocorticoid replacement, especially in cases of bilateral and complete (adrenal rest tumors) adrenalectomy. Oral hydrocortisone is often preferred for children to maximize their growth potential while minimizing the risk for developing iatrogenic Cushing's syndrome.

Congenital Adrenal Hyperplasia: 11Beta-Hydroxylase Deficiency

- 11β-Hydroxylase deficiency is caused by several mutations in the CYP11B1 gene.
- The inherited enzymatic defect (autosomal recessive) results in elevated serum levels of DOC, the principal steroid index of 11β-hydroxylase deficiency [49–53].
- Accounts for approx. 5–8% of all CAH cases, approx. 1 in 200,000 births.
- In Moroccon Jews, the prevalence is approx. 1 in 7,000 births [50, 51].
- Chronic elevation of ACTH due to a deficient cortisol production stimulates the biosynthesis of other mineralocorticoids: 11-deoxycortisol, DOC, and others.
- DOC is a weak mineralocorticoid, but at supraphysiologic levels promotes salt retention, volume expansion, and consequently hypertension.
- Short stature (adult males), hirsutism, advanced bone age, amenorrhea, infertility are some of the most common findings in patients affected by this condition. Males may develop pseudoprecocious puberty (boys are tall as children).
- Biochemical profile: potassium depletion (variable), ↓renin (variable), ↓aldosterone, ↓cortisol, ↑ACTH, ↑11-deoxycortisol, ↑DOC, ↑19-nor-DOC, ↑urinary 17-hydroxy-corticosteroids and DOC, and ↑↑urinary 100*THS/(THE+THF+5αTHF) and 100*THDOC/(THE+THF+5αTHF) ratios [47, 48].
- Other laboratory abnormalities: elevated serum level of 17alpha-hydroxy progesterone (17-OHP) and androstenedione and urinary pregnanetriol.
- Normalization of DOC is an indicator of adequate glucocorticoid therapy which represents the most important therapeutic indication for this condition. Hydrocortisone is frequently used in children to maximize their growth potential while minimizing their risk for developing Cushing's syndrome from overuse of glucocorticoid therapy (i.e., dexamethasone with its longer half-life and higher affinity for the glucocorticoid receptor) In selected patients, bilateral adrenalectomy may be safe and effective in managing blood pressure. In such cases, mineralocorticoid replacement (i.e., fludrocortisone) may be necessary.
- Mutations in the *CYP11B1* gene may not always be found.

Apparent Mineralocorticoid Excess

- 11β-hydroxysteroid dehydrogenase type 2 (11βHSD2) is highly expressed in the kidney where it metabolizes cortisol to cortisone. It is also expressed in all sodium-transporting epithelia.
- A reduced enzymatic activity of 11βHSD2 caused by loss-of-function mutations explains the pathogenesis of the autosomal recessive syndrome of AME which was first described by Ulick et al. in 1979 [54–57].

- Diminished 11βHSD2 activity may be hereditary or acquired.
- Acquired deficiency of this enzyme may result from inhibition by glycyrrhetinic acid which may occur with use of licorice, chewing tobacco, carbenoloxone, and "asam boi" flavor (containing glycyrrhizic acid) if consumed on a daily basis in certain quantities [58].
- Impaired 11βHSD2 activity alters the inactivation of cortisol in the target renal cell leading to above-normal cortisol activity, renal Na retention, and severe hypokalemia.
- The severity of hypertension in patients with AME syndrome seems to correlate with the degree of loss of 11βHSD2 enzyme activity.
- The clinical presentation of AME can include: growth retardation/short stature, hypertension, hypokalemia, and occasional nephrocalcinosis [59, 60].
- A typical case of AME presents with: early hypertension (childhood), hypokalemia, suppressed renin, very low aldosterone levels, and metabolic alkalosis.
- There is a large spectrum of clinical and biochemical features in patients with homozygous mutations of the 11βHSD2 gene; heterozygous individuals usually develop hypertension later in life, have milder biochemical profiles of AME and no phenotypic characteristics of AME [61].
- The biochemical diagnosis can be made by detecting ↑ 24 h urinary-free cortisol/cortisone and ↑urinary (THF+5αTHF)/THE ratios [47, 48].
- Patients diagnosed with AME syndrome respond well to low sodium diet and spironolactone, which blocks binding of both cortisol and aldosterone to the MCR.
- Genetic testing for AME-associated loss-of-function mutations by DNA sequencing of the 11βHSD2 gene may further elucidate the diagnosis.

Licorice-Induced Hypertension

- Licorice has been used for medicinal purposes for many years.
- Licorice or its active component glycyrrhetinic acid may cause hypertension and hypokalemia due to cortisol-mediated activation of the MR by decreasing 11βHSD2 activity [62].
- A detailed dietary history has to be obtained in each patient in the presence of resistant hypertension with associated hypokalemia to exclude the acquired forms of AME.
- Various licorice containing foods, teas, or herbal products (like yokukansan) are available and their individual consumption varies considerably [63]. Possible adverse effects of yokukansan on blood pressure and electrolytes (low K) were reported recently [64]. A daily dose of 10 mg of glycyrrhetinic acid is considered unharmful for most healthy individuals [64]. Glycyrrhizic acid (a component of licorice) is used as a sweetener and also can be found in chewing tobacco products [65, 66].

- Licorice seems to reduce serum testosterone by blocking 17-hydroxysteroid dehydrogenase and 17–20 lyase [67].
- Licorice as a medicinal plant contains not only glycyrrhetinic acid but also compounds with estrogen-like or antiandrogen activity. PTH and calcium levels have been increased in healthy women after 2 months of licorice therapy reflecting its impact on calcium metabolism ([68], see Chap. 9 in this book on the topic Primary Hyperparathyroidism).
- The effects of administration of licorice may be observed after a few days and are reversible in weeks. In some cases, these effects last for months after licorice has been stopped [69, 70].
- Licorice-induced hypertension and hypokalemia are cortisol-dependent and are corrected by the administration of spironolactone [71]. In vitro studies have shown a similar inhibitory dose-dependent activity of both glycyrrhetinic acid and carbenoxolone of the11βHSD2 isoenzyme [70, 72].
- The wide variation of glycyrrhetinic acid effects observed in various people may be due to individual variation to the effects of mineralocorticoids, bioavailability of glycyrrhetinic acid, or sensitivity of 11βHSD2 [73, 74].

Liddle Syndrome

- Autosomal-dominant inherited form of mineralocorticoid hypertension described by Liddle in 1963 [36] in a patient who developed renal failure, underwent cadaveric renal transplant in 1989, and on salt restriction demonstrated normal aldosterone and renin values (previously suppressed).
- This disease is caused by the so-called gain of function mutations in the genes coding for the beta- or gamma-subunit of the renal epithelial sodium channel (expressed in cortical collecting ducts and distal tubule) located on chromosome 16p13.
- The epithelial Na (+) channel (ENaC) and the acid-sensitive ion channel (ASIC) branches of the ENaC/degenerin superfamily of cation channels, have a ubiquitous expression, and have been involved in a variety of disorders [75]. These mutations render a hyperactive renal ENaC due to increased intrinsic activity of ENaC and increasing the number of functioning channels by a lower rate of degradation. As a consequence, there is an increased renal sodium reabsorption with subsequent volume expansion and potassium wasting (through the ROMK K-channel) in the collecting duct.
- Clinical presentation: early severe hypertension (teens), hypokalemia, metabolic alkalosis.
- Commonly, children with this condition are asymptomatic and discovered incidentally at a routine check-up. On the other hand, hypertension resistant to treatment in children may suggest this diagnosis.
- A clinical phenotype with hypertension but without hypokalemia was reported in an Italian family with a βP617L mutation of the beta-subunit of the epithelial sodium channel suggesting the importance of suspecting Liddle syndrome in all cases of early onset hypertension irrespective of K concentrations [76].

- Typical biochemical profile: ↓plasma K, ↑urinary K, ↓plasma renin activity and suppressed aldosterone secretion, ↓urinary THALDO (<2 μg/24 h), normal steroid profile (24-h urine cortisone/cortisol and other ratios), and metabolic alkalosis [47, 48].
- The diagnosis may also be facilitated when hypertension is corrected with a combination of salt restriction (<100 mmol/day) and amiloride/ triamterene.
- Genetic testing (ENaC gene) can identify the disease mutations within 2 (β-subunit *SCNN1B* and γ-subunit *SCNN1G*) of the three subunits of the ENaC channel by direct sequencing (PCR).
- Various types of mutations have been described: missense mutations or deletions/insertions causing premature stop codons, frameshift mutations. Mutations in either beta- or gamma-subunit cause an increased channel number and activity of amiloride-sensitive sodium current by several-fold of this type of ENaC receptor [77–80].
- A heterozygous mutation c.C1852(p.Pro618Ser) in the SCNN1B gene was reported in a Serbian family (son, mother and uncle) in a 13-year-old asymptomatic boy with severe hypertension [81]. The familial history recollected over four generations seems to be concordant with this pathology.
- Another possible role in diagnosing Liddle syndrome may play the sequencing of the Nedd4 gene essential for ENaC trafficking [82].
- Amiloride and triamterene are considered effective in the treatment of this disorder.
- A restricted dietary salt intake is necessary to maintain a good response to the therapy.
- Specific aldosterone antagonists like spironolactone and epleronone play no role in the treatment of this condition because the accelerated rate of sodium transport is independent of the action of aldosterone [83].

Pseudohypoaldosteronism Type 2

- PHA-2 (Gordon syndrome or chloride shunt syndrome) is an autosomal-dominant condition caused by gain-of-function mutations in WNK1 or WNK4 (part of a family of serine–threonine protein kinases) which in turn increase the activity of NaCl cotransporter present in the distal tubule and consequently Na, Cl, and volume extension [84].
- Recently, mutations in the KLHL3, CUL3, and SPAK genes have also been implicated in Gordon syndrome.
- Patients with PHA-2 have short stature, intellectual dysfunction, muscle weakness, low fractional excretion of sodium, hyperchloremic metabolic acidosis, normal aldosterone, and symptoms of severe hypertension.
- Biochemical profile: ↑↑K, hyperchloremic metabolic acidosis, ↓aldosterone, ↓renin, ↓serum HCO_3 (variable in children), hypercalciuria (occasionally), and ↓urinary THALDO [47, 48].

- Genetic testing for WNK1, WNK4, KLHL3, CUL3, SPAK mutations.
- Administration of thiazide diuretics which inhibit salt reabsorption in the distal nephron is the treatment of choice.
- Gordon et al. found that all features could be reversed by very strict dietary salt restriction [38].

Constitutive Activation of the MR (Geller Syndrome)

- This is an autosomal-dominant condition caused by gain-of-function mutations in the MR located on chromosome 4q31.
- The onset of hypertension is before age 20.
- Pregnancy may exacerbate hypertension in patients with this condition because of elevated progesterone levels and altered specificity of the MR receptor with progesterone and traditional MR antagonists now acting as potent MR agonists [45].
- Biochemical profile: normal (!) K, ↓aldosterone, ↓renin, ↓urinary THALDO [47, 48].
- Genetic testing of the MR. A missense mutation S810L located in the hormone-binding domain of the MR has been found in a 15-year-old boy causing hypertension.
- Spironolactone is contraindicated in MR-L810 carriers.

Conclusion

Syndromes of mineralocorticoid excess typically result from overactive amiloride-sensitive sodium channels located in the distal tubule and collecting ducts of the kidney. The effect of such an overactivation which mostly occurs in the condition primary aldosteronism is sodium and water retention with volume expansion and hypertension that is aggravated by a diet high in salt. Biochemically, plasma renin activity is suppressed and hypokalemia may be present. Aldosterone mediates its action through the mineralocorticoid receptor (MR), which regulates salt homeostasis in the kidneys and plays a range of other roles in the vasculature, heart, brain, and adipose tissue.

Apart from aldosterone, the MR is also activated by products of abnormal adrenal steroid biosynthesis, dysregulated metabolism of cortisol in cells that are targets of mineralocorticoids, and activating mutations of the MR or of ion channels that are inducible by the MR to mediate its action. Mineralocorticoid excess can be caused by congenital adrenal hyperplasia due to mutations of the 11beta-hydroxylase and 17alpha-hydroxylase genes, by mutations of the 11βHSD2 gene (AME), mutations of the epithelial sodium channel genes (Liddle syndrome), mutations of the mineralocorticoid receptor gene (Geller syndrome), and pseudohypoaldosteronism-type 2 or Gordon syndrome. Chrousos syndrome (inactivation of the glucocorticoid receptor) can also cause hypertension mediated by increased levels of DOC. Most of these conditions are treated by restricted dietary salt intake. However, some require special therapies including dexamethasone/hydrocortisone (CAH), spironolactone/eplerenone (AME), thiazide diuretics (Liddle and Gordon syndrome), while in others spironolactone and MR antagonists may be contraindicated (Geller syndrome). Understanding the pathophysiology of these rare conditions may help design future molecular targeted therapies, although the mainstay of antihypertensive therapy, reducing the overconsumption of salt in addition to increasing compliance and adherence of patients to therapy will remain [85].

Disclosure Statement

This manuscript represents an update of earlier ones as the subject evolves. The authors own the exclusive intellectual property rights of the present review paper and are free to reproduce it in whole or in part (including figures and tables) in any electronic and/or printed article of which they are authors.

References

1. Van Renterghem C, Lazdunski M. A new non-voltage-dependent, epithelial-like Na+ channel in vascular smooth muscle cells. Pflugers Arch. 1991;419(3–4):401–8.
2. Charmandari E, Sertedaki A, Kino T, Merakou C, Hoffman D, Hatch MM et al. A novel point mutation in the KCNJ5 gene causing familial primary hypoaldosteronism and early onset autosomal dominant hypertension. J Clin Endocrinol Metab 2012;24.
3. Yang J, Fuller PJ. Interactions of the mineralocorticoid receptor—within and without. Mol Cell Endocrinol. 2012;350(2):196–205.
4. Shibata S, Fujita T. Mineralocorticoid receptors in the pathophysiology of chronic kidney diseases and the metabolic syndrome. Mol Cell Endocrinol. 2012;350(2):273–8.
5. Odermatt A, Kratschmar DV. Tissue-specific modulation of mineralocorticoid receptor function by 11β-hydroxysteroid dehydrogenases: an overview. Mol Cell Endocrinol. 2012;350(2):168–86.
6. Kolkhof P, Borden SA. Molecular pharmacology of the mineralocorticoid receptor: prospects for novel therapeutics. Mol Cell Endocrinol. 2012;350(2):310–7.
7. Koch CA. Adrenal cortex, physiology. In: Martini L, editor. Encyclopedia of endocrinology and endocrine diseases. San Diego: Academic; 2004.
8. Hassan-Smith Z, Stewart PM. Inherited forms of mineralocorticoid hypertension. Curr Opin Endocrinol Diabetes Obes. 2011;18(3):177–85.
9. Fields LE, Burt VL, Cutler JA, Hughes J, Roccella EJ, Sorlie P. The burden of adult hypertension in the United States 1999 to 2000: a rising tide. Hypertension. 2004;44(4):398–404.
10. Cutler JA, Sorlie PD, Wolz M, Thom T, Fields LE, Roccella EJ. Trends in hypertension prevalence, awareness, treatment and control rates in United States adults between 1988–1994 and 1999–2004. Hypertension. 2008;52(5):818–27.
11. Calhoun DA, Jones CD, Textor S, Goff DC, Murphy TP, et al. Resistant hypertension: diagnosis, evaluation, and treatment: a scientific statement from the American Heart Association Professional Education Committee of the Council for High Blood Pressure Research. Hypertension. 2008;51:1403–19.

12. Chobanian AV, et al. The Seventh Report of the Joint National Committee on prevention, detection, evaluation, and treatment of high blood pressure. JAMA. 2003;289:2560.
13. Young Jr WF. Endocrine hypertension: then and now. Endocr Pract. 2010;16(5):888–902.
14. Kratzsch J, Wende D, Thiery J, Koch CA. Basal aldosterone-renin-ratio and aldosterone levels in healthy adults during the saline load test. Clin Chem Lab Med. 2007;45–9:A114–5 (German dissertation, Diana Wende, 2008, Leipzig).
15. Mulatero P. A new form of hereditary primary aldosteronism: familial hypoaldosteronism type III. J Clin Endocrinol Metab. 2008;93(8):2972–4.
16. Funder JW, Carey RM, Fardella C, Gomez-Sanchez CE, Mantero F, Stowasser M, et al. Case detection, diagnosis, and treatment of patients with primary aldosteronism: an endocrine society clinical practice guideline. J Clin Endocrinol Metab. 2008;93:3266–81.
17. Cho MJ, Sung EY, Park JA, Lee HD. Congestive heart failure as an initial manifestation of reninoma. J Pediatr Endocrinol Metab. 2011;24(11–12):1085–7.
18. Wong L, Hsu TH, Perlroth MG, Hofmann LV, Haynes CM, Katznelson L. Reninoma: case report and literature review. J Hypertens. 2008;26(2):368–73.
19. Shera AH, Baba AA, Bakshi IH, Lone IA. Recurrent malignant juxtaglomerular cell tumor: a rare cause of malignant hypertension in a child. J Indian Assoc Pediatr Surg. 2011; 16(4):152–4.
20. Gottardo F, Cesari M, Morra A, Gardiman M, Fassina A, Dal Bianco M. A kidney tumor in an adolescent with severe hypertension and hypokalemia: an uncommon case—case report and review of the literature on reninoma. Urol Int. 2010;85(1):121–4.
21. Kondo K, Saruta T, Saito I, Yoshida R, Maruyama H, Matsuki S. Benign desoxycorticosterone-producing adrenal tumor. JAMA. 1976;236(9):1042–4.
22. Sone M, Shibata H, Homma K, Tamura N, Akahira J, Hamada S, et al. Close examination of steroidogenesis disorders in a DOC- and progesterone-producing adrenocortical carcinoma. Endocrine. 2009;35(1):25–33.
23. Kelly WF, O'Hare MJ, Loizou S, Davies D, Laing I. Hypermineralocorticism without excessive aldosterone secretion: an adrenal carcinoma producing deoxycorticosterone. Clin Endocrinol (Oxf). 1982;17(4):353–61.
24. Müssig K, Wehrmann M, Horger M, Maser-Gluth C, Häring HU, Overkamp D. Adrenocortical carcinoma producing 11-deoxycorticosterone: a rare cause of mineralocorticoid hypertension. J Endocrinol Invest. 2005;28(1):61–5.
25. New MI, Geller DS, Fallo F, Wilson RC. Monogenic low rennin hypertension. Trends Endocrinol Metab. 2005;16:92–7.
26. Speiser PW, White PC. Congenital adrenal hyperplasia. N Engl J Med. 2003;349:776–88.
27. Zachmann M, Tassinari D, Prader A. Clinical and biochemical variabilitiy of congenital adrenal hyperplasia due to 11beta-hydroxylase deficiency. J Endocrinol Metab. 1983;56:222–9.
28. Ogawa K, Hara A, Tanabe S, Tamori S, Yoshida H, Pak CH, et al. A case of 17 alpha-hydroxylase deficiency syndrome associated with right adrenal tumor. Clin Exp Hypertens A. 1984;6(4):863–77.
29. Costa-Santos M, Kater CE, Auchus RJ, et al. Two prevalent CYP17 mutations and genotype-phenotype correlations in 24 Brazilian patients with 17-hydroxylase deficiency. J Clin Endocrinol Metab. 2004;89:49–60.
30. Wong SL, Shu SG, Tsai CR. Seventeen alpha-hydroxylase deficiency. J Formos Med Assoc. 2006;105:177–81.
31. Ferrari P. The role of 11β-hydroxysteroid dehydrogenase type 2 in human hypertension. Biochim Biophys Acta. 2010;1802(12):1178–87.
32. New MI, Levine LS, Biglieri EG, Paeira J, Ulick S. Evidence for an unidentified ACTH-induced steroid hormone causing hypertension. J Clin Endocrinol Metab. 1977;44:924–33.
33. Lin-Su K, Zhou P, Arora N, et al. In vitro expression studies of a novel mutation delta299 in a patient affected with apparent mineralocorticoid excess. J Clin Endocrinol Metab. 2004;89:2024–7.

34. Arriza JL, Weinberger C, Cerelli G, Glaser TM, et al. Cloning of the human mineralocorticoid receptor complementary DNA: structural and functional kinship with the glucocorticoid receptor. Science. 1987;237:268–75.
35. Funder JW, Pearce PT, Smith R, Smith AI. Mineralocorticoid action: target tissue specificity is enzyme, not receptor mediated. Science. 1988;242:583–5.
36. Liddle GW, Bledsoe T, Coppage Jr WS. A familial renal disorder simulating primary aldosteronism but with negligible aldosterone secretion. Trans Assoc Am Physicians. 1963;76:199–213.
37. Wilson FH, Disse-Nicodeme S, Choate KA, et al. Human hypertension caused by mutations in WNK kinases. Science. 2001;293:11–4.
38. Gordon RD, Geddes RA, Pawsey CG, O'Halloran MW. Hypertension and severe hyperkalemia associated with suppression of renin and aldosterone and completely reversed by dietary sodium restriction. Australas Ann Med. 1970;19:287–94.
39. Mansfield TA, Simon DB, Farfel Z, et al. Multilocus linkage of familial hyperkalemia and hypertension, pseudohypoaldosteronism type II, to chromosomes 1q31-42 and 17p-q21. Nat Genet. 1997;16:202–5.
40. Kahle KT, Wilson FH, Leng Q, et al. WNK4 regulates the balance between renal NaCl reabsorption and K secretion. Nat Genet. 2003;35:372–6.
41. Klemm SA, Gordon RD, Tunny TJ, Thompson RE. The syndrome of hypertension and hyperkalemia with normal GFR (Gordon's syndrome): is there increased proximal sodium reabsorption ? Clin Invest Med. 1991;14:551–8.
42. Chrousos GP, Vingerhoeds A, Brandon D, et al. Primary cortisol resistance. J Clin Invest. 1982;69:1261–9.
43. Charmandari E, Kino T, Ichijo T, Chrousos GP. Generalized glucocorticoid resistance: clinical aspects, molecular mechanisms, and implications of a rare genetic disorder. J Clin Endocrinol Metab. 2008;93:1563–72.
44. Charmandari E, Kino T. Chrousos syndrome: a seminal report, a phylogenetic enigma and the clinical implications of glucocorticoid signalling changes. Eur J Clin Invest. 2010;40(10):932–42.
45. Geller DS, Farhi A, Pinkerton N, Fradley M, Moritz M, Spitzer A, et al. Activating mineralocorticoid receptor mutation in hypertension exacerbated by pregnancy. Science. 2000;289:119–23.
46. Matthew KA, Manish PP, Thomas HH. Renal and electrolyte disorders : Disordersof the renin-angiotensin-aldosterone system 2010;8:251–271.
47. Ferrari P, Bianchetti MG. Diagnostic investigations in inherited endocrine disorders of sodium regulation. In: Ranke MB, Mullis PE, editors. Diagnostics of endocrine function in children and adolescents. 4th ed. Basel: Karger; 2011. p. 210–34.
48. Shackleton CH. Profiling steroid hormones and urinary steroids. J Chromatogr. 1986;379:91–156.
49. Parsa AA, New MI. Low-renin hypertension of childhood. Endocrinol Metab Clin North Am. 2011;40(2):369–77.
50. White PC, Dupont J, New MI, Leiberman E, Hochberg Z, Rösler A. A mutation in CYP11B1 (Arg-448—His) associated with steroid 11 beta-hydroxylase deficiency in Jews of Moroccan origin. J Clin Invest. 1991;87(5):1664–7.
51. Paperna T, et al. Mutations in CYP11B1 and congenital adrenal hyperplasia in Moroccan Jews. J Clin Endocrinol Metab. 2005;90(9):5463–5.
52. Ben Charfeddine I, Riepe FG, Kahloul N, Kulle AE, Adala L, Mamaï O, et al. Two novel CYP11B1 mutations in congenital adrenal hyperplasia due to steroid 11β hydroxylase deficiency in a Tunisian family. Gen Comp Endocrinol. 2012;175(3):514–8.
53. Melcescu E, Phillips JW, Moll G, Subauste JS, Koch CA. 11-beta-hydroxylase deficiency and other syndromes of mineralocorticoid excess as a rare cause of endocrine hypertension. Horm Metab Res. 2012;44:1–12.
54. Ulick S, et al. A syndrome of apparent mineralocorticoid excess associated with defects in the peripheral metabolism of cortisol. J Clin Endocrinol Metab. 1979;49:757–64.

55. Stewart PM, et al. Syndrome of apparent mineralocorticoid excess: a defect in the cortisol-cortisone shuttle. J Clin Invest. 1988;82:340–9.
56. Knops NB, Monnens LA, Lenders JW, Levtchenko EN. Apparent mineralocorticoid excess: time of manifestation and complications despite treatment. Pediatrics. 2011;127(6):e1610–4.
57. Bailey MA, Paterson JM, Hadoke PW, Wrobel N, Bellamy CO, Brownstein DG, et al. A switch in the mechanism of hypertension in the syndrome of apparent mineralocorticoid excess. J Am Soc Nephrol. 2008;19(1):47–58.
58. Hamidon BB, Jeyabalan V. Exogenously-induced apparent hypermineralocorticoidism associated with ingestion of "asam boi". Singapore Med J. 2006;47(2):156–8.
59. Moudgil A, Rodich G, Jordan SC, Kamil ES. Nephrocalcinosis and renal cysts associated with apparent mineralocorticoid excess syndrome. Pediatr Nephrol. 2000;15(1–2):60–2.
60. Lin-Su K, Zhou P, Arora N, Betensky BP, New MI, Wilson RC. In vitro expression studies of a novel mutation delta299 in a patient affected with apparent mineralocorticoid excess. J Clin Endocrinol Metab. 2004;89(5):2024–7.
61. Morineau G, Sulmont V, Salomon R, Fiquet-Kempf B, Jeunemaitre X, Nicod J, et al. Apparent mineralocorticoid excess:report of six new cases and extensive personal experience. J Am Soc Nephrol. 2006;17:3176–84.
62. Epstein MT, Espiner EA, Donald RA, Hughes H. Liquorice toxicity and the renin–angiotensin–aldosterone axis in man. Br Med J. 1977;1:209–10.
63. Sontia B, Mooney J, Gaudet L, Touyz RM. Pseudohypoaldosteronism, liquorice, and hypertension. J Clin Hypertens (Greenwich). 2008;10(2):153–7.
64. Nishiyama N, Takeshita M, Tanaka K, Miyao M, Mizuno Y. A case of severe hypokalemia caused by a Chinese herbal remedy (Yokukansan) in an 81-year-old woman with dementia. Nihon Ronen Igakkai Zasshi. 2011;48(5):553–7.
65. Stormer FC, Reistad R, Alexander J. Glycyrrhizic acid in liquorice—evaluation of health hazard. Food Chem Toxicol. 1993;31:303–12.
66. Ploeger B, Mensinga T, Sips A, Deerenberg C, Meulenbelt J, DeJongh J. A population physiologically based pharmacokinetic/pharmacodynamic model for the inhibition of 11-beta-hydroxysteroid dehydrogenase activity by glycyrrhetic acid. Toxicol Appl Pharmacol. 2001;170(1):46–55.
67. Armanini D, Mattarello MJ, Fiore C, Bonanni G, Scaroni C, Sartorato P, et al. Licorice reduces serum testosterone in healthy women. Steroids. 2004;69(11–12):763–6.
68. Mattarello MJ, Benedini S, Fiore C, Camozzi V, Sartorato P, Luisetto G, et al. Effect of licorice on PTH levels in healthy women. Steroids. 2006;71(5):403–8.
69. Farese Jr RV, Biglieri EG, Shackleton CH, Irony I, Gomez Fontes R. Licorice-induced hypermineralocorticoidism. N Engl J Med. 1991;325:1223–7.
70. Van Uum SHM, Hermus ARMM, Smits P, Thien T, Lenders JWM. The role of 11b-hydroxysteroid dehydrogenase in the pathogenesis of hypertension. Cardiovasc Res. 1998;38:16–24.
71. Kageyama Y, Suzuki H, Saruta T. Role of glucocorticoid in the development of glycyrrhizin-induced hypertension. Clin Exp Hypertens. 1994;16:761–78.
72. Stewart PM, Wallace AM, Atherden SM, Shearing CH, Edwards CR. Mineralocorticoid activity of carbenoxolone: contrasting effects of carbenoxolone and liquorice on 11 beta-hydroxysteroid dehydrogenase activity in man. Clin Sci. 1990;78:49–54.
73. Nicholls MG, Ramsay LE, Boddy K, Fraser R, Morton JJ, Robertson JI. Mineralocorticoid-induced blood pressure, electrolyte, and hormone changes, and reversal with spironolactone, in healthy men. Metabolism. 1979;28:584–93.
74. Kageyama Y, Suzuki H, Saruta T. Glycyrrhizin induces mineralocorticoid activity through alterations in cortisol metabolism in the human kidney. J Endocrinol. 1992;135:147–52.
75. Qadri YJ, Rooj AK, Fuller CM. ENaCs and ASICs as therapeutic targets. Am J Physiol Cell Physiol. 2012;302(7):C943–65.
76. Rossi E, Farnetti E, Nicoli D, Sazzini M, Perazzoli F, Regolisti G, et al. A clinical phenotype mimicking essential hypertension in a newly discovered family with Liddle's syndrome. Am J Hypertens. 2011;24(8):930–5.

77. Firsov D, Schild L, Gautschi I, Merillat A-M, Schneeberger E, Rossier BC. Cell surface expression of the epithelial Na channel and a mutant causing Liddle syndrome: a quantitative approach. Proc Natl Acad Sci USA. 1996;93:15370–5.
78. Furuhashi M, Kitamura K, Adachi M, Miyoshi T, Wakida N, Ura N, et al. Liddle's syndrome caused by a novel mutation in the proline-rich PY motif of the epithelial sodium channel ß-subunit. J Clin Endocrinol Metab. 2005;90:340–4.
79. Hansson JH, Nelson-Williams C, Suzuki H, Schild L, Shimkets R, Lu Y, et al. Hypertension caused by a truncated epithelial sodium channel γ subunit: genetic heterogeneity of Liddle syndrome. Nat Genet. 1995;11:76–82.
80. Inoue J, Iwaoka T, Tokunaga H, Takamune K, Naomi S, Araki M, et al. A family with Liddle's syndrome caused by a new missense mutation in the ß subunit of the epithelial sodium channel. J Clin Endocrinol Metab. 1998;83:2210–3.
81. Bogdanović R, Kuburović V, Stajić N, Mughal SS, Hilger A, Ninić S, et al. Liddle syndrome in a Serbian family and literature review of underlying mutations. Eur J Pediatr. 2012;171(3):471–8.
82. Abriel H, Loffing J, Rebhun JF, Pratt JH, Schild L, Horisberger J-D, et al. Defective regulation of the epithelial Na(+) channel by Nedd4 in Liddle's syndrome. J Clin Invest. 1993;103:667–73.
83. Warnock DG. Liddle syndrome: an autosomal dominant form of human hypertension. Kidney Int. 1998;53:18–24.
84. Yang CL, Angell J, Mitchell R. Ellison DH:WNK kinases regulate tiazide-sensitive NaCl cotransport. J Clin Invest. 2003;111:1039–45.
85. Suckling RJ, He FJ, Macgregor GA. Altered dietary salt intake for preventing and treating diabetic kidney disease. Cochrane Database Syst Rev. 2010;8(12):CD006763.

Chapter 3
Hypertension in Patients with Cushing's Syndrome

Vitaly Kantorovich, Christian A. Koch, and George P. Chrousos

Abstract Hypertension in patients with Cushing's syndrome (CS) occurs in up to 95% of adult and in half of pediatric cases. It represents a major cardiovascular risk and mortality factor in such patients. Its pathogenesis is incompletely understood and includes an imbalance of factors involved in vasodilation and vasoconstriction. Amongst these are upregulation of the renin–angiotensin system activity, salt and water retention, increased peripheral resistance, increase in production/activity of endothelin-1 and vasopressin, increased reactivity to catecholamines, as well as decline in antioxidants, nitric oxide synthase, and others. Patients with ectopic CS usually have more pronounced hypercortisolism and hypertension than patients with CS of other etiologies. This might in part be caused by a functional state of mineralocorticoid excess due to oversaturation of the 11-beta-hydroxysteroid dehydrogenase type 2 enzyme. In patients with exogenous CS, the prevalence of hypertension is dose-dependent and lower (about 20%) than in those with endogenous CS. The aim of therapy is to normalize blood pressure and to remove the source of glucocorticoid excess with subsequent resolution of hypertension after surgical cure which will occur in almost all children and adolescents, but only in two-thirds of adults. This resolution depends on the age of onset, duration, and degree of glucocorticoid excess, as well as other underlying hypertension risk factors such as obesity, sleep apnea, and insulin resistance. Treatment should include ACE inhibitors and angiotensin II

V. Kantorovich (✉)
Division of Endocrinology and Metabolism, Department of Internal Medicine, University of Arkansas for Medical Sciences, 4301 West Markham Street, Slot #587, Little Rock, AR 72205-7199, USA
e-mail: VKantorovich@uams.edu

C.A. Koch
Division of Endocrinology, University of Mississippi Medical Center, Jackson, MS, USA

G.P. Chrousos
Division of Endocrinology, First Department of Pediatrics, Metabolism and Diabetes, University of Athens Medical School, Children's Hospital Aghia Sophia, Athens, Greece

C.A. Koch and G.P. Chrousos (eds.), *Endocrine Hypertension: Underlying Mechanisms and Therapy*, Contemporary Endocrinology, DOI 10.1007/978-1-60761-548-4_3,

receptor blockers, as well as eplerenone in selected patients (especially those with ectopic CS). Glucocorticoid excess and its effects should be controlled, if necessary with careful use of drugs such as steroidogenesis inhibitors or type II glucocorticoid receptor antagonists.

Keywords Cushing's syndrome • Glucocorticoids • Hypertension • Ectopic ACTH • 11-βHSD system • Endothelins

Introduction

Cushing's syndrome (CS) results from either endogenous or exogenous excess of glucocorticoids. The later is associated with any route of administration (oral, intravenous, inhalation, intranasal, transdermal or rectal) to a threshold dose, equivalent to 5–7.5 mg of oral prednisone. In this context, intra-individual susceptibility to glucocorticoid receptor affinity and duration of action certainly are important. As with other disorders, the prevalence and incidence of endogenous CS depend on sociodemographic and ethnic factors with approximately 2–5 new cases per million of population per annum [1, 2], although milder forms of CS and widely seen iatrogenic cases are underdiagnosed and underreported. The annual incidence can be further subdivided to 1.2–2.4 cases per million coming from pituitary causes and 0.6 cases of CS from adrenal causes [3, 4]. As reviewed in various large series including the one from the National Institutes of Health in Bethesda, MD, USA, signs and/or symptoms in patients with CS are not pathognomonic, although clinical sensitivity has been reported high (>80%) for weight gain, impaired short-term memory, plethora, round face, thin and fragile skin. Specificity (>80%) is thought to be high for osteopenia/fracture, ecchymoses, proximal muscle weakness, and hypertension (see Table. 1 on page 68 of reference [5]).

The prevalence of hypertension in children and adolescents with endogenous CS is up to 60% and in adults it is approx. 80% [2, 6]. Patients with exogenous CS develop hypertension depending on the duration and dose of glucocorticoids administered which may or may not be associated with steroid-induced diabetes mellitus, depending on individual body composition and insulin resistance risk factors. Generally, about 20% of such patients are found to be hypertensive depending on the population studied, i.e., in a global diabetes epidemic, this number may be on the rise and higher in areas such as Mississippi, which has the highest rate of obesity in the United States.

Causes and Diagnosis of Cushing's Syndrome

CS can result from several possible causes:

(a) Pituitary tumor secreting ACTH (approx. 70% of endogenous CS cases in adults and 90% in children)
(b) Any neuroendocrine tumor that secretes either ACTH or CRH (approx. 10%)

(c) Adrenal nodule/adenoma/carcinoma secreting cortisol (4%/10%/5%, respectively)
(d) Iatrogenic (exogenous) use of glucocorticoids

When CS is clinically suspected, it is imperative to both prove the existence and localize it's source, using the following protocol (Fig. 3.1) [13]. Adrenal CS associates with functional autonomy and loss of normal ACTH feedback (ACTH-independence), as well as hypoactivity and atrophy of remaining and contralateral normal adrenal. As a rare exception to this rule, adrenal neuroendocrine tumors (including pheochromocytoma) can secrete ACTH and behave as ectopic CS (see below) [9–12].

Ectopic ACTH secretion usually causes higher glucocorticoid excess than eutopic ACTH oversecretion by an ACTH-oma in the pituitary gland. This explains in part

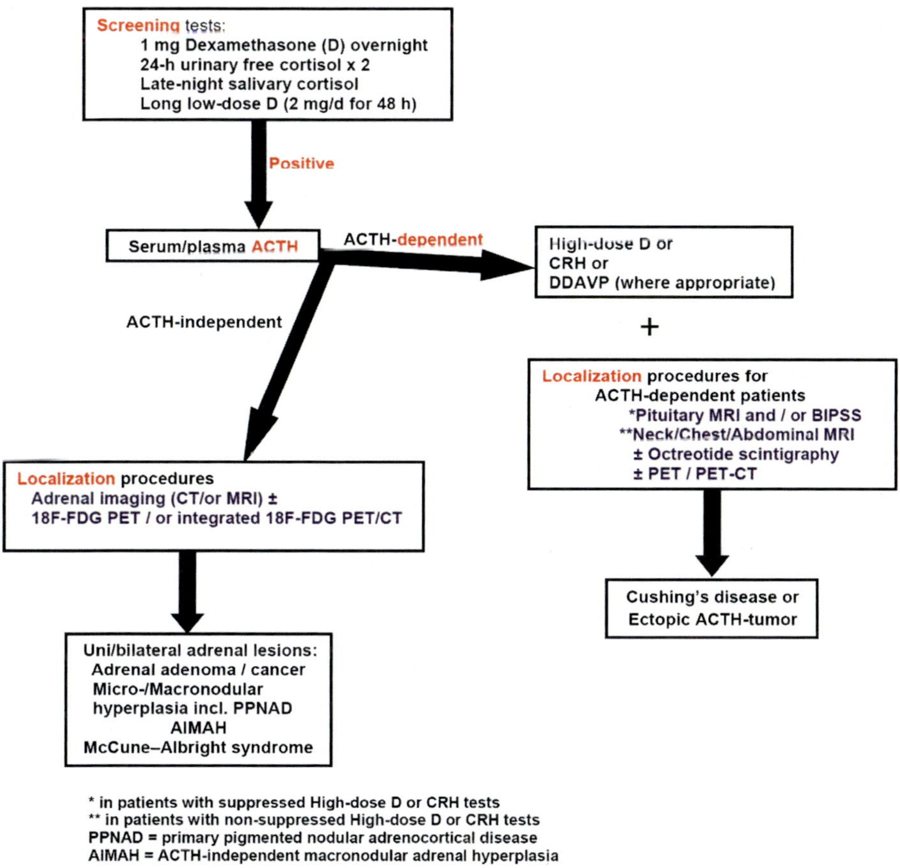

Fig. 3.1 Diagnostic workup for patients with Cushing's syndrome. Modified from Melcescu, Koch. Testing for endocrine hypertension, Chapter 7, In: Leslie De Groot, editor, online http://www.endotext.org; 2012

why patients with ectopic ACTH syndrome usually have a higher prevalence of hypertension and diabetes mellitus than those patients with Cushing's disease [2, 6]. CS is well known to associate with significant morbidity and to increase the mortality rate. The last, assessed as standardized mortality ratio, ranges between 1.7 and 4.1 [3, 4, 14–16], and is driven by associated morbidities which include hypertension, cardio- and cerebrovascular disease, hypercoagulability, diabetes mellitus, and depression. Of significant concern is the fact that mortality remains increased even after patients with CS have successfully been treated [16]. Although hypertension is seen more frequently in patients with Cushing's disease than in those with adrenal CS, the survival rates are better for the first group of patients [17, 18]. Ectopic CS is often caused by neuroendocrine neoplasms, including small cell lung cancer, and the survival rate is expectedly lower than for either of the above [17].

Pathogenesis of Hypertension in Patients with CS

Hypertension is a common clinical feature of CS (sensitivity 74–90%, specificity 83%) but is neither universal nor predictable to the degree of other clinical features of the disease [5]. It is seen in about 80% of adults and up to 60% of children with CS [6, 19, 20]. While after successful cure of CS, hypertension still persists in adults in as many as 30%, in children and adolescents this figure is much more favorable—around 3–4% [21, 22]. Clinical consequences of CS depend on several factors, among these the duration and level of pathologic increase of glucocorticoids. Hypertension will relate mostly to obesity and increased peripheral resistance and sympathetic drive. In patients with ectopic ACTH production by neuroendocrine tumors, marked hyperplasia of the adrenals and a severe increase in various steroids can occur, which will lead to signs of more severe disease with an overall shorter course, more features of mineralocorticoid excess and higher probability of fast overload of functional capacity of 11-beta-hydroxysteroid dehydrogenase (11-βHSD—see below).

In this case, hypertension is seen in up to 95% of cases, while with exogenous glucocorticoids, hypertension is of significantly lower frequency—20%—and correlates with the dose of steroid used [19]. Administration of exogenous glucocorticoids rapidly increases both systolic and, to lesser degree, diastolic blood pressure for hydrocortisone, dexamethasone or ACTH [23, 24]. The establishment of the pathogenesis of CS-related hypertension is based on several lines of evidence: assessment of the phenomenon in patients with CS or chronic treatment with exogenous steroids, studies in healthy volunteers taking ACTH or oral steroids for a limited period of time, and animal studies. The last two have several expected limitations—while short-term hypercortisolemia in healthy people might not represent a long-term multi-organ response, animal studies show significant species variability and might not represent findings relevant to human physiology. For this discussion, we will try to select the most representative data and review additional studies where appropriate.

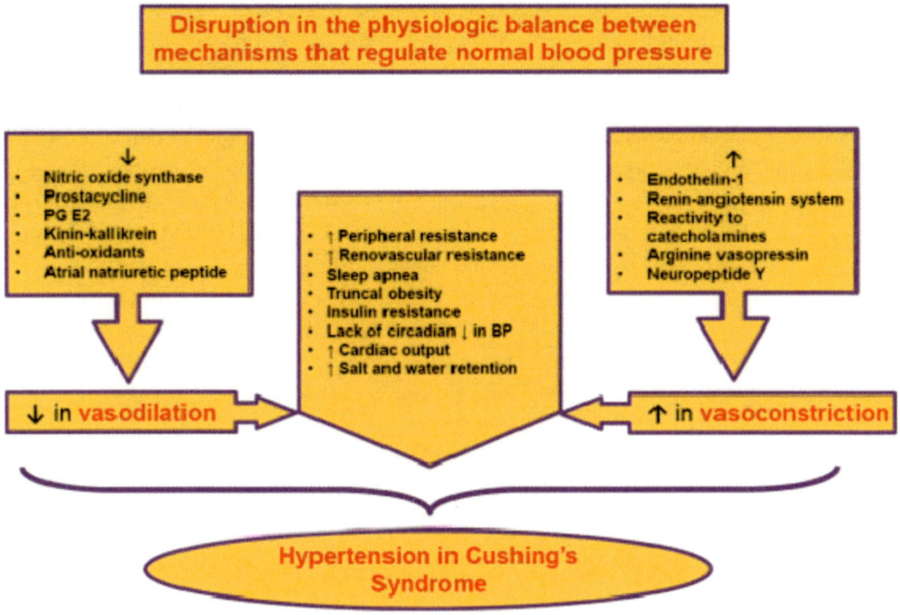

Fig. 3.2 Pathogenic pathways of hypertension development in CS

Causes of hypertension in CS are numerous (Fig. 3.2) and relate to different pathogenesis pathways [6, 25, 26]:

(a) Signaling of glucocorticoids through the mineralocorticoid receptor (MCR)
(b) Signaling of glucocorticoids through the GC receptor (GCR)

- Inhibition of vasodilatation (decrease in nitric oxide synthase, prostacycline, kinin–kallikrein; increase in endothelin-1)
- Activation of the renin–angiotensin system
- Increase in vascular reactivity to catecholamines
- Inhibition of norepinephrine metabolism

(c) Indirect action of glucocorticoids

- Increase in peripheral and renovascular resistance
- Sleep apnea, truncal obesity, insulin resistance
- Lack of circadian decrease in blood pressure

(d) Unrelated to glucocorticoids—lack of hypertension resolution after cure from CS

Actions of Glucocorticoids Through the MCR: A Convenient Culprit

It is common knowledge that glucocorticoids can bind to and signal through the MCR. It is also a well-accepted dogma that the gate-keeping 11-beta-hydroxysteroid dehydrogenase type 2 (11-βHSD2) system is saturable and in case of significantly increased hypercorticolemia glucocorticoids, levels can reach its binding capacity. In case of significant hypercorticolemia, glucocorticoid levels can reach the MCR and act as pure mineralocorticoid (MC), which will expectedly associate with hypertension, as is the case for the syndrome of apparent mineralocorticoid excess (AME). The fact that glucocorticoid levels in patients with CS are significantly higher than normal, which are already at least 100 times higher than the physiologic level of MCs, would suggest that each and every case of CS should associate with clinical signs of severe hyperaldosteronism and appropriately resolve with spironolactone/eplerenone treatment. Unfortunately, this is not the case in most patients with CS and while treatment of CS or administration of GCR antagonist improves hypertension, spironolactone failed to do so [27, 28]. With this apparent conflict in mind, it seems reasonable to review the physiology of this system.

Physiology of the GC/GCR/MCR System: Was it a Faulty Design?

Glucocorticoids are secreted from the zona fasciculata of the adrenal cortex as a part of the hypothalamic–pituitary–adrenal axis under tight control of both hypothalamus and pituitary. The last respond to both environmental and internal stressors, as well as show a robust feedback to cortisol levels. Glucocorticoids act as a ligand for two transcription factors—GR and MR, which belong to the nuclear receptor superfamily. While GR is specific for glucocorticoids, MR is equally affine to both GCs and MCs [29]. Both receptors reside in the cellular cytoplasm and upon activation by the ligand gain capability of nuclear translocation and action as transcription factors (Fig. 3.3).

Although not part of this review, both have an exceedingly complicated co-activation/co-suppression complex, which further affect the action of these factors. There are several differences in physiology of MRs and GRs. The main two are: (a) while GRs are ubiquitously expressed throughout the body, MRs express selective distribution, providing thus "geographic" tissue selectivity—distal nephron of the kidney, colon, salivary, and sweat glands, (b) while GRs are accessible to the ligand at any given time, MRs use a pre-receptor gate keeper 11-βHSD2 (see below) to convert cortisol to cortisone, which lacks the ability to bind to the MR. This assures relative functional selectivity of the MR towards the true mineralocorticoid aldosterone. This process is especially important while keeping in mind the fact that circulating levels of cortisol are about 100–1,000 times higher than those of aldosterone.

Both MRs and GRs are ancient—both descended from an ancestral corticoid receptor (AncCR) by gene duplication over 450 million years ago. Original AncGR was affine to both 11-deoxycorticosterone (aldosterone appeared later in evolution) and cortisol, and could easily be called AncMR, which could probably be more deserving. Series of more prominent changes created GC-specific GCR, while

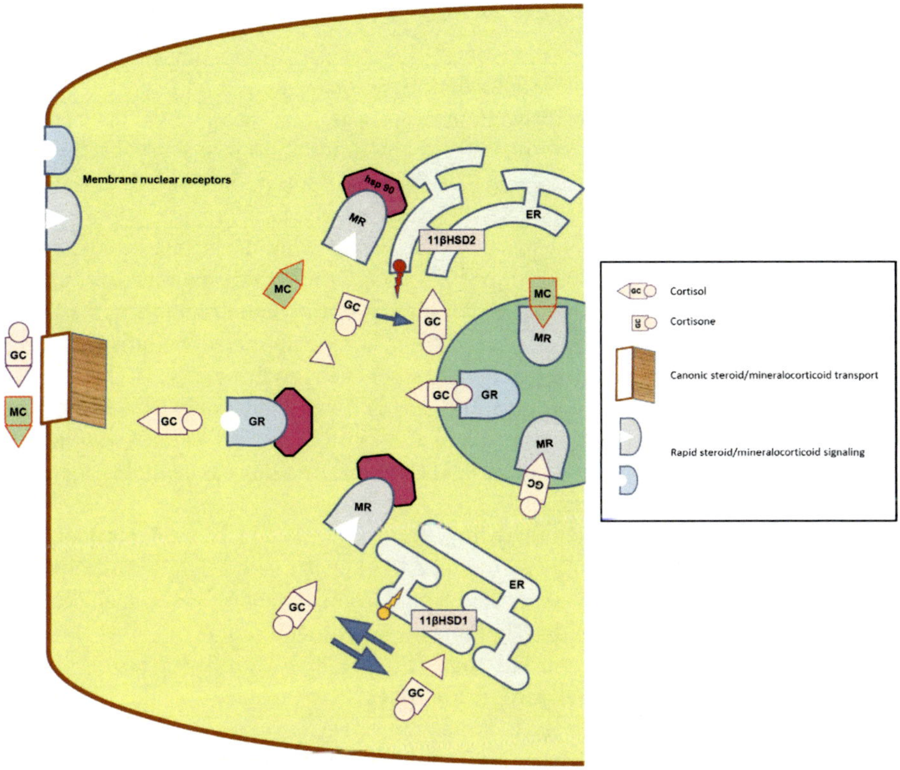

Fig. 3.3 Physiology of intracellular GC and MR transport, binding and signaling. *GC* glucocorticoid, *MC* mineralocorticoid, *GR* glucocorticoid receptor, *MR* mineralocorticoid receptor, *Hsp 90* heat shock protein 90, *ER* endoplasmic reticulum, *11βHSD* hydroxysteroid dehydrogenase

whatever changes happened to the AncGR resulted in MR, which still binds both GRs and MRs with equivalent affinity. While it is hard to fault evolution for lack of imagination or time, specificity of MRs for MCs is maintained through principally different, enzymatic mechanisms rather than the logically expected specificity of the ligand-binding domain [30].

The binding promiscuity of MRs is extensive—it is functionally important for transcriptional activation by both mineralocorticoids (aldosterone and deoxycorticosterone [DOC]) and glucocorticoids (cortisol in humans and corticosterone in rodents), but can actually also bind estrogens. Both GRs and MRs are highly homologous, less at the steroid binding domain, though—56%—which seem not to be able to prevent similar high affinity binding of both MCs and GCs [31]. The canonic—mineralocorticoid action—of MRs is found in the classic MR target epithelial polarized cells—colon, distal nephron, and sweat glands. MR expression in non-epithelial tissues—hippocampus, endothelium, cardiomyocytes, and adipocytes—is the subject of intense interest and research [32].

11-βHSD System: Too Smart to Fail

The existence of functional interconversion between active and inert forms of glucocorticoids (cortisol vs. cortisone in humans, and corticosterone vs. 11-dehydrocorticosterone in rodents, respectively) was characterized in the early 1950s [33]. It was soon discovered that functional activity of the compound was all about possession of a hydroxyl group at C11 [34]. Subsequently, two enzymes were characterized as having 11-βHSD properties—first was what is currently known as 11-βHSD1 and later 11-βHSD2 [35, 36]. Although the term "isoenzymes" is often applied to the pair, other than being 11-β hydroxysteroid dehydrogenases, these two enzymes have very little in common and their nomenclatural division into type 1 and 2 represents the sequence of discovery rather than anything else. Both enzymes are part of the short-chain dehydrogenase superfamily and share only 21% homology, mostly at sites homologous for the rest of the family. For the sake of continuous discussion related to the physiology of the MCR, we first discuss 11-βHSD2 and its relation to glucocorticoid signaling.

11-βHSD2 is a unidirectional dehydrogenase, expressed in mineralocorticoid target tissues—kidneys, colon, salivary gland, and placenta—and tightly co-expressed with MCR. The encoding gene is localized on chromosome 16 (16q22) and the protein consists of 405 amino acids. The enzyme uses nicotinamide adenine dinucleotide (NAD^+) as a cofactor and has high (50 nM K_m) affinity for cortisol [36]. The main functional role is dehydrogenation at C11 of species-specific active GC, while the main existential purpose is protection of MCR from same active GC. The functional importance of the enzyme is underlined by its inherited deficiency—syndrome of AME [37]. Clinically, AME presents with severe early onset hypertension associated with hypokalemia and low levels of both renin and aldosterone. Biochemically, deficiency of either 11-βHSD can be suggested based on the ratio between urinary excretion of A-ring reduced metabolites for both cortisol and cortisone (tetrahydrocortisol/tetrahydrocortisone), as well as the urinary free cortisol/cortisone ratio, the last is thought to be more specific for 11-βHSD2. The disease is caused by mutation in the *11-βHSD2* gene and shows genotype/phenotype correlation, based on the amount of functional enzyme. As a final proof that AME is caused by cortisol ability to signal through the MCR, it readily responds to treatment with spironolactone and/or low salt diet. Another phenomenon is lack of other clinical features of CS, despite increased half-life and thus levels of cortisol, which can be explained by decreased overall secretion through the negative feedback effect [38]. While it is thought that 11-βHSD2 protects MRs from being occupied by glucocorticoids, it has been shown that about 90% of epithelial MRs are occupied by glucocorticoids [39]. This phenomenon occurred in normal conditions—normal levels of endogenous glucocorticoids. In this case, transcriptional activity of the MR-GC complex maintained inactive by high levels of NADH, which activates the corepressor complex [40]. With change in redox that is associated with generation of reactive oxygen species, the MR-GC complex becomes active, changing the glucocorticoid action from antagonist to agonist [41]. The 11-βHSD2, as well as 11-βHSD1, is also expressed in the vascular endothelium, including coronary arteries. Functionally active MRs were described in hippocampus and hypothalamic neurons, as well as cardiomyocytes, adipocytes, and vasculature [32]. One can speculate that in case of significant oxidative stress and decrease in redox potential, the protective capacity of the enzyme will be severely diminished and, at least on the autocrine level, GC will signal through MRs.

11-βHSD1 is a bidirectional microsomal enzyme, highly expressed in glucocorticoid target tissues—liver, lungs, central nervous system, gonads, and adipose tissue. The encoding gene is localized on chromosome 1 (1q32-41) and the protein consists of 292 amino acids. The enzyme depends on NADP(H) as a cofactor and acts as a low affinity both 11-oxo-reductase and dehydrogenase, although reductase seems to be the preferential activity in vivo [33]. The set point, as well as overall activity of 11-βHSD1 also depends on microsomal hexose-6-phosphate dehydrogenase (H6PD), which is responsible for generation and provision of NADPH to 11-βHSD1. The main purpose seems to be provision of active GC to GCR on as needed paracrine fashion. This speculation is based on the following facts [42, 43]:

(a) Intrinsic features of cortisol
   - Circadian variability of levels
   - High binding to cortisol-binding protein
   - Relatively low affinity of GR to cortisol

(b) Intrinsic features of cortisone
   - No circadian variability
   - No significant binding to cortisol-binding protein
   - Relatively constant, significant, and readily available to peripheral issues

(c) Physiology of the paracrine GC system
   - Needed for acute and chronic inflammation
   - Needed for adipocyte maturation
   - Abnormal in obesity and metabolic syndrome

More Causes, Including Imbalance Between Vasoconstrictors and Vasodilators

Administration of synthetic glucocorticoids and ACTH were used extensively to assess the pathogenesis of hypertension in CS. However, the question remains about how much these represent pathophysiology of actual disease, because of relatively high doses, as well as baseline condition, which usually is normal health and acute mode of administration. These last may evoke acute compensatory responses that will significantly modify the process in comparison to actual chronic CS. Additionally, different synthetic glucocorticoids (prednisone, dexamethasone, triamcinolone) have different pharmacodynamics/pharmacokinetic profiles and intrinsic mineralocorticoid activity, which may affect severity and degree of hypertension through induction of additional mechanisms. It was found that oral dexamethasone causes an increase in total calculated peripheral resistance in humans without an increase in cardiac output or heart rate, while in dogs, a higher dose will also add decrease in cardiac output [44, 45]. Both hydrocortisone in humans and ACTH in rats caused hypertension, associated with an increase in both cardiac output and renal vascular resistance, but not total peripheral resistance or heart rate [44–46]. At least with hydrocortisone-induced hypertension in humans, neither β-blocker (atenolol), nor calcium channel blocker (felodipine) affected hypertension, which adds to reservations about clinical relevance of this model, as well as our understanding of this phenomenon [44, 45, 47]. One can argue that an increase in cardiac output and peripheral resistance can relate to an increase in plasma volume and/or fluid/salt retention, but further research shows that this is not the case [27, 28, 48].

Changes in the balance between vasoconstrictors and vasodilators can include different parameters—amount, expression, or sensitivity—and seem to play a significant role in the development of hypertension in patients with CS [6]. The group of vasoconstrictors/vasopressors includes the following: (a) endothelins, (b) angiotensin, (c) arginine vasopressin, (d) catecholamines, (e) neuropeptide Y, and others [6, 49].

Endothelins are potent direct vasoconstrictors and elevated endothelin-1 (Fig. 3.4) levels are found in patients with CS, as well as during treatment with prednisone [50, 51]. Synthetic glucocorticoids can induce catecholamine synthesis through activation of enzymes involved in the process, as well as increased expression of adrenergic receptors in vascular smooth muscles, thus promoting a vasoconstrictive response [49].

The vasodilative side of the equation is represented by (a) nitric oxide, (b) antioxidants, (c) vasodilative eicosanoids (prostacyclin, prostaglandin E2), (d) kallikrein, (e) atrial-natriuretic peptide, and evidence from human or animal studies suggests at least some suppression [2, 6, 28, 52].

Metabolic Syndrome: An Easy Blame

Another way to look at comorbidities of CS, including hypertension, is based on a purely clinical rather than pathophysiologic approach. Metabolic syndrome which includes central obesity, hypertension, insulin resistance, dyslipidemia, closely associates with CS and its morbidity [3, 4]. As with other comorbidities, hypertension seems to persist as part of the metabolic syndrome after resolution of hypercortisolemia with seemingly no difference between different etiologies of CS [53, 54]. Weight gain, especially truncal obesity, obstructive sleep apnea, insulin resistance, loss of circadian BP variability—all by themselves associate with hypertension and do not fully resolve after the treatment of CS and thus can explain, at least in part,

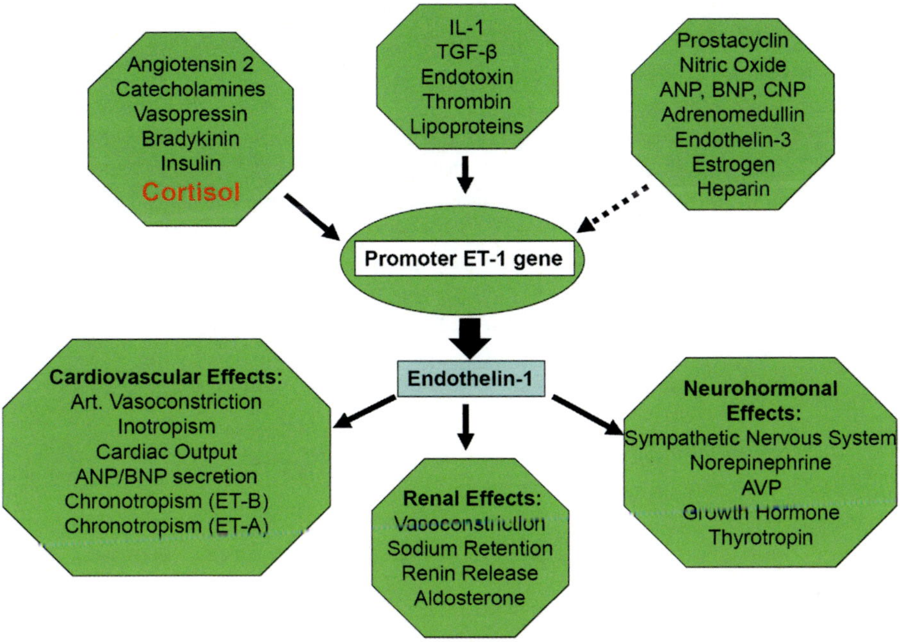

Fig. 3.4 Consequences of disease-related oxidative—stress regarding arteriolar tone. (*Solid arrow*: stimulation, *non-solid arrow*: inhibition), see http://www.endotext.org, Chapter 25. Hormones of the cardiovascular system by Pliquett, Buerke, Paschke, Koch CA. In: Chrousos GP, section editor. Adrenal disease and function; 2011

persistent hypertension after successful treatment. Differently from animal—especially rodent—models of obesity, obese humans show normal or decreased systemic cortisol levels [55]. Thus, while it is known that adiposity associates with local production of cytokines and that cortisol is needed for adipocyte maturation, it seems that it is a paracrine steroid delivery system, based on action of 11-beta-hydroxysteroid dehydrogenase type 1 that delivers the active hormone to the receptor, as both are closely co-expressed in these tissues. The mouse model with overexpression of 11-βHSD1 in white adipose tissue shows the phenotype of metabolic syndrome including hypertension, while obese humans show similar increased activity of 11-βHSD1 in their subcutaneous fat [43, 56].

Treatment

As hypertension in patients with CS depends on many factors including the duration of CS before the diagnosis was made and the individual risk factor profile for hypertension including body composition (adiposity)/insulin sensitivity, family history, age, and others, realistic expectations should be established when setting blood pressure goals and need of antihypertensives. Obviously, the treatment of choice for hypertension that is related to CS includes the elimination of the source of glucocorticoid excess. If the source is exogenous as part of treatment for conditions such as rheumatoid arthritis, lupus, etc, use of lowest therapeutically efficient dose of glucocorticoid should be employed. Concomitant hypertension should be treated by standard antihypertensive therapy as recommended by the Seventh Report of the Joint National Committee on Prevention, Detection, Evaluation, and Treatment of High Blood Pressure.

In patients with endogenous CS, surgical elimination of the source leading to cortisol excess should be pursued. Despite this ambitious goal and surgical cure of such patients, approximately 33% of adult patients remain hypertensive after surgery, whereas children and adolescents become normotensive within 1 year after achieving remission of CS by surgery [2]. This underscores that duration and excess of hypercortisolism in addition to other risk factors for hypertension acquired during lifetime play a role in glucocorticoid-induced hypertension. As children with CS stop growing in height, they will be diagnosed sooner than an adult with CS.

For patients with CS caused by an adrenal tumor, uni- or bilateral adrenalectomy (if both adrenals are tumorous) is recommended. If adrenal cancer is present, additional medical therapy aimed at reducing glucocorticoid excess and destroying cancer cells should be initiated. This might cause adrenal insufficiency if adrenolytic agents such as mitotane are used. Note that after unilateral adrenalectomy for a cortisol-secreting adenoma, the contralateral adrenal gland might be suppressed regarding cortisol production, therefore making it potentially necessary to replace hydrocortisone (and fludrocortisone) for a (short) period of time until the remaining gland is able to secrete sufficient amounts of adrenal hormone(s).

In most patients with newly diagnosed Cushing's disease, transsphenoidal surgery and resection of an ACTH-oma is advised and leads to remission in 70–90% of cases with very low morbidity (perioperative mortality <1.5%, cerebrospinal fluid leak <8%, meningitis <3%, central diabetes insipidus <9%, epistaxis <6%, syndrome of inappropriate secretion of antidiuretic hormone <25%), if performed by an experienced surgeon. However, at 10 years after such surgery, there is a risk of recurrence in up to 30% of patients. Most of these patients benefit from a second pituitary exploration, although further therapy including radiation therapy to the pituitary gland, medical treatment aimed at reducing effects of glucocorticoid excess, and/or bilateral adrenalectomy may be required. Of note, there is a latency period after radiation therapy during which interim medical therapy is generally advised. If rapid control of hypercortisolemia is needed, bilateral adrenalectomy with subsequently lifelong adrenal insufficiency and the need of adrenal hormone replacement (hydrocortisone and fludrocortisone) may have to be performed [57]. For patients with ectopic CS, identification and removal of the source can represent a challenge and may take months to years [10]. During this time period of hypercortisolism most often associated with hypertension, medical therapies to combat both should be started (Fig. 3.5).

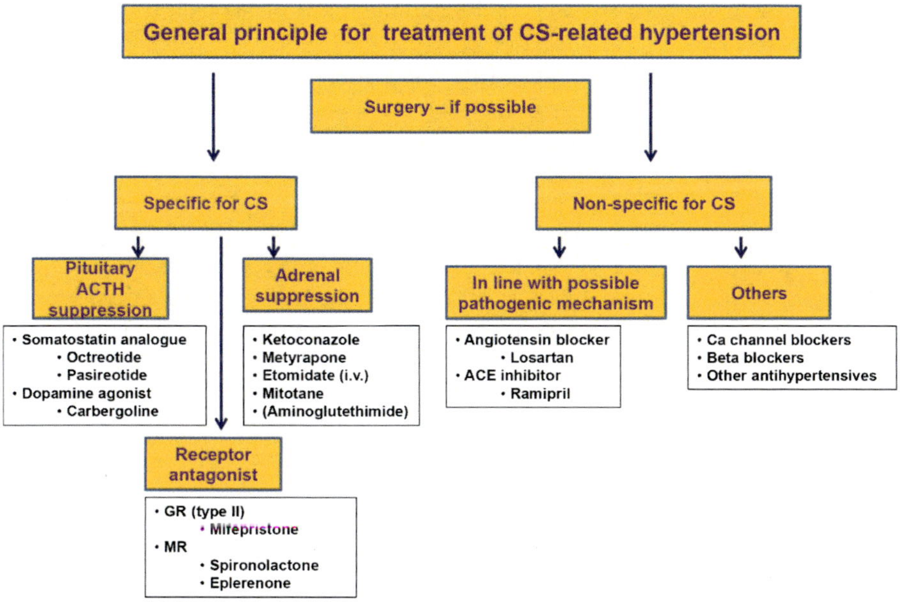

Fig. 3.5 General principles of treating hypertension in CS

Amongst these drugs are steroidogenesis inhibitors including ketoconazole and metyrapone. Ketoconazole as monotherapy decreases cortisol levels in approx. 70% of patients with CS but may lead to elevation of liver enzymes in up to 10% of patients. Metyrapone inhibits 11-beta-hydroxylase and aldosterone synthase and has been used as monotherapy or in combination with ketoconazole with normalization of cortisol levels in approx. 80% of patients. Because of generating a potent mineralocorticoid byproduct, DOC, metyrapone may exacerbate hypertension in addition to increased adrenal androgen synthesis which might lead to virilism in women. Both steroidogenesis inhibitors demonstrate an escape phenomenon related to ACTH secretion which limits their use in long-term treatment. Etomidate is another steroidogenesis inhibitor which can be administered parenterally, therefore being useful in patients with CS who are unable to take oral medications or have to undergo surgical procedures which might limit their oral intake [12].

Mitotane is adrenolytic in addition to inhibiting several steroidogenic enzymes and stored in adipose tissue and therefore has long-term effects with the need of closely monitoring its serum levels and risk to cause lifelong adrenal insufficiency. Aminoglutethimide is no longer available in the United States and showed efficacy in 50% of patients with CS.

Centrally acting agents include cabergoline, a dopamine agonist that is not very effective (approx. 40%) in reducing cortisol levels in patients with Cushing's disease over a 2-year period, and octreotide (primarily binding to somatostatin receptor (SSR) subtype 2) and pasireotide. Pasireotide (SOM230) is an SSR ligand binding to SSRs 1, 2, 3, and 5, that has shown promising results in a phase II trial in patients with Cushing's disease, although one-third of patients had developed hyperglycemia [58].

Recently, a type II glucocorticoid receptor antagonist, mifepristone, has been FDA approved for the use of hyperglycemia in patients with CS. Mifepristone has also been shown to normalize blood pressure in patients with CS [59–61].

Some compounds, as outlined above (see also Fig. 3.5), aim at modulating ACTH release and subsequent cortisol secretion, while others inhibit steroidogenesis or block the action of glucocorticoids at the receptor level. Interestingly, angiotensin-converting enzyme inhibitors (ACEI) and angiotensin II receptor blockers (ARB) can improve hypertension in approx. 50% of patients with Cushing's disease, suggesting an upregulation of the renin–angiotensin system in hypertension related to glucocorticoid excess [2].

Conclusion

Hypertension in patients with CS occurs in up to 95% of adults and half of children. It represents a major cardiovascular risk and mortality factor in such patients. Its pathogenesis is incompletely understood and includes an imbalance of factors involved in vasodilation and vasoconstriction. Amongst these are upregulation of the renin–angiotensin system, salt and water retention, endothelin-1, reactivity to catecholamines, vasopressin, increased peripheral resistance, a decline in antioxidants and nitric oxide synthase, and others. In patients with exogenous CS, the prevalence of hypertension (approximately 20%) is dose-dependent and lower than in those with endogenous CS. The aim of therapy is to normalize blood pressure and remove the source of glucocorticoid excess with resolution of hypertension after surgical cure (almost all children and adolescents but only two-thirds of adults) depending on the age of onset, duration, and amount of glucocorticoid excess and of hypertension in addition to other (underlying) hypertension risk factors such as obesity, sleep apnea, and insulin resistance. Treatment should include ACEI and ARB as well as eplerenone in selected patients (especially those with ectopic CS). Glucocorticoid excess and its effects should be controlled, if necessary with careful use of drugs such as steroidogenesis inhibitors or type II glucocorticoid receptor antagonists.

References

1. Newell-Price J, Bertagna X, Grossman AB, et al. Cushing's syndrome. Lancet. 2006;367:1605–17.
2. Sharma ST, Nieman LN. Cushing's syndrome: all variants, detection, and treatment. Endocrinol Metab Clin North Am. 2011;40(2):379–91.
3. Etxabe J, Vazquez JA. Morbidity and mortality in Cushing's disease: an epidemiological approach. Clin Endocrinol. 1994;40:479–84.
4. Lindholm J, et al. Incidence and late prognosis of Cushing's syndrome: a population-based study. J Clin Endocrinol Metab. 2001;86:117–23.

5. Hall JE, Nieman LK, editors. Handbook of diagnostic endocrinology. Totowa: Humana Press; 2003.
6. Magiakou MA, Smyrnaki P, Chrousos GP. Hypertension in Cushing's syndrome. Best Pract Res Clin Endocrinol Metab. 2006;20:467–82.
7. Robyn JA, Koch CA, Montalto J, Yong A, Warne GL, Batch JA. Cushing's syndrome in childhood and adolescence. J Paediatr Child Health. 1997;33(6):522–7.
8. Koch CA, Bornstein SR, Chrousos GP, Stratakis CA. Primary pigmented nodular adrenocortical dysplasia (PPNAD) within the scope of Carney complex as the etiology of Cushing's syndrome. Med Klin (Munich). 2000;95(4):224–30.
9. Kirkby-Bott J, Brunaud L, Mathonet M, Hamoir E, Kraimps JL, Trésallet C, et al. Ectopic hormone-secreting pheochromocytoma: a francophone observational study. World J Surg. 2012;36(6):1382–8.
10. Singer J, Werner F, Koch CA, Bartels M, Aigner T, Lincke T, et al. Ectopic Cushing's syndrome caused by a well-differentiated ACTH-secreting neuroendocrine carcinoma of the ileum. Exp Clin Endocrinol Diabetes. 2010;118(8):524–9.
11. Uwaifo GI, Koch CA, Hirshberg B, Chen CC, Hartzband P, Nieman LK, et al. Is there a therapeutic role for octreotide in patients with ectopic Cushing's syndrome? J Endocrinol Invest. 2003;26(8):710–7.
12. Krakoff J, Koch CA, Calis KA, Alexander RH, Nieman LK. Use of parenteral propylene glycol-containing etomidate preparation for the long-term management of ectopic Cushing's syndrome. J Clin Endocrinol Metab. 2001;86(9):4104–8.
13. Nieman LK, Biller BM, Findling JW, Newell-Price J, Savage MO, Stewart PM, et al. The diagnosis of Cushing's syndrome: an Endocrine Society clinical practice guideline. J Clin Endocrinol Metab. 2008;93(5):1526–40.
14. Dekkers OM, et al. Mortality in patients treated for Cushing's disease is increased, compared with patients treated for nonfunctioning pituitary macroadenoma. J Clin Endocrinol Metab. 2007;92:976–81.
15. Clayton RN, et al. Mortality and morbidity in Cushing's disease over 50 years in Stoke-on-Trent, UK: audit and meta-analysis of literature. J Clin Endocrinol Metab. 2011;96:632–42.
16. Bolland MJ, et al. Mortality and morbidity in Cushing's syndrome in New Zealand. Clin Endocrinol. 2011;75:436–42.
17. Porterfield JR, et al. Surgery for Cushing's syndrome: an historical review and recent ten-year experience. World J Surg. 2008;32:659–77.
18. Swearingen B, et al. Long-term mortality after transsphenoidal surgery for Cushing's disease. Ann Intern Med. 1999;130:821–4.
19. Baid S, Nieman LK. Glucocorticoid excess and hypertension. Curr Hypertens Rep. 2004; 6:493–9.
20. Magiakou MA, Mastorakos G, Oldfield EH, Gomez MT, Doppman JL, Cutler Jr GB, et al. Cushing's syndrome in children and adolescents, presentation, diagnosis, and therapy. N Engl J Med. 1994;331:629–36.
21. Magiakou MA, Mastorakos G, Zachman K, Chrousos GP. Blood pressure in children and adolescents with Cushing's syndrome before and after surgical cure. J Clin Endocrinol Metab. 1997;82:1734–7.
22. Lodish MB, Sinaii N, Patronas N, Batista DL, Keil M, Samuel J, et al. Blood pressure in pediatric patients with Cushing's Syndrome. J Clin Endocrinol Metab. 2009;94:2002–8.
23. Pirpiris M, et al. Hydrocortisone-indiced hypertension in men. The role of cardiac output. Am J Hypertens. 1993;6:287–94.
24. Connell JM, et al. Effects of ACTH and cortisol administration on blood pressure, electrolyte metabolism, atrial natriuretic peptide and renal function in normal man. J Hypertens. 1987;5:425–33.
25. De Leo M, et al. Cardiovascular disease in Cushing's syndrome. Neuroendocrinology. 2010;92:50–4.
26. Cicala MV, Mantero F. Hypertension in Cushing's syndrome: from pathogenesis to treatment. Neuroendocrinology. 2010;92:44–9.
27. Montrella-Waybill M, et al. Evidence that high dose cortisol-induced Na+ retention in man is not mediated by the mineralocorticoid receptor. J Clin Endocrinol Metab. 1992;72:1060–6.

28. Ong SLH, Whitworth JA. How do glucocorticoids cause hypertension: role of nitric oxide deficiency, oxidative stress, and eicosanoids. Endocrinol Metab Clin N Am. 2011;40:393–407.
29. Pipal JB, Fuller PJ. Structure-function relationships in the mineralocorticoid receptor. J Mol Endocrinol. 2008;41:405–13.
30. Bridgham JT, et al. Evolution of hormone-receptor complexity by molecular exploitation. Science. 2006;312(5770):97–100.
31. Arrizza JL, et al. Cloning of human mineralocorticoid receptor complementary DNA: structural and functional kinship with the glucocorticoid receptor. Science. 1987;237:268–75.
32. De Kloet ER, et al. Brain corticosteroid receptor balance in health and disease. Endocr Rev. 1998;19:269–301.
33. Draper N, Stewart PA. 11β-Hydroxysteroid dehydrogenase and the pre-receptor regulation of corticosteroid hormone action. J Endocrinol. 2005;186:251–71.
34. Amelung D, et al. Conversion of cortisone to compound F. J Clin Endocrinol Metab. 1953;13:1125–6.
35. Agarwal AK, et al. Cloning and expression of rat cDNA encoding corticosteroid 11β-dehydrogenase. J Biol Chem. 1989;264:18939–43.
36. Stewart PM, et al. Human kidney 11β-hydroxysteroid dehydrogenase is a high affinity nicotinamide adenine dinucleotide-dependent enzyme and differs from the cloned "type I" isoform. J Clin Endocrinol Metab. 1994;79:480–4.
37. Ulick S, et al. A syndrome of apparent mineralocorticoid excess associated with defects in the peripheral metabolism of cortisol. J Clin Endocrinol Metab. 1979;49:757–64.
38. Stewart PM, et al. Syndrome of apparent mineralocorticoid excess: a defect in the cortisol-cortisone shuttle. J Clin Invest. 1988;82:340–9.
39. Funder JW and Myles K. Exclusion of corticosterone from epithelial mineralocorticoid receptors is insufficient for selectivity of aldosterone action: in vivo binding studies. Endocrinology. 1996;137:5264–8.
40. Fjeld C, et al. Differential binding of NAD+ and NADH allows the transcriptional corepressor carboxyl-terminal binding protein to serve as a metabolic sensor. Proc Natl Acad Sci USA. 2003;100:9202–7.
41. Ward MR, et al. Eplerenone suppresses constrictive remodeling and collagen accumulation after angioplasty in porcine coronary arteries. Circulation. 2001;104:467–72.
42. Staab CA, Maser E. 11-βHydroxysteroid dehydrogenase type 1 is an important regulator at the interface of obesity and inflammation. J Steroid Mol Biol. 2010;119:56–72.
43. Pereira CD et al. 11-βHydroxysteroid dehydrogenase type 1: relevance of its modulation in the pathophysiology of obesity, the metabolic syndrome and type 2 diabetes mellitus. Diabetes Obes Metab. 2012. doi: 10.1111/j.1463-1326.2012.01582.x.
44. Pirpiris M, et al. Pressor responsiveness in corticosteroid-induced hypertension in humans. Hypertension. 1992;19:567–74.
45. Nakamoto H, et al. Depressor systems contribute to hypertension induced by glucocorticoid excess in dogs. J Hypertens. 1992;10:561–9.
46. Wen C, et al. Hemodynamic profile of corticotrophin-induced hypertension in the rat. J Hypertens. 1999;17:1715–23.
47. Witworth JA, et al. Hemodynamic response to cortisol in man: effects of felodipine. Hypertens Res. 1994;17:137–42.
48. Connell JM, et al. Haemodynamic, hormonal and renal effects of adrenocorticotrophic hormone in sodium-restricted man. J Hypertens. 1988;6:17–23.
49. Peppa M, et al. Hypertension and other morbidities with Cushing's syndrome associated with corticosteroids: a review. Integr Blood Press Control. 2011;4:7–16.
50. Kirilov G, et al. Elevated plasma endothelin as an additional cardiovascular risk factor in patients with Cushing's syndrome. Eur J Endocrinol. 2003;149:549–53.
51. Borcsok I, et al. Glucocorticoids regulate the expression of the humanosteoblastic endothelin A receptor gene. J Exp Med. 1998;188:1563–73.
52. Sala C, et al. Blunted vascular and renal effects of exogenous atrial natriuretic peptide in patients with Cushing's disease. J Clin Endocrinol Metab. 2001;86:1957–61.

53. Colao A, et al. Persistence of increased cardiovascular risk in patients with Cushing's disease after 5 years of successful cure. J Clin Endocrinol Metab. 1999;84:2664–72.
54. Giordano R, et al. Metabolic and cardiovascular outcomes in patients with Cushing's syndrome of different aetiologies during active disease and 1 years after remission. Clin Endocrinol. 2011;75:354–60.
55. Seckl JR, et al. Glucocorticoids and 11-beta-hydroxysteroid dehydrogenase in adipose tissue. Recent Prog Horm Res. 2004;59:359–93.
56. Rask E, et al. Tissue-specific changes in peripheral cortisol metabolism in obese women: increased adipose 11-beta-hydroxysteroid dehydrogenase type 1 activity. J Clin Endocrinol Metab. 2002;87:3330–6.
57. Tritos NA, Biller BM, Swearingen B. Management of Cushing's disease. Nat Rev Endocrinol. 2011;7(5):279–89.
58. Colao A, et al. Pasireotide B2305 Study Group. A 12-month phase 3 study of pasireotide in Cushing's disease. N Engl J Med. 2012;366(10):914–24.
59. Nieman LK, Chrousos GP, Kellner C, Spitz IM, Nisula BC, Cutler GB, et al. Successful treatment of Cushing's syndrome with the glucocorticoid antagonist RU486. J Clin Endocrinol Metab. 1985;61(3):536–40.
60. Castinetti F, Conte-Devolx B, Brue T. Medical treatment of Cushing's syndrome: glucocorticoid receptor antagonists and mifepristone. Neuroendocrinology. 2010;92 Suppl 1:125–30.
61. Fleseriu M, et al. On behalf of the SEISMIC Study Investigators; The SEISMIC Study Investigators include. Mifepristone, a glucocorticoid receptor antagonist produces clinical and metabolic benefits in patients with Cushing's syndrome. J Clin Endocrinol Metab. 2012;97(6):2039–49.

Chapter 4
Primary Generalized Familial and Sporadic Glucocorticoid Resistance (Chrousos Syndrome) and Hypersensitivity

Evangelia Charmandari, Tomoshige Kino, and George P. Chrousos

Abstract The human glucocorticoid receptor (hGR) is a ubiquitously expressed intracellular, ligand-dependent transcription factor, which mediates the action of glucocorticoids and influences physiologic functions essential for life. Alterations in the molecular mechanisms of hGR action modify glucocorticoid signal transduction and alter tissue sensitivity to glucocorticoids. This review summarizes the pathophysiology, molecular mechanisms, and clinical aspects of primary generalized familial and sporadic glucocorticoid resistance (PGGR or Chrousos syndrome) and hypersensitivity (PGGH). The molecular basis of Chrousos syndrome and

Search Strategy and Selection Criteria

We searched PubMed for articles published in English on generalized glucocorticoid resistance and hypersensitivity between 1975 and May 2011, with MeSH terms "generalized glucocorticoid resistance," "generalized glucocorticoid hypersensitivity," "natural glucocorticoid receptor mutations," and "glucocorticoid receptor polymorphisms." A total of 633 articles were identified. The results of these searches were pooled, and subsearches were run with additional MeSH and natural-language terms for the following: "pathophysiology," "molecular mechanisms," "clinical manifestations," "diagnosis," "therapy," and "management." We also reviewed books on generalized glucocorticoid resistance and hypersensitivity published in the same period. We reviewed selected references from articles retrieved by the initial search. Several earlier, commonly referenced key publications have been cited. Relevant references cited in the original source of references were also reviewed.

E. Charmandari (✉) • G.P. Chrousos
Division of Endocrinology and Metabolism, First Department of Pediatrics,
University of Athens Medical School, Children's Hospital Aghia Sophia,
Athens 11527, Greece
e-mail: evangelia.charmandari@googlemail.com

T. Kino
Unit on Molecular Hormone Action, Program in Reproductive and Adult Endocrinology,
Eunice Kennedy Shriver National Institute of Child Health & Human Development,
National Institutes of Health, Bethesda, MD, USA

C.A. Koch and G.P. Chrousos (eds.), *Endocrine Hypertension: Underlying Mechanisms and Therapy*, Contemporary Endocrinology, DOI 10.1007/978-1-60761-548-4_4,

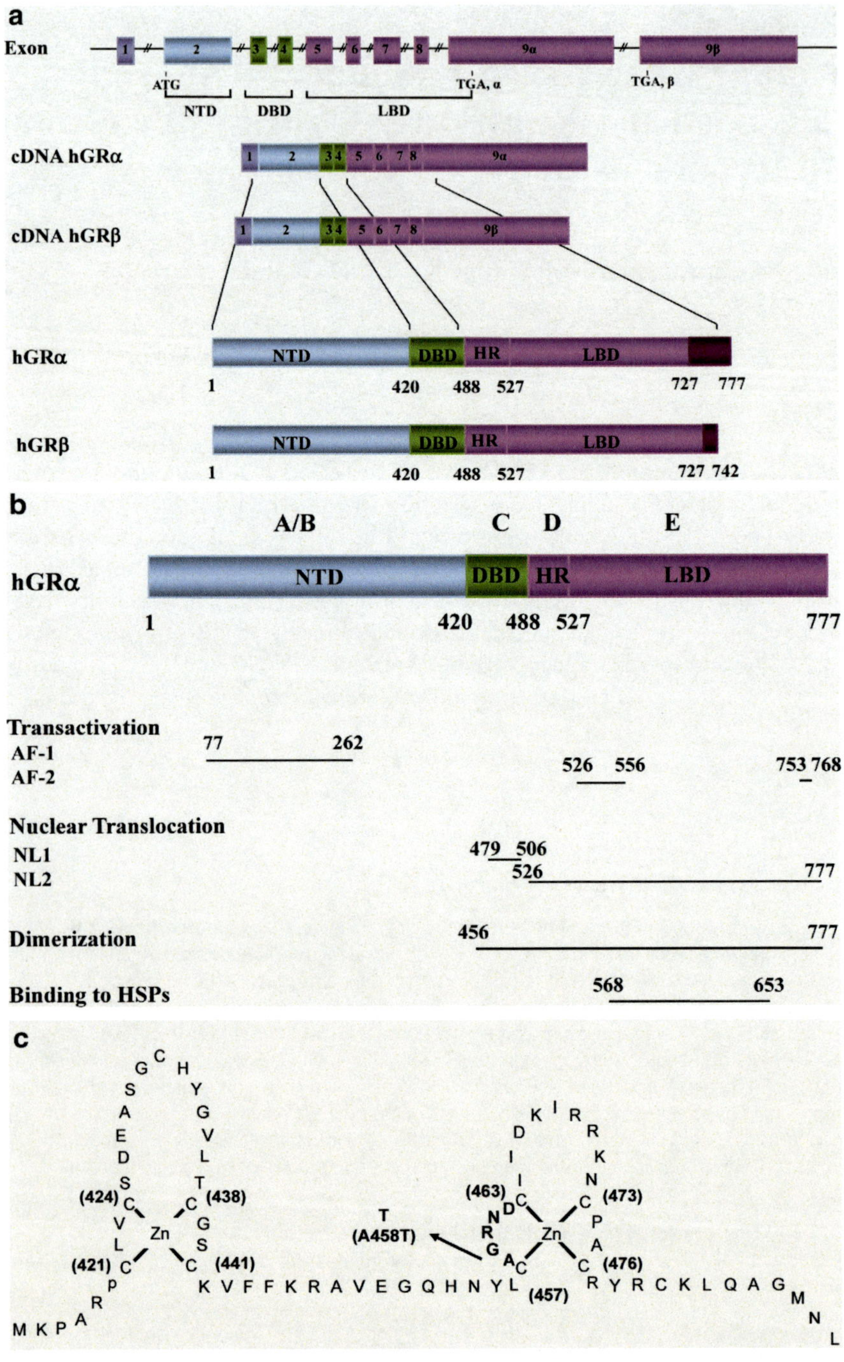

Fig. 4.1 (**a**) Schematic representation of the structure of the human glucocorticoid receptor (hGR) gene. Alternative splicing of the primary transcript gives rise to the two mRNA and protein isoforms, hGRα and hGRβ. (**b**) Functional domains of the hGRα. The functional domains and

PGGH has been ascribed to mutations in the hGR gene, which alter tissue sensitivity to glucocorticoids. The stochastic nature of glucocorticoid signaling pathways in association with the variable effect that hGR gene mutations/polymorphisms might have on glucocorticoid signal transduction indicates that alterations in hGR action may have important implications for many critical biological processes, such as the behavioral and physiologic responses to stress, intermediary metabolism, the immune and inflammatory reaction, as well as growth, development, and reproduction.

Keywords Glucocorticoid receptor • Primary generalized glucocorticoid resistance • Primary generalized glucocorticoid hypersensitivity • Glucocorticoid signal transduction

Introduction

In humans, glucocorticoids regulate a broad spectrum of physiologic functions essential for life and play an important role in the maintenance of basal and stress-related homeostasis [1–3]. Approximately 20% of the genes expressed in human leukocytes are regulated positively or negatively by glucocorticoids [4]. Glucocorticoids are involved in almost every cellular, molecular, and physiologic network of the organism and play a pivotal role in critical biologic processes, such as growth, reproduction, intermediary metabolism, the immune and inflammatory reaction, as well as central nervous system and cardiovascular functions [1, 4]. Furthermore, glucocorticoids represent one of the most widely used therapeutic compounds, often employed in the treatment of inflammatory, autoimmune, and lymphoproliferative disorders [1].

The Human Glucocorticoid Receptor

At the cellular level, the actions of glucocorticoids are mediated by a 94 kDa protein, the glucocorticoid receptor (GR). The human (h) GR belongs to the steroid/thyroid/retinoic acid superfamily of nuclear receptors and functions as a ligand-dependent transcription factor that regulates the expression of glucocorticoid-responsive genes positively or negatively [5–7] (Fig. 4.1a). The hGR cDNA was isolated by expression cloning in 1985 [8]. The hGR gene is one locus on the long arm of chromosome

Fig. 4.1 (continued) subdomains are indicated beneath the linearized protein structures. *AF* activation function; *DBD* DNA-binding domain; *LBD* ligand-binding domain; *NLS* nuclear localization signal. (**c**) Enlargement of part of the DBD showing the amino acid sequence (single letter codes) of the two zinc fingers and the dimerization loop (in *bold*). The A to T mutation at position 458 that could produce a dimerization defective receptor is shown

5 (q31.3) and consists of nine exons. Alternative splicing of the hGR gene in exon 9 generates two highly homologous receptor isoforms, termed α and β. These are identical through amino acid 727, but then diverge, with hGRα having an additional 50 amino acids and hGRβ having an additional, nonhomologous 15 amino acids [3, 5–7] (Fig. 4.1a). The hGRα represents the classic glucocorticoid receptor that functions as a ligand-dependent transcription factor, while the hGRβ does not bind glucocorticoid agonists, has intrinsic, hGRα-independent, gene-specific transcriptional activity, and exerts a dominant negative effect upon the transcriptional activity of hGRα [9, 10].

The human GR is a modular protein composed of distinct regions illustrated in Fig. 4.1b: the amino-terminal A/B region, also called immunogenic or N-terminal domain (NTD), and the C, D, and E regions, which correspond to the DNA-binding domain (DBD), the hinge region, and the ligand-binding domain (LBD), respectively.

The NTD of the hGRα contains a major transactivation domain, termed activation function (AF)-1, which is located between amino acids 77 and 262 of the hGRα and is ligand-independent. The AF-1 plays an important role in the interaction of the receptor with molecules necessary for the initiation of transcription, such as coactivators, chromatin modulators, and basal transcription factors, including RNA polymerase II, TATA-binding protein (TBP), and a host of TBP-associated proteins (TAFIIs) [3, 5, 6].

The DBD of the hGRα corresponds to amino acids 420–480 and contains two zinc finger motifs through which the hGRα binds to specific DNA sequences, the glucocorticoid response elements (GREs) in the promoter region(s) of target genes [5, 6]. The DBD is the most highly conserved domain throughout the steroid receptor family. The two zinc finger motifs are able to tetrahedrally coordinate a zinc atom and are held by four cysteine (Cys) residues (Fig. 4.1c). Only very few amino acids, termed the proximal (P)-box, within the first zinc finger are responsible for specific recognition of the cognate GREs. Another set of amino acids, called the distal (D)-box within the second zinc finger, forms the weak dimerization interface of the DBD. The DBD of the hGRα also contains sequences important for nuclear translocation [5, 6].

The hinge region or region D is a flexible region located between the DBD and LBD. Its amino terminus is an integral part of the DBD and is involved in its dimerization. The hinge region confers structural flexibility in the receptor dimmers, thereby allowing a single receptor dimmer to interact with multiple GREs [5, 6].

The LBD of the hGRα corresponds to amino acids 481–777, binds to glucocorticoids, and plays a critical role in the ligand-induced activation of hGRα. The LBD also contains a second transactivation domain, termed AF-2, which is ligand-dependent, as well as sequences important for receptor dimerization, nuclear translocation, binding to the heat shock proteins (HSPs), and interaction with coactivators [5, 6].

Expressed hGRα is a panel of eight amino-terminal translational isoforms of varying lengths, each of which consists of three subdomains, the NTD, the DBD, and the LBD. These hGRα isoforms differ at their amino-termini and may differentially transduce the glucocorticoid signal to target tissues depending on their selective relative expression and inherent activities. It is likely that similar differential

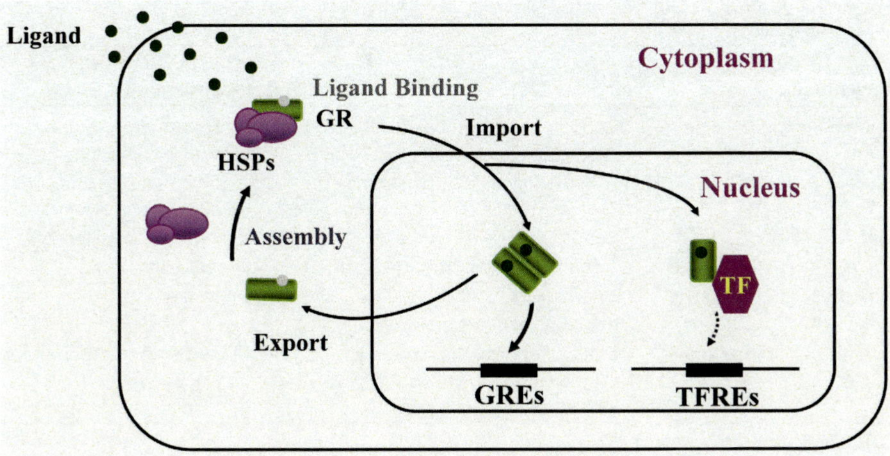

Fig. 4.2 Nucleocytoplasmic shuttling of the glucocorticoid receptor. Upon binding to the ligand, the activated hGRα dissociates from heat shock proteins (HSPs) and translocates into the nucleus, where it homodimerizes and binds to glucocorticoid response elements (GREs) in the promoter region of target genes or interacts with other transcription factors (TFs), such as activator protein-1 (AP-1), nuclear factor-κB (NF-κB), and signal transducer and activator of transcription-5 (STAT5), ultimately modulating the transcriptional activity of respectively GRE- or TFRE-containing genes

cell-specific production and functional differences might also be present between the putative hGRβ translational isoforms [5, 6]. This marked complexity in the transcription/translation of the hGR gene enables target tissues to differentially respond to circulating glucocorticoid concentrations and accounts for the highly stochastic nature of the glucocorticoid signaling pathway [11].

In the absence of ligand, hGRα resides mostly in the cytoplasm of cells as part of a hetero-oligomeric complex, which contains chaperon HSPs 90, 70 and FKBP51, as well as other proteins [7, 11]. Upon ligand-induced activation, the hGRα dissociates from this multiprotein complex and translocates into the nucleus, where it binds as a homodimer to GREs in the promoter regions of target genes and regulates their expression positively or negatively, depending on GRE sequence and promoter context [7, 11] (Fig. 4.2). To initiate transcription, the hGRα uses its transcriptional activation domains, activation function (AF)-1 and AF-2, located in the NTD and LBD, respectively, as surfaces to interact with nuclear receptor coactivators and chromatin-remodeling complexes [12–15]. The ligand-activated hGRα can also modulate gene expression independently of DNA-binding, by interacting, possibly as a monomer, with other transcription factors, such as nuclear factor-κB, activator protein-1, p53, and signal transducers and activators of transcription [7]. Following transcriptional activation or inhibition of glucocorticoid-responsive genes, the hGRα dissociates from the ligand and has a lower affinity for binding to GREs. The unliganded hGRα remains within the nucleus for a considerable length of time and is then exported to the cytoplasm; both within the nucleus and within the cytoplasm the hGRα may be recycled and/or degraded in the proteasome [16] (Fig. 4.2).

Table 4.1 Expected clinical manifestations in tissue-specific glucocorticoid resistance or hypersensitivity[a]

Target tissue	Glucocorticoid hypersensitivity = glucocorticoid excess	Glucocorticoid resistance = glucocorticoid deficiency
Central nervous system	Insomnia, anxiety, depression, defective cognition	Fatigue, somnolence, malaise, defective cognition
Liver	+ Gluconeogenesis, + lipogenesis	Hypoglycemia, resistance to diabetes mellitus
Fat	Accumulation of visceral fat (metabolic syndrome)	Loss of weight, resistance to weight gain
Blood vessels	Hypertension	Hypotension
Bone	Stunted growth, osteoporosis	
Inflammation/immunity	Immune suppression, anti-inflammation, vulnerability to certain infections and tumors	+ Inflammation, + autoimmunity, + allergy

[a]Modified from references [21, 27]

Alterations in the molecular mechanisms of hGRα action may lead to alterations in tissue sensitivity to glucocorticoids, which may take the form of *glucocorticoid resistance* or *glucocorticoid hypersensitivity* and may be associated with significant morbidity [17–19] (Table 4.1). In the present review, we summarize the pathophysiology and molecular mechanisms underlying Chrousos syndrome and primary generalized glucocorticoid hypersensitivity.

Primary Generalized Glucocorticoid Resistance and Hypersensitivity

Clinical Manifestations

Primary generalized familial and sporadic glucocorticoid resistance is a rare, familial or sporadic condition, initially described and elucidated by Chrousos et al. This condition is characterized by generalized, mostly partial, target-tissue insensitivity to glucocorticoids, which leads to compensatory activation of the hypothalamic-pituitary-adrenal (HPA) axis and hypersecretion of adrenocorticotropic hormone (ACTH) in the systemic circulation [20–22]. The latter results in adrenocortical hyperplasia, increased cortisol secretion as a compensation for the reduced action of glucocorticoids at target tissues, and increased production of adrenal steroids with mineralocorticoid [cortisol, deoxycorticosterone (DOC) and corticosterone] and/or androgenic activity [androstenedione, dehydroepiandrosterone (DHEA) and DHEA-sulfate (DHEAS)] [20–22].

The clinical manifestations of PGGR reflect the pathophysiologic alterations described above and primarily include those of mineralocorticoid and/or androgen excess [20–22]. Clinical manifestations of glucocorticoid deficiency might occur, but are rare and were only reported in a young child with hypoglycemic generalized tonic-clonic seizures during the course of a febrile illness [23], in a newborn baby with severe hypoglycemia, excessive fatigability with feeding, increased susceptibility to infections and concurrent growth hormone deficiency [24], and in several adult patients with chronic fatigue [20–22]. Clinical manifestations of mineralocorticoid excess include hypertension and hypokalemic alkalosis. Clinical manifestations of androgen excess include ambiguous genitalia in a karyotypic female at birth and gonadotropin-independent precocious puberty in children of either gender; acne, hirsutism, and hypofertility in both sexes; male-pattern hair loss, menstrual irregularities, and oligo-anovulation in females; and oligospermia in males [20–22]. The clinical spectrum of the condition is broad, ranging from most severe to mild forms, while a number of patients may be asymptomatic, displaying biochemical alterations only [20–22]. This variable clinical phenotype is due to variations in the tissue sensitivity of the glucocorticoid, mineralocorticoid, and/or androgen receptor signaling pathways; variations in the activity of key hormone-inactivating or -activating enzymes, such as the 11β-hydroxysteroid dehydrogenase [25] and other genetic or epigenetic factors, such as the presence of insulin resistance and visceral obesity [21]. In recognition of Professor George P. Chrousos' extensive and groundbreaking research work in this field, it has been proposed that the term "Chrousos Syndrome" is used in place of "Primary Generalized Familial and Sporadic Glucocorticoid Resistance" [26, 27].

Primary generalized glucocorticoid hypersensitivity (PGGH) represents the mirror image of Chrousos syndrome and is characterized by generalized, partial, target-tissue hypersensitivity to glucocorticoids, and compensatory hypoactivation of the HPA axis. To date, there has been only one patient reported with manifestations of tissue-specific glucocorticoid hypersensitivity caused by a novel hGR gene mutation. The patient was a 43-year-old female, who presented with a long-standing history of visceral obesity, hypercholesterolemia, hypertriglyceridemia, diabetes type 2, and hypertension [28] (Table 4.2).

Molecular Mechanisms

hGR Mutations

The molecular basis of Chrousos syndrome has been ascribed primarily to mutations in the hGR gene, which impair the molecular mechanisms of hGR action and decrease tissue sensitivity to glucocorticoids (Table 4.2, Fig. 4.3) [23, 24, 29–41]. The molecular defects that have been elucidated in cases with Chrousos syndrome and have been reported to date are summarized in Table 4.2. We have identified most hGR mutations associated with primary generalized glucocorticoid resistance and have systematically investigated the molecular mechanisms through which these various natural hGR mutants affect glucocorticoid signal transduction in almost all reported cases of generalized glucocorticoid resistance. We studied:

Table 4.2 Mutations of the human glucocorticoid receptor gene causing primary generalized glucocorticoid resistance or hypersensitivity[a]

Mutation position					
References	cDNA	Amino acid	Molecular mechanisms	Genotype	Phenotype
Chrousos et al. [20] Hurley et al. [30]	1922 (A → T)	641 (D → V)	Transactivation ↓ Affinity for ligand ↓ (×3) Nuclear translocation: 22 min Abnormal interaction with GRIP1	Homozygous	Hypertension Hypokalemic alkalosis
Karl et al. [31]	4 bp deletion in exon-intron 6		hGRα number: 50% of control Inactivation of the affected allele	Heterozygous	Hirsutism Male-pattern hair-loss Menstrual irregularities
Malchoff et al. [32]	2185 (G → A)	729 (V → I)	Transactivation ↓ Affinity for ligand ↓ (×2) Nuclear translocation: 120 min Abnormal interaction with GRIP1	Homozygous	Precocious puberty Hyperandrogenism
Karl et al. [29] Kino et al. [33]	1676 (T → A)	559 (I → N)	Transactivation ↓ Decrease in hGR binding sites Transdominance (+) Nuclear translocation: 180 Abnormal interaction with GRIP1	Heterozygous	Hypertension Oligospermia Infertility
Ruiz et al. [34] Charmandari et al. [39]	1430 (G → A)	477 (R → H)	Transactivation ↓ No DNA-binding Nuclear translocation: 20 min	Heterozygous	Hirsutism Fatigue Hypertension
Ruiz et al. [34] Charmandari et al. [39]	2035 (G → A)	679 (G → S)	Transactivation ↓ Affinity for ligand ↓ (×2) Nuclear translocation: 30 min Abnormal interaction with GRIP1	Heterozygous	Hirsutism Fatigue Hypertension
Mendonca et al. [35]	1712 (T → C)	571 (V → A)	Transactivation ↓ Affinity for ligand ↓ (×6) Nuclear translocation: 25 min Abnormal interaction with GRIP1	Homozygous	Ambiguous genitalia Hypertension Hypokalemia Hyperandrogenism

Vottero et al. [36]	2241 (T→G)	747 (I→M)	Transactivation ↓ Transdominance (+) Affinity for ligand ↓ (×2) Nuclear translocation ↓ Abnormal interaction with GRIP1	Heterozygous	Cystic acne Hirsutism Oligo-amenorrhea
Charmandari et al. [38]	2318 (T→C)	773 (L→P)	Transactivation ↓ Transdominance (+) Affinity for ligand ↓ (×2.6) Nuclear translocation: 30 min Abnormal interaction with GRIP1	Heterozygous	Fatigue Anxiety Acne Hirsutism Hypertension
Charmandari et al. [40]	2209 (T→C)	737 (F→L)	Transactivation ↓ Transdominance (time-dependent) (+) Affinity for ligand ↓ (×\1.5) Nuclear translocation: 180 min	Heterozygous	Hypertension Hypokalemia
Nader et al. [23]	2141 (G→A)	7[illegible]4 (R→Q)	Transactivation ↓ Transdominance (+) Affinity for ligand ↓ (×2) Nuclear translocation ↓ Abnormal interaction with GRIP1	Heterozygous	Hypoglycemia Hypokalemia Hypertension Mild clitoromegaly Advanced bone age Precocious pubarche
McMahon et al. [24]	2 bp deletion at nt 2318-9	77[illegible]	Transactivation ↓ Affinity for ligand: absent No suppression of IL-6	Homozygous	Hypoglycemia Fatigability with feeding Hypertension
Zhu Hui-juan et al. [41]	1667 (G→T)	556 (T→I)	Not studied yet	Heterozygous	Adrenal incidentaloma
Charmandari et al. [28]	1201 (G→C)	401 (D→H)	Transactivation ↑ Transdominance (+) Affinity for ligand: N Nuclear translocation: N Interaction with GRIP1: N	Heterozygous	Visceral obesity Hypercholesterolemia Hypertriglyceridemia Hypertension Diabetes type 2

[a]Modified from references [20–22]

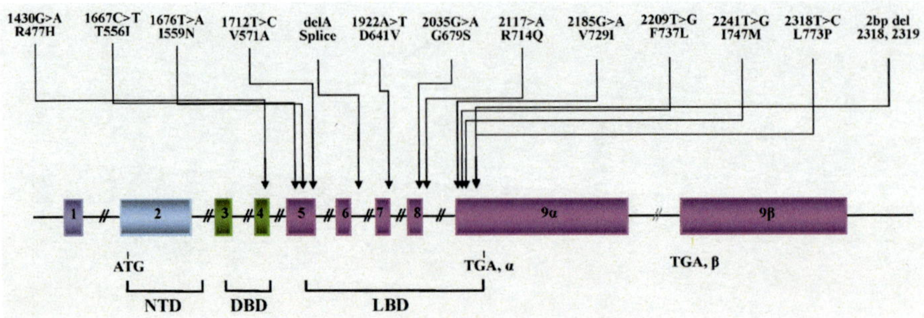

Fig. 4.3 Location of the known mutations of the hGR gene causing Chrousos syndrome. *DBD*: DNA-binding domain; *LBD*: ligand-binding domain; *NTD*: amino terminal domain

(a) the transcriptional activity of the mutant receptors; (b) the ability of the mutant receptors to exert a dominant negative effect upon the wild-type receptor; (c) the affinity of the mutant receptors for the ligand; (d) the subcellular localization of the mutant receptors and their nuclear translocation following exposure to the ligand; (e) the ability of the mutant receptors to bind to GREs; and (f) the interaction of the mutant receptors with the glucocorticoid receptor-interacting protein-1 (GRIP1) coactivator, which belongs to the p160 family of nuclear receptor coactivators and plays an important role in the hGRα-mediated transactivation of glucocorticoid-responsive genes [22, 29–40].

Compared with the wild-type receptor, all mutant receptors demonstrated variable reduction in their ability to transactivate glucocorticoid-responsive genes in response to dexamethasone [29–40]. The mutant receptors hGRαI559N, hGRαF737L, hGRαI747M, and hGRαL773P exerted a dominant negative effect upon the wild-type receptor, which might have contributed to manifestation of the disease at the heterozygote state [29, 33, 35, 37, 40]. All mutant receptors in which the mutations were located in the LBD of the receptor showed a variable reduction in their affinity for the ligand [29–40]. The only mutant receptor that demonstrated normal affinity for the ligand was the hGRαR477H, in which the mutation was located in the DBD [39]. Most pathologic mutant receptors were observed primarily in the cytoplasm of cells in the absence of ligand, except for the hGRαV729I and hGRαF737L receptors, which were localized both in the cytoplasm and the nucleus of cells. Exposure to dexamethasone induced a slow translocation of the mutant receptors into the nucleus, which ranged from 20 to 180 min compared with the wild-type hGRα, which required only 12 min for complete translocation [29–40]. All mutant receptors in which the mutations were located in the LBD preserved their ability to bind to DNA and displayed an abnormal interaction with the GRIP1 coactivator *in vitro* [29–40]. The only mutant receptor that failed to bind to DNA but displayed a normal interaction with the GRIP1 coactivator was the hGRαR477H, in which the mutation was located at the C-terminal zinc finger of the DBD [39].

In the patient with the symptomatology suggestive of PGGH, we identified a novel, heterozygous guanine to cytosine (G→C) substitution at nucleotide position 1201 in exon 2 of the hGR gene, resulting in aspartic acid (D) to histidine (H) substitution at amino acid position 401 in the NTD of the receptor. Functional studies showed that compared with the wild-type hGRα, the hGRαD401H demonstrated a 2.4-fold increase in its ability to transactivate the glucocorticoid-responsive genes and exerted a dominant positive effect upon the wild-type receptor at low concentrations. The mutant receptor hGRαD401H had similar affinity for the ligand and time to nuclear translocation; it preserved its ability to bind to GREs and displayed a normal interaction with the GRIP1 coactivator [28] (Table 4.2).

hGR Polymorphisms

Further to the hGR gene mutations, inter-individual variations in tissue sensitivity to glucocorticoids have been described within the normal population and have been partly attributed to polymorphisms in the hGR gene. Several polymorphisms of the hGR gene have been reported to date [42–44].

The first polymorphism, ER22/23EK, consists of two linked, single-nucleotide mutations in codons 22 and 23 in exon 2 of the hGR gene (rs 6189 and rs 6190). The first nucleotide replacement in codon 22 is silent, not resulting in an amino acid change [GAG to GAA, both coding for glutamic acid (E)], but the second replacement in codon 23 (AGG to AAG) results in arginine (R) to lysine (K) substitution [44, 45]. The ER22/23EK polymorphism results in a small reduction of the transcriptional activation of glucocorticoid-responsive genes compared with the wild-type receptor, but it does not influence transcriptional repression [45]. This polymorphism reduces sensitivity to glucocorticoids, as evidenced by the higher serum cortisol concentrations and the smaller decrease in cortisol concentrations following dexamethasone suppression testing in carriers compared with noncarriers [46] and results in a phenotype that is characterized by a more favorable metabolic profile, leading to longevity. Carriers of the ER22/23EK polymorphism display relative glucocorticoid resistance, lower fasting insulin concentrations and improved insulin sensitivity, lower total and LDL cholesterol concentrations, and lower CRP concentrations [44, 47]. These effects of the ER22/23EK polymorphism suggest a healthier cardiovascular and metabolic profile, which was confirmed in a follow-up study demonstrating an increased survival rate for carriers of this polymorphism over a 4-year period compared with noncarriers [47]. In line with this favorable metabolic profile, the ER22/23EK polymorphism demonstrates significantly higher incidence in the oldest half of the population. At young age, a sexually dimorphic pattern in body composition has been documented in this polymorphism: Male ER22/23EK carriers are taller, have more muscle mass, and are stronger than noncarriers. Female ER22/23EK carriers have smaller waist and hip circumferences and lower body weight [48]. Finally, at older age, carriers of the ER22/23EK polymorphism have lower risk of dementia and fewer white matter lesions in the brain compared to noncarriers [44]. The molecular mechanisms through which the ER22/23EK polymorphism produces the above

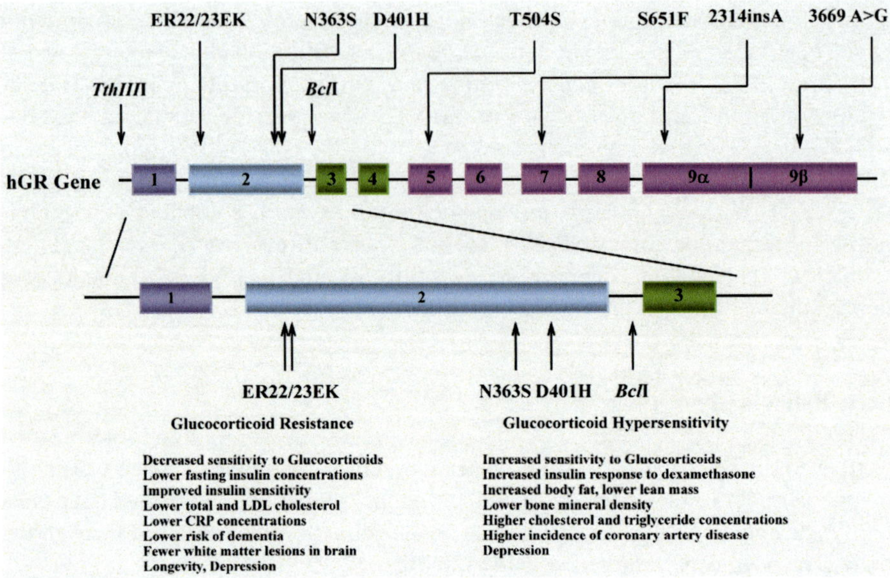

Fig. 4.4 Schematic representation of the hGR gene polymorphisms located in the amino-terminal domain of the receptor and a summary of their clinical associations

effects are likely to involve a higher expression of the hGRα-A (94 kDa) isoform at the expense of the hGRα-B (91 kDa) isoform. Given that the latter isoform has greater transactivational activity, the shift in hGRα-A to hGRα-B expression ratio leads to an overall decrease in transcriptional activity [49] (Fig. 4.4).

Further downstream in exon 2, a polymorphism was identified that changes codon 363 from AAT to AGT (rs 6195), resulting in a serine (N) for asparagine (S) substitution. The N363S polymorphism is associated with higher sensitivity to glucocorticoids *in vivo*, resulting in an increase in the transcriptional activation of glucocorticoid-responsive genes compared with the wild-type receptor, although it does not influence transcriptional repression [45]. The N363S polymorphism is associated with higher sensitivity to glucocorticoids *in vivo*, increased insulin response to exogenous dexamethasone administration [44, 50], higher body mass index (BMI), higher waist-to-hip ratio, a tendency toward lower bone mineral density in trabecular bone, elevated cholesterol and triglyceride concentrations, and higher incidence of coronary artery disease independent of weight [44, 50–56] (Fig. 4.4). The molecular mechanism through which the N363S polymorphism exerts its effects is unknown, but may partly be associated with increased transcriptional activity of the hGR isoform with the N363S replacement. It has been postulated that this polymorphism provides a new serine residue for phosphorylation, whereby protein interactions with transcription cofactors might be altered, as this serine residue is located in the AF-1 transactivation domain.

A frequent *BclI* restriction fragment length polymorphism (rs 41423247) is also associated with increased sensitivity to glucocorticoids, hypertension, visceral adipocity [44, 57, 58], and increased insulin concentrations in obese women [59].

The exact mutation of this polymorphic site was identified as a C→G substitution in intron 2. In the elderly, the G allele of the *BclI* polymorphism is associated with a lower BMI and a tendency towards lower lean body mass, which is likely to arise as a result of the increased sensitivity to glucocorticoids [60, 61] (Fig. 4.4).

The *TthIIII* variant (rs10052957) is a restriction site length polymorphism in the promoter region of the hGR gene, which is not functional by itself [44]. However, the ER22/23EK variant was found to be invariably linked to the *TthIIII* polymorphism. Therefore, associations with glucocorticoid resistance and healthier metabolic profile observed in the *TthIIII* carriers are likely to arise as a result of the ER22/23EK polymorphism.

Finally, a single-nucleotide polymorphism that replaces A with G at the nucleoside 3669 (A3669G) (rs 6198) located in the 3′ end of exon 9β has also been described [62]. This polymorphism does not change the amino acid sequence, but increases the stability of hGRβ mRNA and hGRβ protein expression, leading to greater inhibition of hGRα-induced transcriptional activity and glucocorticoid resistance. The presence of the A3669G allele is associated with reduced central obesity and a more favorable lipid profile in affected subjects [62]. Furthermore, this polymorphism selectively affects the transrepressive activity of the glucocorticoid receptor and is associated with an increased inflammatory state, rheumatoid arthritis, and cardiovascular disease [63–68].

Clinical Evaluation

The first step in evaluating a patient with suspected alterations in tissue sensitivity to glucocorticoids is to obtain a complete personal and family history, with particular attention to evidence suggesting alterations in the activity of the HPA axis. In addition, any evidence suggesting possible CNS dysfunction, such as headaches, visual impairment, or seizures, should be noted. In female subjects, the regularity of menstrual cycles should be documented. In children and adolescents, growth and sexual maturation should be evaluated carefully. The physical examination should include an assessment for signs of hyperandrogenism, virilization, and glucocorticoid excess, as well as a complete neurologic examination. Arterial blood pressure should be recorded and preferably monitored over a 24-h period.

Endocrinologic Evaluation

The concentrations of plasma ACTH, plasma renin activity (recumbent and upright), and aldosterone, as well as those of serum cortisol, testosterone, androstenedione, DHEA, DHEAS, total cholesterol, HDL, LDL, triglycerides, and fasting glucose and insulin should be recorded in the morning. Determination of the 24-h (h) urinary free cortisol (UFC) excretion on two or three consecutive days is central to the diagnosis, given that patients with Chrousos syndrome demonstrate increased 24 h

UFC excretion in the absence of clinical manifestations suggestive of hypercortisolism. In patients with Chrousos syndrome, the rise in serum cortisol and androgen concentrations, as well as in the 24 h UFC excretion, varies considerably depending on the severity of impairment of glucocorticoid signal transduction. In most severe cases, serum cortisol and 24 h UFC concentrations may be, respectively, up to sevenfold higher and 50-fold higher than the upper limit of normal range. Plasma ACTH concentrations may be normal or high in Chrousos syndrome and normal or low in PGGH.

The responsiveness of the HPA axis to exogenous glucocorticoids should also be tested with dexamethasone in patients suspected to have Chrousos syndrome. Increasing doses of dexamethasone (0.3, 0.6, 1.0, 1.5, 2.0, 2.5, 3.0 mg) should be given orally at midnight every other day, and a serum sample should be drawn at 0800h the following morning for determination of serum cortisol and dexamethasone concentrations. The concurrent measurement of serum dexamethasone concentrations is suggested in order to exclude the possibility of non-adherence to treatment, increased metabolic clearance, or decreased absorption of this medication. Affected subjects demonstrate resistance of the HPA axis to dexamethasone suppression, which varies depending on the severity of the condition. The dose of dexamethasone required to suppress serum cortisol concentrations by 50% may be up to 7.5-fold higher than that required to achieve the same degree of HPA axis suppression in normal subjects.

Molecular Studies

Thymidine incorporation assays and dexamethasone-binding assays on peripheral blood mononuclear cells in association with sequencing of the hGR gene are necessary to confirm the diagnosis [28–40]. In Chrousos syndrome, the thymidine incorporation assays reveal resistance to dexamethasone-induced suppression of phytohemaglutinin-stimulated thymidine incorporation, while the dexamethasone-binding assays often show decreased affinity of the hGR receptor for the ligand compared to control subjects [22, 27]. The opposite is true for patients with PGGH. Sequencing of the coding region of the hGR gene, including the intron/exon junctions, will reveal mutations or deletions in most but not all cases with Chrousos syndrome [27, 29–40]. Once a structural defect is determined, it is suggested that functional characterization of the mutant receptor should be undertaken in order to determine the molecular mechanisms through which the mutant hGR impairs glucocorticoid signal transduction.

Management

In Chrousos syndrome, the aim of treatment is to suppress the excess secretion of ACTH, thereby suppressing the increased production of adrenal steroids with mineralocorticoid and androgenic activity. Treatment involves administration of high doses of mineralocorticoid-sparing synthetic glucocorticoids, such as dexamethasone (1–3 mg given once daily at night), which activate the mutant and/or wild-type hGRα and suppress the endogenous secretion of ACTH in affected subjects [20–22]. It is important to achieve adequate suppression of the HPA axis to prevent the development of an ACTH-secreting adenoma in the pituitary gland and an adrenocortical adenoma in the adrenal glands [29]. Long-term dexamethasone treatment should be carefully titrated according to the clinical manifestations and biochemical profile of the affected subjects [20–22]. In PGGH, treatment aims to address the manifestations of glucocorticoid hypersensitivity, such as dyslipidemia, diabetes type 2, and hypertension [28].

Conclusions

The glucocorticoid receptor is a ubiquitously expressed intracellular, ligand-dependent transcription factor, which mediates the action of glucocorticoids and influences physiologic functions essential for life. The stochastic nature of glucocorticoid signaling pathways in association with the variable effect that hGR gene mutations/polymorphisms might have on glucocorticoid signal transduction indicates that alterations in hGR action may have important implications for many critical biological processes, such as the behavioral and physiologic responses to stress, the immune and inflammatory reaction, the process of sleep, as well as basic functions, such as growth and reproduction. In clinical practice, the effects of glucocorticoid treatment may vary considerably between patients and may be partly attributed to mutations or polymorphisms in the hGR gene. Therefore, when the presence of these hGR gene variants is known, the dose of glucocorticoids should be adjusted accordingly to ensure optimal therapy and minimal adverse effects.

Disclosure Statement

The authors have nothing to disclose.
This manuscript represents an update of earlier ones as the subject evolves.
The authors own the exclusive intellectual property rights of the present review paper and they are free to reproduce it in whole or in part (including tables and figures) in any electronic and/or printed article of which they are authors.

References

1. Kino T, Chrousos GP. Glucocorticoid effects on gene expression. In: Steckler T, Kalin NH, Reul JMHM, editors. Handbook of stress and the brain. Amsterdam: Elsevier; 2005. p. 295–311.
2. Chrousos GP, Charmandari E, Kino T. Glucocorticoid action networks–an introduction to systems biology. J Clin Endocrinol Metab. 2004;89:563–4.

3. Chrousos GP. The glucocorticoid receptor gene, longevity, and the complex disorders of western societies. Am J Med. 2004;117:204–7.
4. Galon J, Franchimont D, Hiroi N, Frey G, Boettner A, Ehrhart-Bornstein M, et al. Gene profiling reveals unknown enhancing and suppressive actions of glucocorticoids on immune cells. FASEB J. 2002;16(1):61–71.
5. Zhou J, Cidlowski JA. The human glucocorticoid receptor: one gene, multiple proteins and diverse responses. Steroids. 2005;70(5–7):407–17.
6. Duma D, Jewell CM, Cidlowski JA. Multiple glucocorticoid receptor isoforms and mechanisms of post-translational modification. J Steroid Biochem Mol Biol. 2006;102(1–5):11–21.
7. Nicolaides NC, Galata Z, Kino T, Chrousos GP, Charmandari E. The human glucocorticoid receptor: molecular basis of biologic function. Steroids. 2010;75(1):1–12.
8. Hollenberg SM, Weinberger C, Ong ES, Cerelli G, Oro A, Lebo R, et al. Primary structure and expression of a functional human glucocorticoid receptor cDNA. Nature. 1985;318:635–41.
9. Kino T, Manoli I, Kelkar S, Wang Y, Su YA, Chrousos GP. Glucocorticoid receptor (GR) β has intrinsic, GRα-independent transcriptional activity. Biochem Biophys Res Commun. 2009;381(4):671–5.
10. Oakley RH, Jewell CM, Yudt MR, Bofetiado DM, Cidlowski JA. The dominant negative activity of the human glucocorticoid receptor β isoform specificity and mechanisms of action. J Biol Chem. 1999;274(39):27857–66.
11. Chrousos GP, Kino T. Intracellular glucocorticoid signaling: a formerly simple system turns stochastic. Sci STKE. 2005;2005(304):pe48.
12. McKenna NJ, Lanz RB, O'Malley BW. Nuclear receptor coregulators: cellular and molecular biology. Endocr Rev. 1999;20(3):321–44.
13. McKenna NJ, O'Malley BW. Combinatorial control of gene expression by nuclear receptors and coregulators. Cell. 2002;108:465–74.
14. Auboeuf D, Honig A, Berget SM, O'Malley BW. Coordinate regulation of transcription and splicing by steroid receptor coregulators. Science. 2002;298:416–9.
15. Hittelman AB, Burakov D, Iniguez-Lluhi JA, Freedman LP, Garabedian MJ. Differential regulation of glucocorticoid receptor transcriptional activation via AF-1-associated proteins. EMBO J. 1999;18(19):5380–8.
16. Liu J, DeFranco DB. Protracted nuclear export of glucocorticoid receptor limits its turnover and does not require the exportin 1/CRM1-directed nuclear export pathway. Mol Endocrinol. 2000;14(1):40–51.
17. Chrousos GP. Hormone resistance and hypersensitivity states. In: Chrousos GP, Olefsky JM, Samols E, editors. Modern endocrinology series. Philadelphia: Lippincott, Williams & Wilkins; 2002. p. 542.
18. Kino T, De Martino MU, Charmandari E, Mirani M, Chrousos GP. Tissue glucocorticoid resistance/hypersensitivity syndromes. J Steroid Biochem Mol Biol. 2003;85(2–5):457–67.
19. Chrousos GP, Kino T. Glucocorticoid signaling in the cell: expanding clinical implications to complex human behavioral and somatic disorders. In: Glucocorticoids and mood: clinical manifestations, risk factors, and molecular mechanisms. Proc NY Acad Sci. 2009;1179:153–66.
20. Chrousos GP, Vingerhoeds A, Brandon D, Eil C, Pugeat M, DeVroede M, et al. Primary cortisol resistance in man. A glucocorticoid receptor-mediated disease. J Clin Invest. 1982;69(6):1261–9.
21. Chrousos GP, Detera-Wadleigh SD, Karl M. Syndromes of glucocorticoid resistance. Ann Intern Med. 1993;119(11):1113–24.
22. Charmandari E, Kino T, Ichijo T, Chrousos GP. Generalized glucocorticoid resistance: clinical aspects, molecular mechanisms, and implications of a rare genetic disorder. J Clin Endocrinol Metab. 2008;93(5):1563–72.
23. Nader N, Bachrach BE, Hurt DE, Gajula S, Pittman A, Lescher R, et al. A novel point mutation in the helix 10 of the human glucocorticoid receptor causes generalized glucocorticoid resistance by disrupting the structure of the ligand-binding domain. J Clin Endocrinol Metab. 2010;95(5):2281–5.

24. McMahon SK, Pretorius CJ, Ungerer JP, Salmon NJ, Conwell LS, Pearen MA, et al. Neonatal complete generalized glucocorticoid resistance and growth hormone deficiency caused by a novel homozygous mutation in Helix 12 of the ligand binding domain of the glucocorticoid receptor gene (NR3C1). J Clin Endocrinol Metab. 2010;95(1):297–302.
25. Tomlinson JW, Walker EA, Bujalska IJ, Draper N, Lavery GG, Cooper MS, et al. 11β-hydroxysteroid dehydrogenase type 1: a tissue-specific regulator of glucocorticoid response. Endocr Rev. 2004;25(5):831–66.
26. Charmandari E, Kino T. Chrousos syndrome: a seminal report, a phylogenetic enigma and the clinical implications of glucocorticoid signalling changes. Eur J Clin Invest. 2010;40(10): 932–42.
27. Chrousos G. Q&A: primary generalized glucocorticoid resistance. BMC Med. 2011;9:27.
28. Charmandari E, Ichijo T, Jubiz W, Baid S, Zachman K, Chrousos GP, et al. A novel point mutation in the amino terminal domain of the human glucocorticoid receptor (hGR) gene enhancing hGR-mediated gene expression. J Clin Endocrinol Metab. 2008;93:4963–8.
29. Karl M, Lamberts SW, Koper JW, Katz DA, Huizenga NE, Kino T, et al. Cushing's disease preceded by generalized glucocorticoid resistance: clinical consequences of a novel, dominant-negative glucocorticoid receptor mutation. Proc Assoc Am Physicians. 1996;108(4):296–307.
30. Hurley DM, Accili D, Stratakis CA, Karl M, Vamvakopoulos N, Rorer E, et al. Point mutation causing a single amino acid substitution in the hormone binding domain of the glucocorticoid receptor in familial glucocorticoid resistance. J Clin Invest. 1991;87(2):680–6.
31. Karl M, Lamberts SW, Detera-Wadleigh SD, Encio IJ, Stratakis CA, Hurley DM, et al. Familial glucocorticoid resistance caused by a splice site deletion in the human glucocorticoid receptor gene. J Clin Endocrinol Metab. 1993;76(3):683–9.
32. Malchoff DM, Brufsky A, Reardon G, McDermott P, Javier EC, Bergh CH, et al. A mutation of the glucocorticoid receptor in primary cortisol resistance. J Clin Invest. 1993;91(5):1918–25.
33. Kino T, Stauber RH, Resau JH, Pavlakis GN, Chrousos GP. Pathologic human GR mutant has a transdominant negative effect on the wild-type GR by inhibiting its translocation into the nucleus: importance of the ligand-binding domain for intracellular GR trafficking. J Clin Endocrinol Metab. 2001;86(11):5600–8.
34. Ruiz M, Lind U, Gafvels M, Eggertsen G, Carlstedt-Duke J, Nilsson L, et al. Characterization of two novel mutations in the glucocorticoid receptor gene in patients with primary cortisol resistance. Clin Endocrinol (Oxf). 2001;55(3):363–71.
35. Mendonca BB, Leite MV, de Castro M, Kino T, Elias LL, Bachega TA, et al. Female pseudohermaphroditism caused by a novel homozygous missense mutation of the GR gene. J Clin Endocrinol Metab. 2002;87(4):1805–9.
36. Vottero A, Kino T, Combe H, Lecomte P, Chrousos GP. A novel, C-terminal dominant negative mutation of the GR causes familial glucocorticoid resistance through abnormal interactions with p160 steroid receptor coactivators. J Clin Endocrinol Metab. 2002;87(6):2658–67.
37. Charmandari E, Kino T, Vottero A, Souvatzoglou E, Bhattacharyya N, Chrousos GP. Natural glucocorticoid receptor mutants causing generalized glucocorticoid resistance: molecular genotype, genetic transmission and clinical phenotype. J Clin Endocrinol Metab. 2004;89(4): 1939–49.
38. Charmandari E, Raji A, Kino T, Ichijo T, Tiulpakov A, Zachman K, et al. A novel point mutation in the ligand-binding domain (LBD) of the human glucocorticoid receptor (hGR) causing generalized glucocorticoid resistance: the importance of the C terminus of hGR LBD in conferring transactivational activity. J Clin Endocrinol Metab. 2005;90(6):3696–705.
39. Charmandari E, Kino T, Ichijo T, Zachman K, Alatsatianos A, Chrousos GP. Functional characterization of the natural human glucocorticoid receptor (hGR) mutants hGRαR477H and hGRαG679S associated with generalized glucocorticoid resistance. J Clin Endocrinol Metab. 2006;91(4):1535–43.
40. Charmandari E, Kino T, Ichijo T, Jubiz W, Mejia L, Zachman K, et al. A novel point mutation in helix 11 of the ligand-binding domain of the human glucocorticoid receptor gene causing generalized glucocorticoid resistance. J Clin Endocrinol Metab. 2007;92(10):3986–90.

41. Zhu HJ, Dai YF, Wang O, Li M, Lu L, Zhao WG, et al. Generalized glucocorticoid resistance accompanied with an adrenocortical adenoma and caused by a novel point mutation of human glucocorticoid receptor gene. Chin Med J (Engl). 2011;124(4):551–5.
42. Lamberts SW, Huizenga AT, de Lange P, de Jong FH, Koper JW. Clinical aspects of glucocorticoid sensitivity. Steroids. 1996;61(4):157–60.
43. Smit P, Russcher H, de Jong FH, Brinkmann AO, Lamberts SW, Koper JW. Differential regulation of synthetic glucocorticoids on gene expression levels of glucocorticoid-induced leucine zipper and interleukin-2. J Clin Endocrinol Metab. 2005;90(5):2994–3000.
44. van Rossum EF, Lamberts SW. Polymorphisms in the glucocorticoid receptor gene and their associations with metabolic parameters and body composition. Recent Prog Horm Res. 2004;59:333–57.
45. Russcher H, Smit P, van den Akker EL, van Rossum EF, Brinkmann AO, de Jong FH, et al. Two polymorphisms in the glucocorticoid receptor gene directly affect glucocorticoid-regulated gene expression. J Clin Endocrinol Metab. 2005;90(10):5804–10.
46. van Rossum EF, Koper JW, Huizenga NA, Uitterlinden AG, Janssen JA, Brinkmann AO, et al. A polymorphism in the glucocorticoid receptor gene, which decreases sensitivity to glucocorticoids in vivo, is associated with low insulin and cholesterol levels. Diabetes. 2002; 51(10):3128–34.
47. van Rossum EF, Feelders RA, van den Beld AW, Uitterlinden AG, Janssen JA, Ester W, et al. Association of the ER22/23EK polymorphism in the glucocorticoid receptor gene with survival and C-reactive protein levels in elderly men. Am J Med. 2004;117(3):158–62.
48. van Rossum EF, Voorhoeve PG, te Velde SJ, Koper JW, de Waal HA Delemarre-van, Kemper HC, Lamberts SW. The ER22/23EK polymorphism in the glucocorticoid receptor gene is associated with a beneficial body composition and muscle strength in young adults. J Clin Endocrinol Metab. 2004;89(8):4004–9.
49. Russcher H, van Rossum EF, de Jong FH, Brinkmann AO, Lamberts SW, Koper JW. Increased expression of the glucocorticoid receptor-A translational isoform as a result of the ER22/23EK polymorphism. Mol Endocrinol. 2005;19(7):1687–96.
50. Huizenga NA, Koper JW, De Lange P, Pols HA, Stolk RP, Burger H, et al. A polymorphism in the glucocorticoid receptor gene may be associated with and increased sensitivity to glucocorticoids in vivo. J Clin Endocrinol Metab. 1998;83(1):144–51.
51. Lin RC, Wang XL, Dalziel B, Caterson ID, Morris BJ. Association of obesity, but not diabetes or hypertension, with glucocorticoid receptor N363S variant. Obes Res. 2003;11(6):802–8.
52. Di Blasio AM, van Rossum EF, Maestrini S, Berselli ME, Tagliaferri M, Podestà F, et al. The relation between two polymorphisms in the glucocorticoid receptor gene and body mass index, blood pressure and cholesterol in obese patients. Clin Endocrinol (Oxf). 2003;59(1):68–74.
53. Roussel R, Reis AF, Dubois-Laforgue D, Bellanné-Chantelot C, Timsit J, Velho G. The N363S polymorphism in the glucocorticoid receptor gene is associated with overweight in subjects with type 2 diabetes mellitus. Clin Endocrinol (Oxf). 2003;59(2):237–41.
54. Dobson MG, Redfern CP, Unwin N, Weaver JU. The N363S polymorphism of the glucocorticoid receptor: potential contribution to central obesity in men and lack of association with other risk factors for coronary heart disease and diabetes mellitus. J Clin Endocrinol Metab. 2001;86(5):2270–4.
55. Lin RC, Wang XL, Morris BJ. Association of coronary artery disease with glucocorticoid receptor N363S variant. Hypertension. 2003;41(3):404–7.
56. Szabó V, Borgulya G, Filkorn T, Majnik J, Bányász I, Nagy ZZ. The variant N363S of glucocorticoid receptor in steroid-induced ocular hypertension in Hungarian patients treated with photorefractive keratectomy. Mol Vis. 2007;13:659–66.
57. Rosmond R, Chagnon YC, Holm G, Chagnon M, Pérusse L, Lindell K, et al. A glucocorticoid receptor gene marker is associated with abdominal obesity, leptin, and dysregulation of the hypothalamic-pituitary-adrenal axis. Obes Res. 2000;8(3):211–8.
58. Ukkola O, Pérusse L, Chagnon YC, Després JP, Bouchard C. Interactions among the glucocorticoid receptor, lipoprotein lipase and adrenergic receptor genes and abdominal fat in the québec family study. Int J Obes Relat Metab Disord. 2001;25(9):1332–9.

59. Weaver JU, Hitman GA, Kopelman PG. An association between a BclI restriction fragment length polymorphism of the glucocorticoid receptor locus and hyperinsulinaemia in obese women. J Mol Endocrinol. 1992;9(3):295–300.
60. van Rossum EF, Koper JW, van den Beld AW, Uitterlinden AG, Arp P, Ester W, et al. Identification of the bcli polymorphism in the glucocorticoid receptor gene: association with sensitivity to glucocorticoids in vivo and body mass index. Clin Endocrinol (Oxf). 2003;59(5):585–92.
61. Melcescu E, Griswold M, Xiang L, Belk S, Montgomery D, Bray M, et al. Prevalence and cardiometabolic associations of the glucocorticoid receptor gene polymorphisms N363S and Bcli in obese and non-obese black and white Mississippians. Hormones (Athens). 2012;11(2):166–77.
62. Syed AA, Irving JA, Redfern CP, Hall AG, Unwin NC, White M, et al. Association of glucocorticoid receptor polymorphism A3669G in exon 9beta with reduced central adiposity in women. Obesity (Silver Spring). 2006;14(5):759–64.
63. Lee EB, Kim JY, Lee YJ, Song YW. Glucocorticoid receptor polymorphisms in Korean patients with rheumatoid arthritis. Ann Rheum Dis. 2005;64(3):503–4.
64. van den Akker EL, Russcher H, van Rossum EF, Brinkmann AO, de Jong FH, Hokken A, et al. Glucocorticoid receptor polymorphism affects transrepression but not transactivation. J Clin Endocrinol Metab. 2006;91(7):2800–3.
65. van den Akker EL, Nouwen JL, Melles DC, van Rossum EF, Koper JW, Uitterlinden AG, et al. Staphylococcus aureus nasal carriage is associated with glucocorticoid receptor gene polymorphisms. J Infect Dis. 2006;194(6):814–8.
66. van den Akker EL, Koper JW, van Rossum EF, Dekker MJ, Russcher H, de Jong FH, et al. Glucocorticoid receptor gene and risk of cardiovascular disease. Arch Intern Med. 2008;168(1):33–9.
67. Otte C, Wüst S, Zhao S, Pawlikowska L, Kwok PY, Whooley MA. Glucocorticoid receptor gene, low-grade inflammation, and heart failure: the heart and soul study. J Clin Endocrinol Metab. 2010;95(6):2885–91.
68. Geelhoed JJ, van Duijn C, van Osch-Gevers L, Steegers EA, Hofman A, Helbing WA, et al. Glucocorticoid receptor-9beta polymorphism is associated with systolic blood pressure and heart growth during early childhood. The generation r study. Early Hum Dev. 2011;87(2): 97–102.

Chapter 5
Congenital Adrenal Hyperplasia

Smita B. Abraham and Deborah P. Merke

Abstract Of the six known types of congenital adrenal hyperplasia (CAH), 11β(beta)-hydroxylase deficiency and 17α(alpha)-hydroxylase deficiency are distinct in that patients suffer from hypertension. Impaired cortisol synthesis results in ACTH driven mineralocorticoid excess in both disorders. Interestingly, the mineralocorticoid hormones that are responsible for the development of hypertension in 11β(beta)-hydroxylase deficiency and 17α(alpha)-hydroxylase deficiency are not identical. In addition, the degree of blood pressure elevation does not directly correlate with known mineralocorticoid hormone levels suggesting that unknown factors may contribute to the development of hypertension in these forms of CAH. Hypertension is not pathognomonic of CAH due to 21-hydroxylase deficiency, but patients with the classic form of the disease have been found to commonly have blood pressure elevation in some studies. Several contributing factors have been proposed including an association with glucocorticoid and mineralocorticoid treatment regimens and obesity.

Treatment of hypertension in patients with 11β(beta)-hydroxylase deficiency and 17α(alpha)-hydroxylase deficiency is most successful if the disorder is diagnosed early and glucocorticoid therapy is started early in life. A mineralocorticoid receptor antagonist is an excellent therapeutic option if glucocorticoid replacement

S.B. Abraham (✉)
The *Eunice Kennedy Shriver* National Institute of Child Health and Human Development, National Institutes of Health, Building 10, Room 1-3140, 10 Center Drive, Bethesda, MD 20892, USA
e-mail: baids@mail.nih.gov

D.P. Merke
The *Eunice Kennedy Shriver* National Institute of Child Health and Human Development, National Institutes of Health Clinical Center, National Institutes of Health,, Bethesda, MD, USA

C.A. Koch and G.P. Chrousos (eds.), *Endocrine Hypertension: Underlying Mechanisms and Therapy*, Contemporary Endocrinology, DOI 10.1007/978-1-60761-548-4_5,

does not resolve the hypertension. For patients with 21-hydroxylase deficiency, one class of anti-hypertensive treatment has not been identified as standard of care as the pathophysiology of the hypertension is unclear. Treatment with an anti-hypertensive medication that will not interfere with volume status is preferred.

Patients with CAH due to 11β(beta)-hydroxylase deficiency, 17α(alpha)-hydroxylase deficiency, and 21-hydroxylase deficiency are at risk for hypertension, a major risk factor for cardiovascular disease. Careful screening for hypertension, and early pharmacologic therapy should be implemented. The interplay between hormonal imbalances and the development of hypertension requires further study. Future longitudinal studies to assess cardiovascular events, morbidity, and mortality are needed and will lead to improved therapeutic strategies.

Keywords Congenital Adrenal Hyperplasia • Enzymatic deficiencies • 11β(beta)-hydroxylase deficiency • Hypertension • 17α(alpha)-hydroxylase deficiency • 21-Hydroxylase deficiency • mineralocorticoid excess

Introduction

Congenital adrenal hyperplasia (CAH) is a group of autosomal recessive diseases in which the synthesis of cortisol is impaired. There are six known types of CAH. Four are caused by enzymatic deficiencies in the cortisol biosynthetic pathway: 21-hydroxylase, 11β(beta)-hydroxylase, 17α(alpha)-hydroxylase, and 3β(beta)-hydroxysteroid dehydrogenase; one is caused by a defect in an electron donor, P450 oxidoreductase (POR); and, lastly, lipoid CAH is due to impairment of a transporter protein, steroidogenic acute regulatory protein. CAH caused by 21-hydroxylase deficiency is the most common form of the disease, comprising approximately 95% of cases. The second most common form of CAH is caused by 11β(beta)-hydroxylase deficiency and the remaining types of CAH are quite rare. Hypertension (HTN) is characteristic of 11β(beta)-hydroxylase and 17α(alpha)-hydroxylase deficiencies. Recently, studies have suggested that pediatric and adult patients with 21-hydroxylase deficiency commonly have hypertension and subsequently are at risk of developing cardiovascular disease.

The Fourth Report on the Diagnosis, Evaluation, and Treatment of High Blood Pressure in Children and Adolescents defines hypertension in children as: average systolic blood pressure (SBP) and/or diastolic blood pressure (DBP) that is ≥95th percentile for gender, age, and height on ≥3 occasions [1]. SBP and DBP <90th percentile for gender, age, and height is considered normal. Those children with SBP or DBP ≥90th but less than 95th percentile are categorized as high normal and at risk for developing hypertension [1].

High blood pressure in childhood is considered a risk factor for high blood pressure in adulthood [1]. In adults aged 18 and older, the Seventh Report of the Joint National Committee on Prevention, Detection, Evaluation, and Treatment of High Blood Pressure (JNC 7) classifies optimal blood pressure as less than 120/80 mmHg;

pre-HTN as 120–139/80–89 mmHg; stage 1 HTN as 140–159/90–99 mmHg; stage 2 HTN as 160–179/100–109; and stage 3 HTN as ≥180/110 mmHg [2]. This classification is based on an average of two or more properly measured, seated blood pressure readings on each of two or more office visits [2].

In this chapter, hypertension in CAH due to 11β(beta)-hydroxylase, 17α(alpha)-hydroxylase, and 21-hydroxylase deficiency will be reviewed.

11β(Beta)-Hydroxylase Deficiency

Epidemiology

CAH due to 11β(beta)-hydroxylase deficiency is an autosomal recessive disorder occurring in approximately 1:100,000 to 1:200,000 live births in non-consanguineous populations [3]. It is reported to be more common (1/5–7,000) in the Moroccan Jewish population [4].

Genetics

In humans, 11β(beta)-hydroxylase consists of two isoenzymes, encoded by two homologous genes, *CYP11B1* and *CYP11B2*, that are part of the mitochondrial cytochrome p450 super family [5]. Both the *CYP11B1* and *CYP11B2* genes have been mapped to chromosome 8 (8q22) and lie approximately 40 kb apart. *CYP11B1* and *CYP11B2* have 95 and 90% of their respective coding and noncoding regions identical [6]; however, the promoter regions of both genes are significantly different implying different regulatory mechanisms at the transcription level [3, 7]. CAH due to 11β(beta)-hydroxylase deficiency is caused by mutations in *CYP11B1*. *CYP11B2* encodes aldosterone synthase which 11-hydroxylates, 18-hydroxylates, and 18-oxidizes [8] deoxycorticosterone (DOC) to aldosterone and is primarily regulated by angiotensin II and potassium. Mutations of *CYP11B2* result in corticosterone methyloxidase deficiency or isolated aldosterone deficiency which is not a form of CAH and will not be discussed here.

At least 50 different *CYP11B1* mutations have been identified. These mutations are distributed over the entire coding region but tend to cluster in exons 2, 6, 7, and 8 [9, 10] with the most common mutation found to be R448H. The majority of cases are severe (or classic), but a mild or non-classic form of the disease has been described [11, 12]. Genotype–phenotype correlation has not been well studied. However, recent functional studies of various *CYP11B1* mutations accurately predicted phenotype; partially inactivating mutations resulted in non-classic 11β(beta)-hydroxylase deficiency [11].

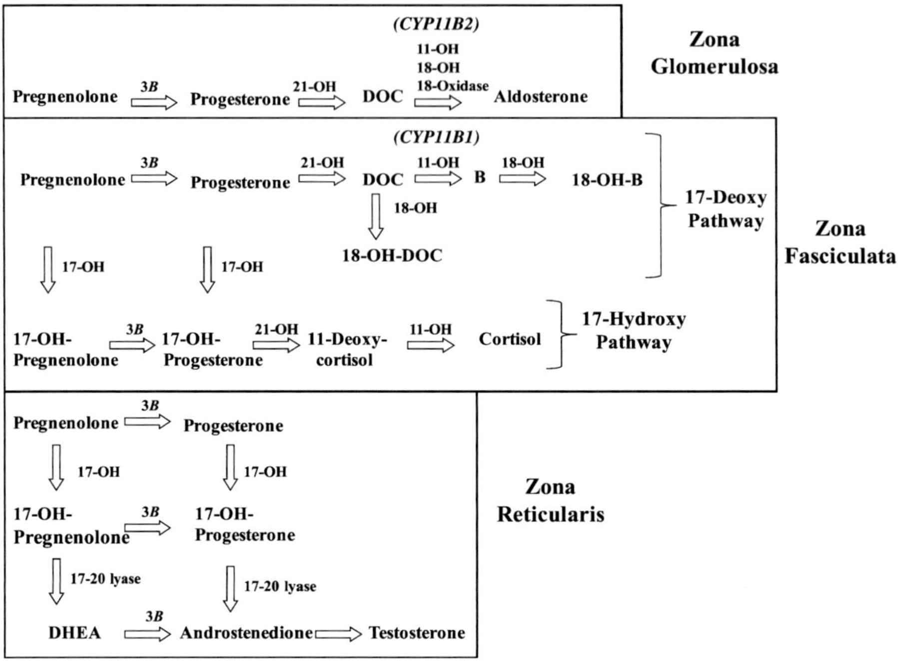

Fig. 5.1 Pathway of adrenal steroid biosynthesis. The enzymes responsible for each biosynthetic step are above or adjacent to *arrows*. Each *box* represents a respective zone of the adrenal cortex. Three steps in aldosterone synthesis are mediated by a single gene, *CYP11B2*. 11β(beta)-hydroxylase and some 18-hydroxylase activity are mediated by *CYP11B1*. 3β 3β(beta)-hydroxysteroid dehydrogenase; 21-OH 21-hydroxylase; 11-OH 11β(beta)-hydroxylase; 18-OH 18-hydroxylase; 17-OH 17α(alpha)-hydroxylase; DOC deoxycorticosterone; B corticosterone; 18-OH-DOC 18-hydroxydeoxycorticosterone; 18-OH-B 18-hydroxycorticosterone

Pathophysiology

CYP11B1 encodes the enzyme 11β(beta)-hydroxylase which converts 11-DOC to corticosterone in the 17-deoxy pathway and 11-deoxycortisol to cortisol in the 17-hydroxy pathway (Fig. 5.1). The 11β(beta)-hydroxylase enzyme also exhibits weak 18-hydroxylase activity. Both pathways are active in the zona fasciculata [13] and are primarily under ACTH regulation. *CYP11B2* is exclusively expressed and has strong activity in the zona glomerulosa [10]. When DOC is converted to aldosterone, the same steroid molecule probably remains bound to the enzyme for all three conversions without the release of intermediate products [3]. CAH due to 11β(beta)-hydroxylase deficiency results in a lack of systemic cortisol which stimulates ACTH production from the pituitary and subsequently causes increased androgen production as adrenal steroid biosynthesis is shunted to unimpeded androgen producing pathways. In addition, there is a build-up of precursors proximal to the 11β(beta)-hydroxylase step, most notably 11-deoxycortisol and DOC (Fig. 5.1, Table 5.1).

Table 5.1 Comparison of congenital adrenal hyperplasia disorders associated with hypertension

	11β(beta)-hydroxylase deficiency	17α(alpha)-hydroxylase deficiency	21-Hydroxylase deficiency
Gene	*CYP11B1*	*CYP17A1*	*CYP21A2*
Etiology of hypertension	Mineralocorticoid excess	Mineralocorticoid excess	Multifactorial: treatment-related, obesity-related, unknown hormonal imbalances
Laboratory findings	↑ DOC, ↑ 11-deoxycortisol DOC	↑ DOC	17-OH-progesterone
	↓↓ B	↑ B	
	↓↓ 18-OH derivatives	↑ 18-OH derivatives	
	↓↓ Aldosterone	↓↓ Aldosterone	↓ or Nl Aldosterone
Clinical features at diagnosis	Genital ambiguity (XX)	Delayed puberty in phenotypic female (XX, XY)	Genital ambiguity (XX)
	Precocious virilization (XY)	Possible genital ambiguity (XY)	Precocious virilization (XY) ± salt losing adrenal crisis

DOC deoxycorticosterone; B corticosterone; Nl normal

Clinical Presentation

Increased androgen production in utero causes virilization resulting in ambiguous genitalia evident at birth in genetic females. Internal structures are normal for female. Males do not have obvious signs at birth but present with precocious virilization in the first few years of life. In both genders, excess androgen production postnatally may lead to premature secondary sexual characteristics including early appearance of pubic, axillary, and facial hair, acne, deepening of voice, and rapid skeletal growth. Although 11β(beta)-hydroxylase deficiency results in mineralocorticoid excess, there have been reports of transient salt wasting in newborns [14], presumably due to the unique physiology of the newborn which includes mineralocorticoid resistance. Males diagnosed as toddlers, usually have hypertension at presentation, in addition to the signs and symptoms of androgen excess. This initial hypertension usually resolves with glucocorticoid therapy.

Chronic low renin hypertension occurs in approximately 2/3 of patients with 11β(beta)-hydroxylase deficiency. Onset of hypertension typically occurs in later childhood and although it has been reported, it occurs rarely in infancy [15]. The degree of hypertension is often mild to moderate, but can become malignant as there are reports of retinopathy, retinal vein occlusion, cardiomyopathy, and left ventricular hypertrophy [7, 16, 17]. Pediatric patients may have elevated blood pressure primarily during acute illnesses, when the adrenal is stimulated, but then remain normotensive when well (personal experience DPM).

The incidence of non-classic 11β(beta)-hydroxylase deficiency is quite rare. Blood pressure may be normal or mildly elevated in these patients [18].

Physiology of Hypertension in 11β(beta)-Hydroxylase Deficiency

DOC is a weak mineralocorticoid; however, its level can rise up to 60 times normal in patients with 11β(beta)-hydroxylase deficiency [19]. Accumulation of DOC, or other mineralocorticoid hormones, causes a net sodium retaining effect and extracellular fluid volume expansion which eventually leads to an increase in total peripheral vascular resistance and hypertension. In addition, mineralocorticoid hormones have a positive inotropic effect resulting in increased stroke volume and cardiac output which also contribute to the development of hypertension [13]. Suppression of the renin-angiotensin system due to mineralocorticoid excess results in low plasma renin activity and aldosterone levels although the ability to synthesize aldosterone is unimpaired.

Intuitively, it would seem that the accumulation of DOC could be the sole cause of HTN in patients with 11β(beta)-hydroxylase deficiency. However, there are several factors that argue against this: (1) elevations in blood pressure, suppressed plasma renin activity and hypokalemia, present variably in this patient population; [7, 10, 14] (2) suppression of DOC does not always result in resolution of hypertension; [14] and (3) elevation in blood pressure does not correlate with DOC levels [12, 14, 20]. It is hypothesized that there are unidentified mineralocorticoid metabolites contributing to the development of hypertension in patients with this type of CAH [3, 14, 15].

Diagnosis of 11β(beta)-Hydroxylase Deficiency

Diagnosis of 11β(beta)-hydroxylase deficiency is evident by the steroid pattern produced in response to chronic elevation of ACTH and is based primarily on elevation of 11-deoxycortisol. In general, the following hormones are elevated in 11β(beta)-hydroxylase deficiency: (1) non-11β(beta)-hydroxylated products including 11-deoxycortisol, DOC, 17-hydroxyprogesterone and androstenedione; (2) tetrahydro-11-deoxycortisol (THS) and tetrahydrodeoxycorticosterone (THDOC), the principal urinary metabolites of serum 11-deoxycortisol and DOC, respectively; and (3) urinary 17-ketosteroids (reflecting elevated androgen levels) [10].

17α(alpha)-Hydroxylase Deficiency

Epidemiology

Classic 17α(alpha)-hydroxylase deficiency is an autosomal recessive disorder that is very rare. However, 17α(alpha)-hydroxylase deficiency, as opposed to 11β(beta)-hydroxylase deficiency, is the second most common form of CAH in Brazil, where a founder effect likely accounts for the majority of cases [13, 21].

Genetics

The *CYP17A1* gene consists of eight exons and is located on chromosome 10 (10q24.3) [22]. It encodes the cytochrome P450c17 α enzyme which is present in both the adrenal glands and the gonads. Over 70 mutations have been identified in the *CYP17A1* gene [23]. Frequently reoccurring mutations are seen in four populations: (1) Brazilians; (2) Canadian Mennonites; (3) Japanese; and (4) East Asians. However, mutational hot spots have not been identified in most other large populations [23].

Pathophysiology

Unlike other steroidogenic enzymes, P450c17α is responsible for catalyzing two reactions in the steroidogenic pathway. First, as 17α(alpha)-hydroxylase, it 17-hydroxylates pregnenolone and progesterone, reactions that are necessary for cortisol production. Second, as 17, 20 lyase, it transforms 17-hydroxypregnenolone to DHEA and 17-hydroxyprogesterone to androstenedione which are reactions necessary for sex steroid production (Fig. 5.1).

17α(alpha)-hydroxylase and 17, 20 lyase are expressed in the zona fasciculata, zona reticularis, testicular leydig cells, and ovarian theca cells [24]. They are not found in the zona glomerulosa. Mutations in the *CYP17A1* gene can result in one of three types of deficiencies: (1) isolated 17α(alpha)-hydroxylase deficiency; (2) combined 17α(alpha)-hydroxylase and 17, 20 lyase deficiencies; or (3) isolated 17, 20 lyase deficiency. It is difficult to differentiate isolated 17α(alpha)-hydroxylase deficiency from combined 17α(alpha)-hydroxylase and 17, 20 lyase deficiencies and isolated 17, 20 lyase deficiency is rare [25, 26]. Classic "17α(alpha)-hydroxylase deficiency" refers to the combined 17α(alpha)-hydroxylase and 17, 20 lyase deficiencies resulting in loss of glucocorticoid and sex steroid production [27].

Blockage of 17α(alpha)-hydroxylase activity shunts steroid production to the 17-deoxy pathway resulting in an increase of DOC, corticosterone (B), 18-hydroxycorticosterone (18-OH-B), and 18-hydroxydeoxycorticosterone (18-OH-DOC). Corticosterone is a weak glucocorticoid and can substitute cortisol action. However, because corticosterone is not as potent as cortisol, high serum levels are required before negative feedback inhibition will reduce pituitary gland production of ACTH [13]. This leads to an ACTH driven increased production of mineralocorticoid hormones causing hypertension in patients with 17α(alpha)-hydroxylase deficiency (Table 5.1).

Clinical Presentation

CAH patients with classic 17α(alpha)-hydroxylase deficiency suffer from lack of glucocorticoid and sex steroid production. However, patients do not suffer from adrenal insufficiency because overproduction of corticosterone allows for normal endogenous glucocorticoid activity. Therefore, the enzyme deficiency is often not detected until adolescence when patients present as females with delayed puberty.

Hypergonadotropic hypogonadism is characteristic in this patient population. 46XX patients do not enter puberty and present with primary amenorrhea and sexual infantilism. 46XY patients may present early in life with ambiguous genitalia or sexual infantilism, but often are phenotypic females at birth and may not be identified as 46XY until adolescence [28]. In contrast to CAH patients with 21- and 11β(beta)-hydroxylase deficiencies, these patients do not suffer from restricted growth, but are often tall presenting with eunuchoid proportions [26].

Significant variations in sexual development have been described in patients with 17α(alpha)-hydroxylase deficiency indicating some sex steroid production. A wide range in the degree of virilization of 46XY patients and, the presence of menses and breast development in 46XX patients have been described [26, 29, 30].

While elevations in mineralocorticoid hormone levels are present since birth, hypertension and hypokalemia are not typically the presenting symptoms in these patients. Hypertension has been reported as early as infancy and as late as the fifth decade of life, but is most often detected at the time of diagnosis when patients present with delayed puberty. There is considerable variation in the severity of hypertension. Blood pressure can range from normotensive to malignant hypertension associated with end-organ disease [26, 28, 31]. The same variable presentation is true for hypokalemia.

The variability in sexual development and the wide range of effects on blood pressure and potassium are possibly due to distinct genetic mutations resulting in differing degrees of enzyme activity or other unknown environmental or genetic factors [29, 32]. Interestingly, the severity and degree of hypertension does not correlate with the degree of hypogonadism [26].

Physiology of Hypertension in 17α(alpha)-Hydroxylase Deficiency

Similar to patients with 11β(beta)-hydroxylase deficiency, patients with17α(alpha)-hydroxylase deficiency have low renin hypertension. Mineralocorticoid excess leads to suppression of plasma renin activity and decreased aldosterone production. In 17α(alpha)-hydroxylase deficiency, DOC undergoes both 18-hydroxylation and 19-hydroxylation [33, 34] leading to production of 18-OH-B, 18-OH-DOC, and 19-nor-deoxycorticosterone (19-nor-DOC). This is distinct from 11β(beta)-hydroxylase deficiency, where DOC is not significantly hydroxylated at the 11 or 18 positions. Thus, DOC levels are much greater in 11β(beta)-hydroxylase deficiency than in 17α(alpha)-hydroxylase deficiency [29]. The metabolite, 19-nor-DOC, is thought to be a more potent mineralocorticoid than DOC and contributes significantly to the development of hypertension [13]. Interestingly, there are reported cases of patients with 17α(alpha)-hydroxylase deficiency who have normal or even elevated aldosterone levels [26, 29]. The cause of this physiological paradox is unclear.

Diagnosis of 17α(alpha)-Hydroxylase Deficiency

Diagnosis of 17α(alpha)-hydroxylase deficiency is made by detecting markedly elevated levels of the 17-deoxysteroids including progesterone, DOC, and corticosterone at baseline and also upon ACTH stimulation testing [21]. Plasma 17-hydroxyprogesterone and androgen levels and urinary pregnanetriol and 17-ketosteroid levels are low to undetectable. Distinguishing 17 from 11β(beta)-hydroxylase deficiency can be done by calculating the corticosterone to DOC ratio which is negligible in the latter.

21-Hydroxylase Deficiency

Epidemiology

CAH due to 21-hydroxylase deficiency is typically divided into three phenotypic categories: classic severe (associated with mineralocorticoid deficiency, "salt losing"), simple virilizing ("non-salt losing"), and mild or non-classic (NC). Data pooled from 13 countries shows an overall incidence of 1/15,000 live births where approximately 67% are salt losing and 33% are non-salt losing [35]. Similarly, the incidence in the United States amongst Caucasians is 1/15,500, but is lower in the African-American population (1/42,000) [36]. Newborn screening does not accurately detect NC CAH; however, the limited data available suggest an incidence of approximately 1/1,000 in the Caucasian population [37, 38].

Two isolated populations are known to have an increased incidence of 21-hydroxylase deficiency: the Yupik Eskimos of Alaska (1/280) [39] and the people of the French island of La Réunion (1/2,100). Brazil and the Philippines are also areas of increased frequency [40]. NC CAH is more frequent in Hispanic, Yugoslavic, and eastern European Jewish populations [38].

Genetics

The gene encoding 21-hydroxylase is located on the short arm of chromosome 6p21.3 within the HLA histocompatibility complex class III region [41]. There are two highly homologous 21-hydroxylase genes that sit approximately 30 kb apart: *CYP21A2 (CYP21B)* is the active gene and *CYP21A1P (CYP21A, CYP21P)* is the inactive pseudogene [42]. Recombination events between the active and inactive gene occur frequently accounting for up to 95% of the mutations associated with this enzyme [43–45].

There are several different mutations in the 21-hydroxylase gene resulting in a wide range of genotypes and associated phenotypes. The majority of patients are compound heterozygotes meaning that they have different mutations on the two alleles. The clinical phenotype results from the less severely mutated allele and is thus dictated by the residual 21-hydroxylase activity [35].

Pathophysiology

CAH due to 21-hydroxylase deficiency is characterized by cortisol deficiency with or without mineralocorticoid deficiency. Similar to 11β(beta)-hydroxylase deficiency, low or absent cortisol levels drive increased ACTH production which, in turn, stimulates adrenal androgen steroidogenesis. Impairment of cortisol biosynthesis allows steroid precursors to be shunted into the unimpeded androgen production pathways resulting in androgen excess (Fig. 5.1, Table 5.1).

Clinical Presentation

The classic form of 21-hydroxylase deficiency presents in early childhood. Females with classic salt losing CAH or classic non-salt losing CAH present with ambiguous genitalia at birth due to excess androgen exposure in utero. Similar to 11β(beta)-hydroxylase deficiency, the internal female structures are normal. Male infants do not have signs of CAH at birth except possible mild hyperpigmentation and penile enlargement. Prior to the advent of neonatal screening programs, the diagnosis was dependent on the severity of the mineralocorticoid deficiency with severe deficiency presenting at approximately 2 weeks of life with weight loss, dehydration, hyponatremia, vomiting, and possibly shock. Males with the simple virilizing, non-salt losing classic form, if not detected by neonatal screening, present with signs of early virilization at approximately age 2–4 years.

NC CAH patients typically present with signs of androgen excess in school-aged children, adolescence, or early adulthood. Males with NC CAH are often asymptomatic. Females may present with hirsutism, oligo- or amenorrhea with polycystic ovaries and acne alone or in combination [35, 46]. These patients do not have cortisol deficiency.

Hypertension is not pathognomonic of CAH due to 21-hydroxylase deficiency. Mineralocorticoid deficiency or normal mineralocorticoid production is the norm, unlike the mineralocorticoid excess characteristic of 11β(beta)-hydroxylase and 17α(alpha)-hydroxylase deficiency. In 2003, Roche et al. performed a study evaluating 24-h ambulatory blood pressure and obesity in 38 children (range 6.1–18.2 years) with classic salt losing 21-hydroxylase deficiency. Mean daytime SBPs were significantly higher than those of the reference population and 58% of patients, both males and females, had systolic hypertension. Mean DBP was also elevated and 24% had diastolic hypertension. In this study, CAH patients also had a higher BMI than the reference population and BMI was significantly correlated with SBP, especially in females [47].

Since then, several small studies have looked at the incidence and prevalence of hypertension in this population including salt losers and non-salt losers. Nebesio et al. found 5/91 (5.5%; two female infants, one 6-year-old female, one 12-year-old male, and one unknown age female) patients with hypertension that required anti-hypertensive treatment [48]. In a German study of 55 children, Volkl et al. found approximately 11% of patients to have blood pressures in the hypertensive range and a significantly greater percentage of CAH patients to have blood pressures above the 50th percentile compared to a reference population [49]. One small study of 11 children reported 1 patient with daytime systolic hypertension and 6 with nocturnal hypertension [50].

Conversely, there are several studies of pediatric and adult patients that did not observe an increased prevalence of hypertension in patients with classic CAH due to 21-hydroxylase deficiency [51–55]. In addition, data collection methods for the reference population in the study by Roche et al. had limitations in that single blood pressure measurements were used as opposed to the more accurate 24-h ambulatory monitoring [49].

Pathophysiology of Hypertension in 21-Hydroxylase Deficiency

The discrepant findings regarding hypertension in patients with classic 21-hydroxylase deficiency likely result from the multiple potential causes of increased blood pressure in these patients. Several hypotheses have been proposed.

Supraphysiologic glucocorticoid treatment may lead to elevation in blood pressure. Glucocorticoids activate the mineralocorticoid receptor at high doses and the affinity of cortisol for the mineralocorticoid receptor is at least equal to or greater than that of aldosterone [56]. However, metabolism of cortisol by 11β-hydroxysteroid dehydrogenase to inactive metabolites protects against excessive binding of glucocorticoid to mineralocorticoid receptors [57, 58]. Multiple studies have shown no correlation between glucocorticoid dose and blood pressure [47–50, 54, 55]. While the dose itself may play an indirect and/or minor role in the development of hypertension in these patients, other factors related to glucocorticoid treatment may contribute, including the type of glucocorticoid (i.e., long-acting vs. short-acting), the fact that current replacement regimens cannot replace the normal physiological rhythm of cortisol [59], and patient variability in glucocorticoid sensitivity and metabolism. Moreover, the dose, regimen, and non-physiologic nature of the mineralocorticoid replacement therapy could be a contributing factor.

A second hypothesis is that there is a relationship between blood pressure and known or unknown adrenal metabolites that may be elevated in 21-hydroxylase deficiency. Blood pressure has not been shown to be correlated with the typical biomarkers including plasma renin activity, androstenedione, 17-hydroxyprogesterone, or 24-h urine pregnanetriol [47–49].

A third possibility is that obesity is a major contributor to the development of hypertension in patients with 21-hydroxylase deficiency. An increased prevalence of obesity and a positive association between BMI and blood pressure in this population has been reported [47, 49, 54].

A possible mechanism of obesity-induced hypertension in the general population is increased sympathetic activity in part modulated by increased leptin levels [60]. Interestingly, CAH patients with classic 21-hydroxylase deficiency have been found to have hyperleptinemia which may play a role in the development of elevated blood pressure [61]. These patients also suffer from adrenomedullary hypofunction which contributes to elevated leptin [62]. The effect of epinephrine deficiency on regulation of the sympathetic nervous system appears negligible but is largely unknown [63]. Also, patients with the classic salt losing phenotype do not produce aldosterone. The complex interplay between obesity hormones and the sympathetic nervous system still needs considerable investigation to help elucidate the mechanisms underlying the development of hypertension in this patient population.

Diagnosis of 21-Hydroxylase Deficiency

Basal or ACTH-stimulated levels of 17-hydroxyprogesterone >1,200 ng/dL (36 nmol/L) are diagnostic of 21-hydroxylase deficiency. Patients with the classic (severe) form often have basal levels >8,000 ng/dL (242 nmol/L).

Treatment of Hypertension

Glucocorticoid therapy in patients with CAH allows for reduction in ACTH levels and subsequently reduction in steroid precursor levels including DOC and DOC metabolites for patients with 11β(beta)-hydroxylase deficiency or 17α(alpha)-hydroxylase deficiency and androgens in patients with 11β(beta)-hydroxylase deficiency or 21-hydroxylase deficiency.

In adults and children, the goal of therapy is to reduce the ACTH drive.

Avoiding glucocorticoid excess is also key in the treatment plan. In children, use of hydrocortisone versus dexamethasone, a more potent glucocorticoid, is appropriate as there is less chance of negative effects on growth and bone density. In adults, dexamethasone or prednisone use is more common and the goal is to use the lowest dose possible (usually 0.25–0.5 or 5–7.5 mg, respectively). Dexamethasone is preferable in patients with either 11β(beta)-hydroxylase deficiency or 17α(alpha)-hydroxylase deficiency due to the lack of mineralocorticoid activity.

In patients with either 11β(beta)-hydroxylase deficiency or 17α(alpha)-hydroxylase deficiency, reduction in mineralocorticoid allows for natriuresis, diuresis, and normalization of plasma volume and potassium which should allow for normalization of blood pressure. Plasma renin activity also normalizes and stimulation of aldosterone production through the separate 11β(beta)-hydroxylase/18 hydroxylase/18 oxidase system (*CYP11B2*) in the zona glomerulosa can occur.

While hypertension does improve with glucocorticoid therapy in patients with either 11β(beta)-hydroxylase deficiency or 17α(alpha)-hydroxylase deficiency, it is not always completely reversible [31]. Many factors affect whether or not the blood pressure can be normalized including: (1) imperfect glucocorticoid dosing (supraphysiologic doses often needed; dosing not able to follow diurnal rhythm of cortisol or blood pressure); (2) duration of hypertension; (3) severity of hypertension; and (4) patient compliance with treatment and follow-up. Duration and severity of blood pressure prior to treatment may lead to irreparable damage of the vasculature [64]. If glucocorticoid therapy does not control blood pressure elevation, then treatment with anti-hypertensive medications according to The Fourth Report on the Diagnosis, Evaluation, and Treatment of High Blood Pressure in Children and Adolescents is indicated [1]. Anti-hypertensive medications that have anti-mineralocorticoid properties should be considered first line therapy [29]. It should be noted that it may take months to years for the renin-angiotensin system to normalize; thus, care must be taken to avoid hypovolemic crises in these patients prior to recovery of the renin-angiotensin system [13].

In patients with 21-hydroxylase deficiency and hypertension, evaluation of fludrocortisone therapy should be performed. Plasma renin activity should be measured and the goal is to keep it in the mid-normal range. A suppressed value reflects overtreatment and would indicate that a fludrocortisone dose reduction is warranted. Weight reduction and nutrition counseling should be pursued for obesity and the lowest possible glucocorticoid dose should be used. Chronic hypertension that is unresponsive to fludrocortisone dose adjustment should be treated according to The Fourth Report on the Diagnosis, Evaluation, and Treatment of High Blood Pressure in Children and Adolescents for children and the JNC 7 for adults.

Bilateral adrenalectomy has been performed successfully for rare select cases of CAH due to 11β(beta)-hydroxylase deficiency with severe hypertension that failed medical management [65, 66]. A surgical approach should be considered with caution since patients with 11β(beta)-hydroxylase deficiency are not mineralocorticoid deficient but following bilateral adrenalectomy would be mineralocorticoid deficient, thus, at increased risk for adrenal crisis.

Patients with CAH due to 11β(beta)-hydroxylase deficiency, 17α (alpha)-hydroxylase deficiency, and 21-hydroxylase deficiency are at risk for hypertension, and hypertension is a major risk factor for cardiovascular disease. Early diagnosis and frequent monitoring will allow for early detection and treatment of blood pressure elevation.

Conclusion

The study of mineralocorticoid excess and the development of hypertension in the 11β(beta) and 17α(alpha)-hydroxylase deficiency syndromes has led to a greater understanding of adrenal steroid biosynthesis. However, there is still much more to be learned as the complete pathophysiologic mechanism underlying the cause of hypertension, especially in 11β(beta)-hydroxylase deficiency, remains elusive.

Likewise, hypertension in CAH due to 21-hydroxylase deficiency, once thought not to occur, is an entity which requires a significant amount of investigation to determine the etiology and, ultimately, the most effective therapeutic options.

Future longitudinal studies to assess the incidence of hypertension, cardiovascular events, and the effectiveness of pharmacologic interventions are needed. Many unanswered questions remain regarding the interplay between hormonal imbalances and the development of hypertension, but early intervention will lead to improved patient outcome.

Regardless of the cause of hypertension, it is critical that blood pressure be monitored regularly in all adult and pediatric patients with CAH. Early detection and treatment of CAH and hypertension are the greatest tools available to physicians in preventing the significant comorbidities associated with these diseases.

Acknowledgments This work was supported by The Intramural Research Programs of The *Eunice Kennedy Shriver* National Institute of Child Health and Human Development (NICHD) and the National Institutes of Health Clinical Center.

References

1. National High Blood Pressure Education Program Working Group on High Blood Pressure in Children and Adolescents. The fourth report on the diagnosis, evaluation, and treatment of high blood pressure in children and adolescents. Pediatrics. 2004;114(2 Suppl 4th Report):555–76.
2. Chobanian AV, Bakris GL, Black HR, et al. Seventh report of the Joint National Committee on Prevention, Detection, Evaluation, and Treatment of High Blood Pressure. Hypertension. 2003;42(6):1206–52.
3. White PC, Curnow KM, Pascoe L. Disorders of steroid 11 beta-hydroxylase isozymes. Endocr Rev. 1994;15(4):421–38.
4. Rosler A, Leiberman E, Cohen T. High frequency of congenital adrenal hyperplasia (classic 11 beta-hydroxylase deficiency) among Jews from Morocco. Am J Med Genet. 1992;42(6): 827–34.
5. Suhara K, Gomi T, Sato H, Itagaki E, Takemori S, Katagiri M. Purification and immunochemical characterization of the two adrenal cortex mitochondrial cytochrome P-450-proteins. Arch Biochem Biophys. 1978;190(1):290–9.
6. Mornet E, Dupont J, Vitek A, White PC. Characterization of two genes encoding human steroid 11 beta-hydroxylase (P-450(11) beta). J Biol Chem. 1989;264(35):20961–7.
7. Peter M, Dubuis JM, Sippell WG. Disorders of the aldosterone synthase and steroid 11beta-hydroxylase deficiencies. Horm Res. 1999;51(5):211–22.
8. Levine LS, Rauh W, Gottesdiener K, et al. New studies of the 11 beta-hydroxylase and 18-hydroxylase enzymes in the hypertensive form of congenital adrenal hyperplasia. J Clin Endocrinol Metab. 1980;50(2):258–63.
9. Curnow KM, Slutsker L, Vitek J, et al. Mutations in the CYP11B1 gene causing congenital adrenal hyperplasia and hypertension cluster in exons 6, 7, and 8. Proc Natl Acad Sci USA. 1993;90(10):4552–6.
10. Nimkarn S, New MI. Steroid 11beta- hydroxylase deficiency congenital adrenal hyperplasia. Trends Endocrinol Metab. 2008;19(3):96–9.
11. Parajes S, Loidi L, Reisch N, et al. Functional consequences of seven novel mutations in the CYP11B1 gene: four mutations associated with nonclassic and three mutations causing classic 11{beta}-hydroxylase deficiency. J Clin Endocrinol Metab. 2010;95(2):779–88.

12. de Simone G, Tommaselli AP, Rossi R, et al. Partial deficiency of adrenal 11-hydroxylase. A possible cause of primary hypertension. Hypertension. 1985;7(2):204–10.
13. Kater CE, Biglieri EG. Disorders of steroid 17 alpha-hydroxylase deficiency. Endocrinol Metab Clin North Am. 1994;23(2):341–57.
14. Zachmann M, Tassinari D, Prader A. Clinical and biochemical variability of congenital adrenal hyperplasia due to 11 beta-hydroxylase deficiency. A study of 25 patients. J Clin Endocrinol Metab. 1983;56(2):222–9.
15. Cerame BI, New MI. Hormonal hypertension in children: 11beta-hydroxylase deficiency and apparent mineralocorticoid excess. J Pediatr Endocrinol Metab. 2000;13(9):1537–47.
16. Chabre O, Portrat-Doyen S, Chaffanjon P, et al. Bilateral laparoscopic adrenalectomy for congenital adrenal hyperplasia with severe hypertension, resulting from two novel mutations in splice donor sites of CYP11B1. J Clin Endocrinol Metab. 2000;85(11):4060–8.
17. Hague WM, Honour JW. Malignant hypertension in congenital adrenal hyperplasia due to 11 beta-hydroxylase deficiency. Clin Endocrinol (Oxf). 1983;18(5):505–10.
18. Joehrer K, Geley S, Strasser-Wozak EM, et al. CYP11B1 mutations causing non-classic adrenal hyperplasia due to 11 beta-hydroxylase deficiency. Hum Mol Genet. 1997;6(11):1829–34.
19. Spoudeas HA, Slater JD, Rumsby G, Honour JW, Brook CG. Deoxycorticosterone, 11 beta-hydroxylase and the adrenal cortex. Clin Endocrinol (Oxf). 1993;39(2):245–51.
20. Rosler A, Leiberman E, Sack J, et al. Clinical variability of congenital adrenal hyperplasia due to 11 beta-hydroxylase deficiency. Horm Res. 1982;16(3):133–41.
21. Costa-Santos M, Kater CE, Auchus RJ. Two prevalent CYP17 mutations and genotype-phenotype correlations in 24 Brazilian patients with 17-hydroxylase deficiency. J Clin Endocrinol Metab. 2004;89(1):49–60.
22. Matteson KJ, Picado-Leonard J, Chung BC, Mohandas TK, Miller WL. Assignment of the gene for adrenal P450c17 (steroid 17 alpha-hydroxylase/17,20 lyase) to human chromosome 10. J Clin Endocrinol Metab. 1986;63(3):789–91.
23. Krone N, Arlt W. Genetics of congenital adrenal hyperplasia. Best Pract Res Clin Endocrinol Metab. 2009;23(2):181–92.
24. Sahakitrungruang T, Tee MK, Speiser PW, Miller WL. Novel P450c17 mutation H373D causing combined 17alpha-hydroxylase/17,20-lyase deficiency. J Clin Endocrinol Metab. 2009;94(8):3089–92.
25. Geller DH, Auchus RJ, Mendonca BB, Miller WL. The genetic and functional basis of isolated 17,20-lyase deficiency. Nat Genet. 1997;17(2):201–5.
26. Yanase T, Simpson ER, Waterman MR. 17 alpha-hydroxylase/17,20-lyase deficiency: from clinical investigation to molecular definition. Endocr Rev. 1991;12(1):91–108.
27. Biglieri EG, Herron MA, Brust N. 17-hydroxylation deficiency in man. J Clin Invest. 1966;45(12):1946–54.
28. Peter M, Sippell WG, Wernze H. Diagnosis and treatment of 17-hydroxylase deficiency. J Steroid Biochem Mol Biol. 1993;45(1–3):107–16.
29. Auchus RJ. The genetics, pathophysiology, and management of human deficiencies of P450c17. Endocrinol Metab Clin North Am. 2001;30(1):101–19; vii.
30. Dhir V, Reisch N, Bleicken CM, et al. Steroid 17alpha-hydroxylase deficiency: functional characterization of four mutations (A174E, V178D, R440C, L465P) in the CYP17A1 gene. J Clin Endocrinol Metab. 2009;94(8):3058–64.
31. Mantero F, Opocher G, Rocco S, Carpene G, Armanini D. Long-term treatment of mineralocorticoid excess syndromes. Steroids. 1995;60(1):81–6.
32. Winter JS, Couch RM, Muller J, et al. Combined 17-hydroxylase and 17,20-desmolase deficiencies: evidence for synthesis of a defective cytochrome P450c17. J Clin Endocrinol Metab. 1989;68(2):309–16.
33. Griffing GT, Wilson TE, Holbrook MM, et al. Plasma and urinary 19-Nor-deoxycorticosterone in 17{alpha}-hydroxylase deficiency syndrome. J Clin Endocrinol Metab. 1984;59(5):1011–5.
34. Melby JC. Endocrine hypertension. J Clin Endocrinol Metab. 1989;69(4):697–703.
35. Merke DP, Bornstein SR. Congenital adrenal hyperplasia. Lancet. 2005;365(9477):2125–36.

36. Therrell Jr BL, Berenbaum SA, Manter-Kapanke V, et al. Results of screening 1.9 million Texas newborns for 21-hydroxylase-deficient congenital adrenal hyperplasia. Pediatrics. 1998;101(4 Pt 1):583–90.
37. Fitness J, Dixit N, Webster D, et al. Genotyping of CYP21, linked chromosome 6p markers, and a sex-specific gene in neonatal screening for congenital adrenal hyperplasia. J Clin Endocrinol Metab. 1999;84(3):960–6.
38. Speiser PW, Dupont B, Rubinstein P, Piazza A, Kastelan A, New MI. High frequency of nonclassical steroid 21-hydroxylase deficiency. Am J Hum Genet. 1985;37(4):650–67.
39. Pang S, Murphey W, Levine LS, et al. A pilot newborn screening for congenital adrenal hyperplasia in Alaska. J Clin Endocrinol Metab. 1982;55(3):413–20.
40. Therrell BL. Newborn screening for congenital adrenal hyperplasia. Endocrinol Metab Clin North Am. 2001;30(1):15–30.
41. Dupont B, Oberfield SE, Smithwick EM, Lee TD, Levine LS. Close genetic linkage between HLA and congenital adrenal hyperplasia (21-hydroxylase deficiency). Lancet. 1977; 2(8052–8053):1309–12.
42. White PC, New MI, Dupont B. Structure of human steroid 21-hydroxylase genes. Proc Natl Acad Sci U S A. 1986;83(14):5111–5.
43. Concolino P, Mello E, Zuppi C, Capoluongo E. Molecular diagnosis of congenital adrenal hyperplasia due to 21-hydroxylase deficiency: an update of new CYP21A2 mutations. Clin Chem Lab Med. 2010;48(8):1057–62.
44. Lee H. CYP21 mutations and congenital adrenal hyperplasia. Clin Genet. 2001;59(5):293–301.
45. Werkmeister JW, New MI, Dupont B, White PC. Frequent deletion and duplication of the steroid 21-hydroxylase genes. Am J Hum Genet. 1986;39(4):461–9.
46. Moran C, Azziz R, Carmina E, et al. 21-Hydroxylase-deficient nonclassic adrenal hyperplasia is a progressive disorder: a multicenter study. Am J Obstet Gynecol. 2000;183(6):1468–74.
47. Roche EF, Charmandari E, Dattani MT, Hindmarsh PC. Blood pressure in children and adolescents with congenital adrenal hyperplasia (21-hydroxylase deficiency): a preliminary report. Clin Endocrinol (Oxf). 2003;58(5):589–96.
48. Nebesio TD, Eugster EA. Observation of hypertension in children with 21-hydroxylase deficiency: a preliminary report. Endocrine. 2006;30(3):279–82.
49. Volkl TM, Simm D, Dotsch J, Rascher W, Dorr HG. Altered 24-hour blood pressure profiles in children and adolescents with classical congenital adrenal hyperplasia due to 21-hydroxylase deficiency. J Clin Endocrinol Metab. 2006;91(12):4888–95.
50. de Silva KS, Kanumakala S, Brown JJ, Jones CL, Warne GL. 24-hour ambulatory blood pressure profile in patients with congenital adrenal hyperplasia–a preliminary report. J Pediatr Endocrinol Metab. 2004;17(8):1089–95.
51. Falhammar H, Filipsson H, Holmdahl G, et al. Metabolic profile and body composition in adult women with congenital adrenal hyperplasia due to 21-hydroxylase deficiency. J Clin Endocrinol Metab. 2007;92(1):110–6.
52. Mooij CF, Kapusta L, Otten BJ. Claahsen-van der Grinten HL. Blood pressure in the first year of life in children with congenital adrenal hyperplasia due to 21-hydroxylase deficiency: a pilot study. Horm Res Paediatr. 2010;74(5):328–32.
53. Sartorato P, Zulian E, Benedini S, et al. Cardiovascular risk factors and ultrasound evaluation of intima-media thickness at common carotids, carotid bulbs, and femoral and abdominal aorta arteries in patients with classic congenital adrenal hyperplasia due to 21-hydroxylase deficiency. J Clin Endocrinol Metab. 2007;92(3):1015–8.
54. Ubertini G, Bizzarri C, Grossi A, et al. Blood pressure and left ventricular characteristics in young patients with classical congenital adrenal hyperplasia due to 21-hydroxylase deficiency. Int J Pediatr Endocrinol. 2009;2009:383610.
55. Hoepffner W, Herrmann A, Willgerodt H, Keller E. Blood pressure in patients with congenital adrenal hyperplasia due to 21-hydroxylase deficiency. J Pediatr Endocrinol Metab. 2006; 19(5):705–11.
56. Arriza JL, Weinberger C, Cerelli G, et al. Cloning of human mineralocorticoid receptor complementary DNA: structural and functional kinship with the glucocorticoid receptor. Science. 1987;237(4812):268–75.

57. Edwards CR, Stewart PM, Burt D, et al. Localisation of 11 beta-hydroxysteroid dehydrogenase–tissue specific protector of the mineralocorticoid receptor. Lancet. 1988;2(8618):986–9.
58. Funder JW, Pearce PT, Smith R, Smith AI. Mineralocorticoid action: target tissue specificity is enzyme, not receptor, mediated. Science. 1988;242(4878):583–5.
59. Verma S, Vanryzin C, Sinaii N, et al. A pharmacokinetic and pharmacodynamic study of delayed- and extended-release hydrocortisone (Chronocort) vs. conventional hydrocortisone (Cortef) in the treatment of congenital adrenal hyperplasia. Clin Endocrinol (Oxf). 2010;72(4):441–7.
60. Rahmouni K, Correia ML, Haynes WG, Mark AL. Obesity-associated hypertension: new insights into mechanisms. Hypertension. 2005;45(1):9–14.
61. Charmandari E, Weise M, Bornstein SR, et al. Children with classic congenital adrenal hyperplasia have elevated serum leptin concentrations and insulin resistance: potential clinical implications. J Clin Endocrinol Metab. 2002;87(5):2114–20.
62. Riepe FG, Krone N, Krüger SN, et al. Absence of exercise-induced leptin suppression associated with insufficient epinephrine reserve in patients with classic congenital adrenal hyperplasia due to 21-hydroxylase deficiency. Exp Clin Endocrinol Diabetes. 2006;114(3):105–10.
63. Merke DP, Chrousos GP, Eisenhofer G, et al. Adrenomedullary dysplasia and hypofunction in patients with classic 21-hydroxylase deficiency. N Engl J Med. 2000;343(19):1362–8.
64. Colao A, Pivonello R, Spiezia S, et al. Persistence of increased cardiovascular risk in patients with Cushing's disease after five years of successful cure. J Clin Endocrinol Metab. 1999; 84(8):2664–72.
65. Kacem M, Moussa A, Khochtali I, Nabouli R, Morel Y, Zakhama A. Bilateral adrenalectomy for severe hypertension in congenital adrenal hyperplasia due to 11beta-hydroxylase deficiency: long term follow-up. Ann Endocrinol (Paris). 2009;70(2):113–8.
66. Van Wyk JJ, Ritzen EM. The role of bilateral adrenalectomy in the treatment of congenital adrenal hyperplasia. J Clin Endocrinol Metab. 2003;88(7):2993–8.

Chapter 6
Adrenal Incidentalomas and Arterial Hypertension

Theodora Pappa, Gregory Kaltsas, George Piaditis, and George P. Chrousos

Abstract In the last decades, the prevalence of arterial hypertension, a well-established cardiovascular risk factor, in the general population has substantially been increased. The same holds true for "adrenal incidentalomas" (AI), inapparent adrenal masses detected in approximately 5–10% of patients undergoing imaging of the abdomen for non-adrenal-related diseases. Once excluding the possibility of adrenal lesions being malignant, the clinician has to identify the subgroup of AI that exhibit autonomy of cortisol, aldosterone, or catecholamine secretion, states that are all associated with the development of hypertension. As these entities are usually found in the subclinical form, their clinical significance is not precisely known, and the follow-up and proper management of such patients has not been exactly clarified. In this chapter we attempt to delineate the relation between arterial hypertension and subclinical states of hormone overproduction in AI, such as subclinical Cushing's syndrome, autonomous aldosterone secretion, silent pheochromocytomas, and apparently nonfunctioning lesions. The detailed diagnostic and therapeutic algorithms of the separate overt syndromes are presented in the relevant chapters.

Keywords Adrenal incidentaloma • Subclinical Cushing's syndrome • Primary aldosteronism • Silent pheochromocytoma • Nonfunctioning adrenal incidentaloma • Arterial hypertension

---

T. Pappa • G. Piaditis
Endocrinology Department and Diabetes Center, Athens General Hospital "G. Gennimatas", Athens, Greece

G. Kaltsas
Department of Pathophysiology, Laikon General Hospital, Athens University Medical School, Athens, Greece

G.P. Chrousos (✉)
Division of Endocrinology, Metabolism and Diabetes, First Department of Pediatrics, University of Athens Medical School, Children's Hospital Aghia Sophia, Athens, Greece
e-mail: chrousog@mail.nih.gov

C.A. Koch and G.P. Chrousos (eds.), *Endocrine Hypertension: Underlying Mechanisms and Therapy*, Contemporary Endocrinology, DOI 10.1007/978-1-60761-548-4_6,

Introduction

The term adrenal incidentaloma (AI) is used to describe clinically inapparent adrenal masses discovered serendipitously in the course of diagnostic testing or treatment for conditions unrelated to adrenal disease [1]. The term AI is considered rather an "umbrella" definition that includes many different entities sharing a common discovery pathway. Given the aging population and the technological advances in radiology, it is anticipated that AI will become an even more frequent issue in clinical practice. This is the reason why some regard AI as a by-product of modern technology [1]. Clinicians dealing with such lesions are faced with two major questions; firstly whether the adrenal adenoma harbors a benign or malignant potential, and secondly, whether the tumor is functioning or not. Until recently, algorithms for the management of AI were based on expert opinions [2, 3], but recently the Italian Association of Clinical Endocrinologists (AME) has issued a position statement synthesizing existing literature data and providing clinical recommendations for AI diagnosis, treatment, and follow-up [4].

The prevalence of AI in autopsy studies ranges from 1 to almost 9%, whereas in radiological reports it is over 10% increasing with age, obesity, and the presence of hypertension [5–10].

Adrenal imaging with either computed tomography (CT) or magnetic resonance (MR) using specific criteria of lipid content and contrast washout exerts a very high sensitivity in differentiating benign from malignant lesions (Fig. 6.1) [11]. Assessment of AI secretory status includes biochemical testing for autonomous cortisol, aldosterone, and catecholamine secretion. Hormonal evaluation may not be performed in AI with typical characteristics of a myelolipoma or an adrenal cyst [7, 12].

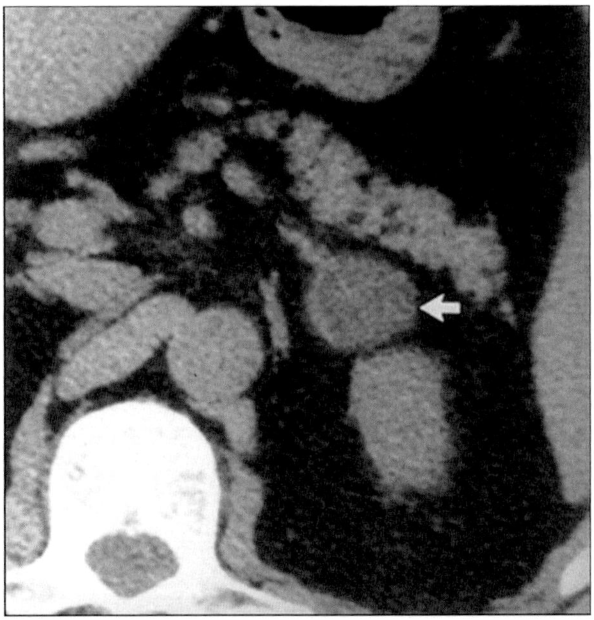

Fig. 6.1 Computerized tomography of a benign adrenocortical adenoma of the left adrenal (*arrow*). Reprinted with permission from Androulakis et al. [19]

Table 6.1 Cumulative data on the prevalence of arterial hypertension in studies of patients harboring an adrenal incidentaloma

First author	Study population	Prevalence of AH Number of patients (%)	References
Fernandez-Real, *Clin Endocrinol* 1998	NFAI	20/64 (31)	[14]
Barzon, *JCEM* 1999	AI	41/75 (55)	[15]
Mantero, *JCEM* 2000	AI	362/863 (41)	[16]
	SCS	38/92 (41)	
Rossi, *JCEM* 2000	AI	24/50 (48)	[17]
	SCS	11/12 (92)	
Midorikawa, *Clin Endocrinol* 2001	AI	7/12 (58)	[27]
Tauchmanovà, *JCEM* 2002	SCS	17/28 (61)	[28]
Terzolo, *Eur J Endocrinol* 2005	AI	113/210 (54)	[30]
	SCS	8/23 (35)	
Erbil, *World J Surg* 2006	SCS	7/11 (63)	[31]
Comlekci, *Endocrine* 2010	AI	207/376 (55)	[32]
Giordano, *Eur J Endocrinol* 2010	AI	73/118 (61)	[33]
	NFAI	59/102 (58)	
	SCS	13/16 (81)	
Terzolo, *Clin Endocrinol* 1998	AI	19/53 (36)	[37]
Piaditis, *Clin Endocrinol* 2009	AI	41/83 (49)	[39]
Libè, *Eur J Endocrinol* 2002	AI	35/64 (55)	[44]
Bernini, *Br J Cancer* 2005	AI	76/115 (66)	[45]
Vassilatou, *Clin Endocrinol* 2009	NFAI	32/57 (56)	[47]
	SCS	15/20 (75)	
Reincke, *JCEM* 1992	SCS	7/8 (88)	[49]
Bernini, *Eur J Endocrinol* 2003	AI	10/15 (67)	[50]
	SCS	5/6 (83)	
Mitchell, *Surgery* 2007	SCS	8/9 (89)	[51]
Tsuiki, *Endocr J* 2008	SCS	9/20 (45)	[52]
Sereg, *Eur J Endocrinol* 2009	NFAI	93/113 (82)	[53]
Chiodini, *JCEM* 2010	AI	62/108 (57)	[54]
	SCS	24/41 (59)	
Toniato, *Ann Surg* 2009	SCS	33/45 (73)	[55]
Wagnerova, *Neoplasma* 2009	AI	51/92 (55)	[102]
Yilmaz, *J Endocrinol Invest* 2009	NFAI	6/32 (20)	[103]

AI adrenal incidentaloma; *SCS* subclinical Cushing's syndrome; *NFAI* non-functioning adrenal incidentaloma; *AH* arterial hypertension

Arterial hypertension (AH) is a prevailing, but not an innocent bystander in the aging population. The prevalence of AH increases with advanced age [13]. Several studies have reported an increased prevalence of arterial hypertension, diabetes mellitus and/or glucose intolerance, hyperlipidemia, and obesity in AI patients, reaching up to 54%, 66%, 36%, and 28%, respectively [14–18]. The reported incidence of AH in studies investigating patients with AI ranges between 36 and 67% and is cumulatively depicted in Table 6.1. However, there is a wide variation in the reported prevalence due to the different inclusion criteria, methodology used, and cut-offs employed.

The adverse metabolic and cardiovascular profile observed in AI has initiated the search for potential links between AH and other potentially adverse metabolic parameters [15, 18, 19]. This is reinforced further by the presence of surrogate markers of cardiovascular dysfunction even in patients with apparently nonfunctioning AI. Such patients have worse indices of left ventricle hypertrophy and diastolic function compared to normotensive lean subjects, whereas hypertensive AI patients have the most impaired cardiac morphology and function [20]. Additionally, patients with nonfunctioning AI have significantly lower flow-mediated dilation, a marker of endothelial function, compared to age, sex, and body mass index (BMI)-matched control group [21]. Furthermore, early atherosclerotic changes such as increased carotid intima-media thickness are found in nonfunctioning AI subjects [22].

The scope of this chapter is to provide an update on current literature concerning the relation of arterial hypertension with AI.

Subclinical Cushing's syndrome

Cushing's syndrome (CS) is accompanied by increased morbidity and mortality attributed mostly to a higher cardiovascular disease (CVD) risk. Among other metabolic features, AH is frequently found in subjects with CS, especially in adults (80%), and less commonly in the pediatric population [23–25]. Even in subclinical cases, the incidence of AH in AI-related subclinical Cushing's syndrome (SCS) is high in several clinical reports varying from 35% up to 92% [16–18, 26–33]. Overt or subtle hypercortisolism is associated with hypertension through the activation of the mineralocorticoid receptor, following saturation of the 11 beta-hydroxysteroid dehydrogenase 2 (11βHSD2) enzyme, that inactivates cortisol to cortisone in the renal cortex (*see below*). SCS refers to a state of altered hormonal secretory dynamics and autonomous glucocorticoid production without apparent clinical signs and symptoms. The term "subclinical" is preferred to "preclinical," since the majority of cases do not develop overt Cushing's syndrome (CS) after prolonged follow-up. The absence of Cushing's phenotype rests in clinical judgment, but even for experienced clinicians it may be difficult to attribute a sign to hypercortisolism or the other encountered entities such as the metabolic syndrome (MS). SCS is the most common finding when evaluating an incidentally discovered adrenal mass and its prevalence has been reported to vary from 5 to 56%, but its clinical significance is not as yet fully defined [8, 17, 29, 34–39]. Biochemical tests applied to diagnose hypercortisolism include 24-h urinary-free cortisol (UFC), midnight salivary cortisol, and dexamethasone suppression test (DST). Lowering cortisol cut-off levels following the DST, the proposed screening test in AI, is anticipated to reveal more cases of SCS. Measurement of ACTH and dehydroepiandrosterone (DHEAS) levels has also been proposed, but the ideal strategy to detect SCS in AI is not yet established and controversy exists between European and American Societies [40, 41]. Recently, it was suggested that the cost-effectiveness of extensive evaluation for SCS should be reappraised [42]. Diagnostic algorithms for Cushing's syndrome have been published by the Endocrine Society and are explicitly reviewed in the relevant book chapter [43].

Current literature suggests that progression of SCS to overt Cushing's syndrome is uncommon, whereas occasionally resolution of functional alterations has also been observed [8, 15, 17, 37, 44–48]. Patients with SCS appear to harbor an unfavorable metabolic profile with increased frequency of arterial hypertension, diabetes mellitus, central adiposity, and dyslipidemia [16–18, 26–33]. This raises the question whether surgical management is indicated in AI bearing subtle cortisol overproduction. It should be stressed, however, that there is scant data supporting the increased CVD morbidity and mortality in AI patients exhibiting SCS. These associations have favored the implementation of surgical therapy that led to some improvement of AH and other metabolic parameters in SCS patients. However, as long-term results are lacking, definite conclusions are probably arbitrary [15, 17, 29, 31, 33, 49–54]. In the only randomized trial up to now, Toniato et al. demonstrated a significant improvement of AH in the patients' group treated surgically compared to those managed conservatively [55]. In that study, 12 out of 18 surgically treated SCS patients (67%) exhibited stabilization or improvement of their blood pressure control, whereas in the conservatively managed group 12 out of 15 hypertensives required change or increase of their antihypertensive medication. However, the final therapeutic approach is based on an individualized basis, taking into consideration the surgical risk, expense, and outcome of laparoscopic adrenalectomy compared to life-style modification and pharmacological intervention. Some advocate that the surgical approach should be employed for young patients with AI associated with an unfavorable metabolic profile that is unresponsive to medical treatment [4, 41]. In case of surgical management, postoperative glucocorticoid coverage is used until recovery of the adrenal function [56]. In every case, surgical or medical management of hypercortisolism is necessary in order to lower or—when possible—normalize blood pressure and thus ameliorate the CVD risk profile of patients with CS.

Pathophysiological Link Between Hypercortisolism and AH

The "dipping" phenomenon, the fall of blood pressure at nighttime, was suggested to be the link between hypercortisolism and AH, as it was markedly lower in CS compared to subjects with essential hypertension without CS. Furthermore, this abnormality was resolved with the treatment of CS [57]. As previously stated, excessive cortisol production in CS results in substrate saturation of the 11βHSD2 enzyme, responsible for the inactivation of cortisol to cortisone in the renal cortex, but also in vascular endothelial cells and vascular smooth muscle cells [58]. This results in spillover of cortisol and binding with the mineralocorticoid receptor, thus inducing sodium reabsorption from the renal tubule, volume expansion, and finally hypertension [24]. However, spironolactone administration, a mineralocorticoid receptors antagonist, did not prevent the development of hypertension [59]. Therefore, cortisol-induced hypertension cannot be solely interpreted by the mineralocorticoid effect of cortisol and it is likely that other factors may also be implicated [60].

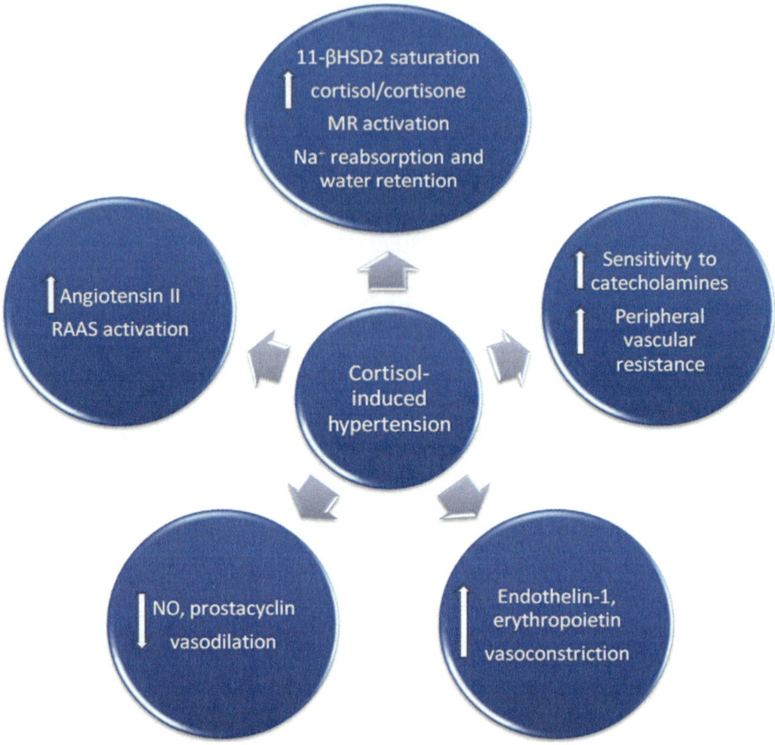

Fig. 6.2 Proposed pathogenetic mechanisms of cortisol-induced hypertension. *11-βHSD2* 11-beta-hydroxysteroid dehydrogenase type 2; *MR* mineralocorticoid receptor; *Na⁺* sodium; *RAAS* renin–angiotensin–aldosterone system; *NO* nitric oxide

According to animal data, glucocorticoids enhance angiotensin II production and up-regulate its receptors in both the brain and periphery [61, 62]. Besides activation of the renin–angiotensin–aldosterone system (RAAS), it appears that glucocorticoids decrease vasodilation by inhibiting the production of nitric oxide (NO) and prostacyclin [63]. Defective transport of L-arginine, a precursor of NO synthesis, as well as inhibition, uncoupling, and increased inactivation of NO synthase are thought to participate in cortisol-induced hypertension [64]. Glucocorticoid-induced oxidative stress hypertension has also been implicated through the stimulation of the nicotinamide adenine dinucleotide phosphate (NADPH) oxidase pathway and an imbalance between reactive oxygen species (ROS) production and degradation [64]. Vasoconstrictive substances, such as endothelin-1 and erythropoietin, are also elevated in hypercortisolism states [65, 66]. Given the discrepancy of animal and human data, further studies are warranted to identify the exact role of these substances. Moreover, clinical studies in healthy subjects have demonstrated that glucocorticoids enhance the sensitivity of the vasculature to catecholamines, induce peripheral vascular resistance, and increase arterial blood pressure [67]. Figure 6.2 illustrates a summary of the underlying mechanisms in cortisol-induced hypertension.

Primary Aldosteronism: Autonomous Aldosterone Secretion

Primary aldosteronism (PA) is the syndrome resulting from autonomous aldosterone secretion (AAS) leading to hypokalemia, endothelial dysfunction, arterial stiffness, cardiovascular hypertrophy, and fibrosis placing PA patients at a significant CVD risk [68, 69]. The vast majority of cases are due to an aldosterone-producing adrenal adenoma (APA) and bilateral adrenal hyperplasia or idiopathic PA (IPA). The differential diagnosis is crucial, since APA is cured with unilateral adrenalectomy, whereas the treatment of choice for IHA includes antihypertensive medication targeting the RAAS. Early diagnosis and tailored treatment is pivotal in the prevention or regression of CVD alterations induced by aldosterone overproduction.

In adult hypertensives the prevalence of PA is estimated to be approximately 13% [70], whereas its prevalence is increased with the severity of AH [71]. According to the Primary Aldosteronism Prevalence in Hypertensives (PARY) Study, the prevalence of PA was 11.2% with APA comprising 43% of the cases [72]. PA appears to be the most frequent cause of endocrine AH and, as a result, all hypertensive patients diagnosed with an AI should undergo testing for PA. The initial diagnostic tool to screen for PA is the aldosterone/renin ratio (ARR), i.e., the ratio of plasma aldosterone levels (ng/dL) divided by the plasma renin activity (PRA) (ng/mL/h). The most widely used cut-off values are 20–30 [73]. However, sensitivity of the test ranges widely mainly due to the PRA induced wide variation of ARR [74]. It has therefore been suggested that clinicians do not rely solely to a single ARR to diagnose patients with suspected PA [70]; and that repeated measurements of the ARR should be obtained [75]. The oral saline loading, the saline infusion, the fludrocortisone with salt loading test, and the captopril challenge test are second-line tests used to confirm or exclude the presence of PA. Guidelines for the diagnosis of PA have been issued by Endocrine Society [73] and a concise update on the diagnosis and treatment of PA is included in a previous chapter of this book, where the reader is referred for a detailed literature review.

The prevalence of PA in patients bearing an AI has been estimated to range from 1 up to 24% depending on the hormonal test used to diagnose PA [16, 26, 34, 36, 39, 76–79]. However, it should be acknowledged that the cut-off value of the screening and the confirmatory test exploited in the diagnostic process is a major determinant of the estimated prevalence of PA and an important guide to further testing. We have recently found an increased prevalence of AAS among hypertensive patients (31%) and in subjects with unilateral adrenal adenomas (24%) [39, 80]. Similar results were found when investigating patients with incidentally discovered bilateral adrenal masses [81]. This higher than previously described prevalence of PA was attributed to the methodology used as cut-off values were obtained from normotensive subjects with normal adrenal morphology [39]. Furthermore, the confirmatory saline infusion test of PA was modified with prior dexamethasone administration to eliminate the effect of adrenocorticotropin hormone (ACTH) on aldosterone secretion [80]. The above features underline the need to take into consideration the methodology used when interpreting study findings on the prevalence of PA. The clinical significance of subtle AAS forms remains unknown, but data from the Framingham Offspring showed that normotensive subjects with high aldosterone levels, yet in the normal range, were at increased risk for the development of AH [82].

Pathophysiological Mechanism of Aldosterone-Induced Hypertension

Aldosterone is well known to act via the mineralocorticoid receptor to promote renal sodium retention. Additionally, it augments angiotensin II activity and can thus lead to endothelial dysfunction and impaired vascular resistance. One should also consider the significant paracrine actions of aldosterone in the central nervous system, the myocardium, and the brain independent of the circulating aldosterone levels [83–85]. It is possible that these mechanisms may mediate an alternative pathway to aldosterone-induced hypertension.

Pheochromocytoma

Pheochromocytomas (PHEO), tumors arising from catecholamine-producing chromaffin cells in the adrenal medulla, are an uncommon cause of AH [86]. The classical constellation includes hypertension, headaches, palpitations, and diaphoresis. Timely diagnosis of this "great mimicker" and effective treatment is critical in order to avoid or attenuate the long-term consequences on the cardiovascular, cerebrovascular, and renal system. Besides imaging studies, biochemical screening tests include blood and urine measurements of catecholamines and their metabolic products (adrenaline, noradrenaline and metanephrine, normetanephrine and vanillylmandelic acid, respectively) with fractionated metanephrine and normetanephrine being the preferred initial choice [87].

PHEO may be a rare cause of AH, but when occurs the vast majority of patients have AH related to excessive catecholamine production. AH may be sustained or paroxysmal (50% and 45%, respectively) and occasionally patients may have paroxysms of AH in a setting of sustained hypertension. Until recently, only few patients with PHEO (5–15%) were considered to have normal arterial pressure [88]. Several factors influence the phenotypic characteristics of AH in patients with PHEO, such as the amount of catecholamines produced by the tumor and their secretory pattern [89]. Excessive norepinephrine secretion is considered to induce vasoconstriction, thus resulting in sustained hypertension. Epinephrine hypersecretion is commonly associated with paroxysmal hypertension and is more frequently encountered in PHEO patients with multiple endocrine neoplasia 2 (MEN-2) syndromes [89]. Albeit a minority, patients harboring a very small, familial, or dopamine-producing PHEO may have normal arterial pressure. These subjects represent a special, not negligible, subgroup of PHEO patients with atypical symptoms that may be diagnosed in the evaluation of an incidentally discovered adrenal mass.

Lately, due to increased awareness and with the advent of imaging techniques, the prevalence of incidentally identified, "subclinical" PHEO is rising [8, 16, 26, 35, 90–97]. A PHEO prevalence of 10% has been reported among patients undergoing operation for an adrenal incidentaloma [98]. In an Italian study, PHEO were found to comprise 3.4% of AIs and half of these incidentally diagnosed PHEO had no elevations of blood pressure [16]. Lee et al. found borderline elevation of urinary or plasma metanephrine levels in 24% of patients with an AI, and among them, one third were diagnosed to have subclinical or asymptomatic PHEO according to pathological examination [99]. The authors proposed repeating biochemical testing along with iodine-131-meta-iodobenzylguanidine (MIBG) scanning or preoperative alpha-blockade in AI subjects with marginal elevation of metanephrine levels. In alignment with the previous studies, in a German cohort of 201 PHEOs, almost 30% of them were incidental findings confirming the need for evaluation of PHEO in all AI patients [100]. In a further study, incidental discovery of a PHEO was associated with older age and lower catecholamine concentrations compared to symptomatic patients [95], in agreement with the findings of Grozinsky-Glasberg et al. in their study in clinically silent PHEOs [101].

Nonfunctioning Adrenal Incidentalomas

The majority of AI is not hormonally active, but increasing evidence is emerging concerning an increased CVD risk in patients with NFAIs. The prevalence of AH, diabetes mellitus, fatty liver disease, and dyslipidemia is higher in NFAI subjects compared to the general population [102, 103] whereas recently an increased prevalence of insulin resistance in NFAIs was reported [104]. However, it should be stressed that the classification of AI as nonfunctioning relies on the cut-off values applied in their hormonal evaluation. It is highly probable that lowering the cut-offs used to identify autonomous adrenal steroid production will identify more AI with subtle hormonal overproduction and decrease the prevalence of the up to now recognized NFAIs. The beneficial effect of adrenalectomy in NFAIs on AH and other metabolic markers demonstrated in two studies may suggest that NFAIs harbor an increased CVD risk [17, 50]. However, controversy exists as a further study showed no improvement in blood pressure control and no difference in cardio- and cerebrovascular morbidity [53].

The design of the clinical studies evaluating the metabolic status of AI patients and the inconsistency of data from studies evaluating the outcome of adrenalectomy does not permit the optimal characterization of the relation between AI and the parameters of the metabolic syndrome as causal. An interesting approach was introduced by Reincke et al., who showed a mitogenic effect of insulin on adrenal cancer cells in vitro and proposed that sustained hyperinsulinemia may lead to adrenocortical tumorigenesis [105]. The therapeutic dilemmas in AI can only be solved with longitudinal, properly controlled studies that will assess the evolution of various metabolic parameters, like AH, diabetes, hyperlipidemia, but most importantly should address the role of adrenalectomy—if any—in "hard" outcomes, like major CVD events and mortality.

Conclusions

SCS is the most frequently encountered hormonal abnormality when evaluating a patient with an AI and appears to follow a relatively indolent course without progression to overt disease. The association of hypertension with SCS is very strong and consistent. In most, but not all, studies a marked improvement of AH is observed following surgical treatment, but this cannot at the present time be translated in reduction of CVD risk. Therefore, the ideal management of SCS patients, surgical or pharmacological, remains a debate. Primary aldosteronism is considered the most common cause of endocrine hypertension. The emerging data on the role of aldosterone in the heart and the vasculature renewed the interest in PA. Controversy exists regarding the suitable screening test and its cut-off value that will not miss patients with AAS yet not at the cost of a high false-positive number. Concerning pheochromocytomas, a change in their initial presentation is reported with a growing number of these chromaffin-cell tumors being discovered incidentally, the so-called silent pheochromocytomas. Early identification and establishing the correct diagnosis in these borderline cases is critical for the preoperative medical blockade of the patients to prevent a life-threatening hypertensive crisis intra-operatively. The clustering of parameters of the metabolic syndrome, like AH, diabetes, and dyslipidemia, even in NFAIs raises important questions regarding the pathogenesis and the appropriate management of these until now considered hormonally silent adrenal lesions.

Broadening our knowledge on the subclinical hormone overproduction in adrenal incidentalomas is a very interesting scientific field that is anticipated to gain increasing attention in the years to come. Clarifying if and in what extent subclinical hormonal excess is depicted in the general health status of a patient with an AI and thus identifying those patients that will benefit most from a more aggressive, surgical management rather than a conservative, observatory approach is a conundrum waiting to be solved.

References

1. NIH state-of-the-science statement on management of the clinically inapparent adrenal mass ("incidentaloma"). NIH Consens State Sci Statements. 2002;19:1–25.
2. Terzolo M, Reimondo G, Bovio S, et al. Management of adrenal incidentalomas. Exp Clin Endocrinol Diabetes. 2007;115:166–70.
3. Young Jr WF. Clinical practice. The incidentally discovered adrenal mass. N Engl J Med. 2007;356:601–10.

4. Terzolo M, Stigliano A, Chiodini I, et al. Italian Association of Clinical Endocrinologists. AME position statement on adrenal incidentaloma. Eur J Endocrinol. 2011;164:851–70.
5. Kloos RT, Gross MD, Francis IR, et al. Incidentally discovered adrenal masses. Endocr Rev. 1995;16:460–84.
6. Young Jr WF. Management approaches to adrenal incidentalomas. A view from Rochester, Minnesota. Endocrinol Metab Clin North Am. 2000;29:159–85.
7. Grumbach MM, Biller BM, Braunstein GD, et al. Management of the clinically inapparent adrenal mass ("incidentaloma"). Ann Intern Med. 2003;138:424–9.
8. Barzon L, Sonino N, Fallo F, et al. Prevalence and natural history of adrenal incidentalomas. Eur J Endocrinol. 2003;149:273–85.
9. Mansmann G, Lau J, Balk E, et al. The clinically inapparent adrenal mass: update in diagnosis and management. Endocr Rev. 2004;25:309–40.
10. Bovio S, Cataldi A, Reimondo G, et al. Prevalence of adrenal incidentaloma in a contemporary computerized tomography series. J Endocrinol Invest. 2006;29:298–302.
11. Hamrahian AH, Ioachimescu AG, Remer EM, et al. Clinical utility of noncontrast computed tomography attenuation value (hounsfield units) to differentiate adrenal adenomas/hyperplasias from nonadenomas: Cleveland Clinic experience. J Clin Endocrinol Metab. 2005;90:871–7.
12. Young Jr WF. Adrenal causes of hypertension: pheochromocytoma and primary aldosteronism. Rev Endocr Metab Disord. 2007;8:309–20.
13. Burt VL, Whelton P, Roccella EJ, et al. Prevalence of hypertension in the US adult population. Results from the Third National Health and Nutrition Examination Survey, 1988–1991. Hypertension. 1995;25:305–13.
14. Fernández-Real JM, Engel WR, Simó R, et al. Study of glucose tolerance in consecutive patients harbouring incidental adrenal tumours. Study Group of Incidental Adrenal Adenoma. Clin Endocrinol (Oxf). 1998;49:53–61.
15. Barzon L, Scaroni C, Sonino N, et al. Risk factors and long-term follow-up of adrenal incidentalomas. J Clin Endocrinol Metab. 1999;84:520–6.
16. Mantero F, Terzolo M, Arnaldi G, et al. A survey on adrenal incidentaloma in Italy. Study Group on Adrenal Tumors of the Italian Society of Endocrinology. J Clin Endocrinol Metab. 2000;85:637–44.
17. Rossi R, Tauchmanova L, Luciano A, et al. Subclinical Cushing's syndrome in patients with adrenal incidentaloma: clinical and biochemical features. J Clin Endocrinol Metab. 2000;85:1440–8.
18. Terzolo M, Pia A, Alì A, et al. Adrenal incidentaloma: a new cause of the metabolic syndrome? J Clin Endocrinol Metab. 2002;87:998–1003.
19. Androulakis II, Kaltsas G, Piaditis G, et al. The clinical significance of adrenal incidentalomas. Eur J Clin Invest. 2011;41:552–60.
20. Ermetici F, Dall'Asta C, Malavazos AE, et al. Echocardiographic alterations in patients with non-functioning adrenal incidentaloma. J Endocrinol Invest. 2008;31:573–7.
21. Erbil Y, Ozbey N, Barbaros U, et al. Cardiovascular risk in patients with nonfunctional adrenal incidentaloma: myth or reality? World J Surg. 2009;33:2099–105.
22. Yener S, Genc S, Akinci B, et al. Carotid intima media thickness is increased and associated with morning cortisol in subjects with non-functioning adrenal incidentaloma. Endocrine. 2009;35:365–70.
23. Ross EJ, Linch DC. Cushing's syndrome–killing disease: discriminatory value of signs and symptoms aiding early diagnosis. Lancet. 1982;2:646–9.
24. Stewart PM, Walker BR, Holder G, et al. 11 Beta-hydroxysteroid dehydrogenase activity in Cushing's syndrome: explaining the mineralocorticoid excess state of the ectopic adrenocorticotropin syndrome. J Clin Endocrinol Metab. 1995;80:3617–20.
25. Magiakou MA, Mastorakos G, Zachman K, et al. Blood pressure in children and adolescents with Cushing's syndrome before and after surgical care. J Clin Endocrinol Metab. 1997;82:1734–8.
26. Barzon L, Scaroni C, Sonino N, et al. Incidentally discovered adrenal tumors: endocrine and scintigraphic correlates. J Clin Endocrinol Metab. 1998;83:55–62.

27. Midorikawa S, Sanada H, Hashimoto S, et al. The improvement of insulin resistance in patients with adrenal incidentaloma by surgical resection. Clin Endocrinol (Oxf). 2001;54:797–804.
28. Tauchmanovà L, Rossi R, Biondi B, et al. Patients with subclinical Cushing's syndrome due to adrenal adenoma have increased cardiovascular risk. J Clin Endocrinol Metab. 2002;87:4872–8.
29. Emral R, Uysal AR, Asik M, et al. Prevalence of subclinical Cushing's syndrome in 70 patients with adrenal incidentaloma: clinical, biochemical and surgical outcomes. Endocr J. 2003;50:399–408.
30. Terzolo M, Bovio S, Pia A, et al. Midnight serum cortisol as a marker of increased cardiovascular risk in patients with a clinically inapparent adrenal adenoma. Eur J Endocrinol. 2005;153:307–15.
31. Erbil Y, Ademoğlu E, Ozbey N, et al. Evaluation of the cardiovascular risk in patients with subclinical Cushing syndrome before and after surgery. World J Surg. 2006;30:1665–71.
32. Comlekci A, Yener S, Ertilav S, et al. Adrenal incidentaloma, clinical, metabolic, follow-up aspects: single centre experience. Endocrine. 2010;37:40–6.
33. Giordano R, Marinazzo E, Berardelli R, et al. Long-term morphological, hormonal, and clinical follow-up in a single unit on 118 patients with adrenal incidentalomas. Eur J Endocrinol. 2010;162:779–85.
34. Caplan RH, Strutt PJ, Wickus GG. Subclinical hormone secretion by incidentally discovered adrenal masses. Arch Surg. 1994;129:291–6.
35. Osella G, Terzolo M, Borretta G, et al. Endocrine evaluation of incidentally discovered adrenal masses (incidentalomas). J Clin Endocrinol Metab. 1994;79:1532–9.
36. Mantero F, Masini AM, Opocher G, et al. Adrenal incidentaloma: an overview of hormonal data from the National Italian Study Group. Horm Res. 1997;47:284–9.
37. Terzolo M, Osella G, Alì A, et al. Subclinical Cushing's syndrome in adrenal incidentaloma. Clin Endocrinol (Oxf). 1998;48:89–97.
38. Terzolo M, Bovio S, Reimondo G, et al. Subclinical Cushing's syndrome in adrenal incidentalomas. Endocrinol Metab Clin North Am. 2005;34:423–39.
39. Piaditis GP, Kaltsas GA, Androulakis II, et al. High prevalence of autonomous cortisol and aldosterone secretion from adrenal adenomas. Clin Endocrinol (Oxf). 2009;71:772–8.
40. Tabarin A, Bardet S, Bertherat J, et al. French Society of Endocrinology Consensus. Exploration and management of adrenal incidentalomas. French Society of Endocrinology Consensus. Ann Endocrinol (Paris). 2008;69:487–500.
41. Zeiger MA, Thompson GB, Duh QY, et al; American Association of Clinical Endocrinologists; American Association of Endocrine Surgeons. The American Association of Clinical Endocrinologists and American Association of Endocrine Surgeons medical guidelines for the management of adrenal incidentalomas. Endocr Pract. 2009;15 Suppl 1:1–20.
42. Cawood TJ, Hunt PJ, O'Shea D, et al. Recommended evaluation of adrenal incidentalomas is costly, has high false-positive rates and confers a risk of fatal cancer that is similar to the risk of the adrenal lesion becoming malignant; time for a rethink? Eur J Endocrinol. 2009;161:513–27.
43. Nieman LK, Biller BM, Findling JW, et al. The diagnosis of Cushing's syndrome: an Endocrine Society Clinical Practice Guideline. J Clin Endocrinol Metab. 2008;93:1526–40.
44. Libè R, Dall'Asta C, Barbetta L, et al. Long-term follow-up study of patients with adrenal incidentalomas. Eur J Endocrinol. 2002;147:489–94.
45. Bernini GP, Moretti A, Oriandini C, et al. Long-term morphological and hormonal follow-up in a single unit on 115 patients with adrenal incidentalomas. Br J Cancer. 2005;92:1104–9.
46. Bülow B, Jansson S, Juhlin C, et al. Adrenal incidentaloma—follow-up results from a Swedish prospective study. Eur J Endocrinol. 2006;154:419–23.
47. Vassilatou E, Vryonidou A, Michalopoulou S, et al. Hormonal activity of adrenal incidentalomas: results from a long-term follow-up study. Clin Endocrinol (Oxf). 2009;70:674–9.
48. Yener S, Ertilav S, Secil M, et al. Prospective evaluation of tumor size and hormonal status in adrenal incidentalomas. J Endocrinol Invest. 2010;33:32–6.

49. Reincke M, Nieke J, Krestin GP, et al. Preclinical Cushing's syndrome in adrenal "incidentalomas": comparison with adrenal Cushing's syndrome. J Clin Endocrinol Metab. 1992;75:826–32.
50. Bernini G, Moretti A, Iacconi P, et al. Anthropometric, haemodynamic, humoral and hormonal evaluation in patients with incidental adrenocortical adenomas before and after surgery. Eur J Endocrinol. 2003;148:213–9.
51. Mitchell IC, Auchus RJ, Juneja K, et al. "Subclinical Cushing's syndrome" is not subclinical: improvement after adrenalectomy in 9 patients. Surgery. 2007;142:900–5.
52. Tsuiki M, Tanabe A, Takagi S, et al. Cardiovascular risks and their long-term clinical outcome in patients with subclinical Cushing's syndrome. Endocr J. 2008;55:737–45.
53. Sereg M, Szappanos A, Toke J, et al. Atherosclerotic risk factors and complications in patients with non-functioning adrenal adenomas treated with or without adrenalectomy: a long-term follow-up study. Eur J Endocrinol. 2009;160:647–55.
54. Chiodini I, Morelli V, Salcuni AS, et al. Beneficial metabolic effects of prompt surgical treatment in patients with an adrenal incidentaloma causing biochemical hypercortisolism. J Clin Endocrinol Metab. 2010;95:2736–45.
55. Toniato A, Merante-Boschin I, Opocher G, et al. Surgical versus conservative management for subclinical Cushing syndrome in adrenal incidentalomas: a prospective randomized study. Ann Surg. 2009;249:388–91.
56. Eller-Vainicher C, Morelli V, Salcuni AS, et al. Post-surgical hypocortisolism after removal of an adrenal incidentaloma: is it predictable by an accurate endocrinological work-up before surgery? Eur J Endocrinol. 2010;162:91–9.
57. Zacharieva S, Orbetzova M, Stoynev A, et al. Circadian blood pressure profile in patients with Cushing's syndrome before and after treatment. J Endocrinol Invest. 2004;27:924–30.
58. Hatakeyama H, Inaba S, Miyamori I. 11Beta-hydroxysteroid dehydrogenase in cultured human vascular cells. Possible role in the development of hypertension. Hypertension. 1999;33:1179–84.
59. Montrella-Waybill M, Clore JN, Schoolwerth AC, et al. Evidence that high dose cortisol-induced Na+ retention in man is not mediated by the mineralocorticoid receptor. J Clin Endocrinol Metab. 1991;72:1060–6.
60. Whitworth JA, Mangos GJ, Kelly JJ. Cushing, cortisol, and cardiovascular disease. Hypertension. 2000;36:912–6.
61. Sato A, Suzuki H, Murakami M, et al. Glucocorticoid increases angiotensin II type 1 receptor and its gene expression. Hypertension. 1994;23:25–30.
62. Shelat SG, King JL, Flanagan-Cato LM, et al. Mineralocorticoids and glucocorticoids cooperatively increase salt intake and angiotensin II receptor binding in rat brain. Neuroendocrinology. 1999;69:339–51.
63. Axelrod L. Inhibition of prostacyclin production mediates permissive effect of glucocorticoids on vascular tone. Perturbations of this mechanism contribute to pathogenesis of Cushing's syndrome and Addison's disease. Lancet. 1983;1:904–6.
64. Ong SL, Whitworth JA. How do glucocorticoids cause hypertension: role of nitric oxide deficiency, oxidative stress, and eicosanoids. Endocrinol Metab Clin North Am. 2011;40: 393–407.
65. Kelly JJ, Martin A, Whitworth JA. Role of erythropoietin in cortisol-induced hypertension. J Hum Hypertens. 2000;14:195–8.
66. Kirilov G, Tomova A, Dakovska L, et al. Elevated plasma endothelin as an additional cardiovascular risk factor in patients with Cushing's syndrome. Eur J Endocrinol. 2003;149: 549–53.
67. Pirpiris M, Sudhir K, Yeung S, et al. Pressor responsiveness in corticosteroid-induced hypertension in humans. Hypertension. 1992;19:567–74.
68. Rossi GP, Di Bello V, Ganzaroli C, et al. Excess aldosterone is associated with alterations of myocardial texture in primary aldosteronism. Hypertension. 2002;40:23–7.
69. Farquharson CA, Struthers AD. Aldosterone induces acute endothelial dysfunction in vivo in humans: evidence for an aldosterone-induced vasculopathy. Clin Sci (Lond). 2002;103:425–31.

70. Schwartz GL, Turner ST. Screening for primary aldosteronism in essential hypertension: diagnostic accuracy of the ratio of plasma aldosterone concentration to plasma renin activity. Clin Chem. 2005;51:386–94.
71. Mosso L, Carvajal C, González A, et al. Primary aldosteronism and hypertensive disease. Hypertension. 2003;42:161–5.
72. Rossi GP, Bernini G, Caliumi C, et al; PAPY Study Investigators. A prospective study of the prevalence of primary aldosteronism in 1,125 hypertensive patients. J Am Coll Cardiol. 2006;48:2293–300.
73. Funder JW, Carey RM, Fardella C, et al; Endocrine Society. Case detection, diagnosis, and treatment of patients with primary aldosteronism: an endocrine society clinical practice guideline. J Clin Endocrinol Metab. 2008;93:3266–81.
74. Schwartz GL, Chapman AB, Boerwinkle E, et al. Screening for primary aldosteronism: implications of an increased plasma aldosterone/renin ratio. Clin Chem. 2002;48:1919–23.
75. Gordon RD. The challenge of more robust and reproducible methodology in screening for primary aldosteronism. J Hypertens. 2004;22:251–5.
76. Stowasser M. Primary aldosteronism: revival of a syndrome. J Hypertens. 2001;19:363–6.
77. Bernini G, Moretti A, Argenio G, et al. Primary aldosteronism in normokalemic patients with adrenal incidentalomas. Eur J Endocrinol. 2002;146:523–9.
78. Cicala MV, Sartorato P, Mantero F. Incidentally discovered masses in hypertensive patients. Best Pract Res Clin Endocrinol Metab. 2006;20:451–66.
79. Vierhapper H. Determination of the aldosterone/renin ratio in 269 patients with adrenal incidentaloma. Exp Clin Endocrinol Diabetes. 2007;115:518–21.
80. Gouli A, Kaltsas G, Tzonou A, Gouli A, Kaltsas G, Tzonou A, et al. High prevalence of autonomous aldosterone secretion among patients with essential hypertension. Eur J Clin Invest. 2011. doi:doi: 10.1111/j.1365-2362.2011.02531.x.
81. Androulakis II, Kaltsas GA, Markou A, et al. The functional status of incidentally discovered bilateral adrenal lesions. Clin Endocrinol (Oxf). 2011. doi:doi: 10.1111/j.1365-2265.2011.04013.x.
82. Vasan RS, Evans JC, Larson MG, et al. Serum aldosterone and the incidence of hypertension in nonhypertensive persons. N Engl J Med. 2004;351:33–41.
83. Hatakeyama H, Miyamori I, Fujita T, et al. Vascular aldosterone. Biosynthesis and a link to angiotensin II-induced hypertrophy of vascular smooth muscle cells. Biol Chem. 1994;269:24316–20.
84. Gómez-Sánchez EP, Zhou M, Gomez-Sanchez CE. Mineralocorticoids, salt and high blood pressure. Steroids. 1996;61:184–8.
85. Rocha R, Funder JW. The pathophysiology of aldosterone in the cardiovascular system. Ann N Y Acad Sci. 2002;970:89–100.
86. Ariton M, Juan CS, AvRuskin TW. Pheochromocytoma: clinical observations from a Brooklyn tertiary hospital. Endocr Pract. 2000;6:249–52.
87. Pacak K, Eisenhofer G. An assessment of biochemical tests for the diagnosis of pheochromocytoma. Nat Clin Pract Endocrinol Metab. 2007;3:744–5.
88. Zelinka T, Eisenhofer G, Pacak K. Pheochromocytoma as a catecholamine producing tumor: implications for clinical practice. Stress. 2007;10:195–203.
89. Manger WM, Gifford Jr RW, Hoffman BB. Pheochromocytoma: a clinical and experimental overview. Curr Probl Cancer. 1985;9:1–89.
90. Bernini GP, Vivaldi MS, Argenio GF, et al. Frequency of pheochromocytoma in adrenal incidentalomas and utility of the glucagon test for the diagnosis. J Endocrinol Invest. 1997;20:65–71.
91. Kasperlik-Zeluska AA, Rosłonowska E, Słowinska-Srzednicka J, et al. Incidentally discovered adrenal mass (incidentaloma): investigation and management of 208 patients. Clin Endocrinol (Oxf). 1997;46:29–37.
92. Mannelli M, Ianni L, Cilotti A, et al. Pheochromocytoma in Italy: a multicentric retrospective study. Eur J Endocrinol. 1999;141:619–24.

93. Noshiro T, Shimizu K, Watanabe T, et al. Changes in clinical features and long-term prognosis in patients with pheochromocytoma. Am J Hypertens. 2000;13:35–43.
94. Bülow B, Ahrén B; Swedish Research Council Study Group of Endocrine Abdominal Tumours. Adrenal incidentaloma—experience of a standardized diagnostic programme in the Swedish prospective study. J Intern Med. 2002;252:239–46.
95. Amar L, Servais A, Gimenez-Roqueplo AP, et al. Year of diagnosis, features at presentation, and risk of recurrence in patients with pheochromocytoma or secreting paraganglioma. J Clin Endocrinol Metab. 2005;90:2110–6.
96. Kasperlik-Zaluska AA, Roslonowska E, Slowinska-Srzednicka J, et al. 1,111 patients with adrenal incidentalomas observed at a single endocrinological center: incidence of chromaffin tumors. Ann N Y Acad Sci. 2006;1073:38–46.
97. Adler JT, Mack E, Chen H. Isolated adrenal mass in patients with a history of cancer: remember pheochromocytoma. Ann Surg Oncol. 2007;14:2358–62.
98. Angeli A, Osella G, Alì A, et al. Adrenal incidentaloma: an overview of clinical and epidemiological data from the National Italian Study Group. Horm Res. 1997;47:279–83.
99. Lee JA, Zarnegar R, Shen WT, et al. Adrenal incidentaloma, borderline elevations of urine or plasma metanephrine levels, and the "subclinical" pheochromocytoma. Arch Surg. 2007;142:870–3.
100. Kopetschke R, Slisko M, Kilisli A, et al. Frequent incidental discovery of phaeochromocytoma: data from a German cohort of 201 phaeochromocytoma. Eur J Endocrinol. 2009;161: 355–61.
101. Grozinsky-Glasberg S, Szalat A, Benbassat CA, et al. Clinically silent chromaffin-cell tumors: tumor characteristics and long-term prognosis in patients with incidentally discovered pheochromocytomas. J Endocrinol Invest. 2010;33:739–44.
102. Wagnerova H, Dudasova D, Lazurova I. Hormonal and metabolic evaluation of adrenal incidentalomas. Neoplasma. 2009;56:521–5.
103. Yilmaz H, Tütüncü NB, Sahin M. Two-year follow-up of thirty-two non-functional benign adrenal incidentalomas. J Endocrinol Invest. 2009;32:913–6.
104. Peppa M, Boutati E, Koliaki C, et al. Insulin resistance and metabolic syndrome in patients with nonfunctioning adrenal incidentalomas: a cause-effect relationship? Metabolism. 2010;59:1435–41.
105. Reincke M, Fassnacht M, Väth S, et al. Adrenal incidentalomas: a manifestation of the metabolic syndrome? Endocr Res. 1996;22:757–61.

Chapter 7
Pheochromocytoma: Unmasking the Chameleon

Jeremyjones F. Robles, Leilani B. Mercado-Asis, and Karel Pacak

Abstract Pheochromocytomas and extraadrenal paragangliomas are functional tumors of the neuroendocrine system. They can secrete excessive amounts of catecholamines and although signs and symptoms may vary, generally they present as hypertension accompanied by sympathetic signs and symptoms.

Plasma or urine metanephrines are reliable biochemical tests that are sensitive to detect patients with biochemically active tumors. CT-scan and MRI are anatomic imaging tests that remain vital for accurate pre-operative assessment. Functional imaging can be diagnostic and therapeutic; it enables detection of tumor extent and assesses possible response to therapy.

Focus on genetic studies for familial predisposition for early detection is now at the forefront of research. Identification of *SDHB* mutations warrants aggressive treatment because of the propensity of these tumors for metastases with poor prognosis.

Surgery remains the cornerstone of treatment with potential cure for benign tumors and palliative management. Long-term follow-up is necessary to detect recurrences and metastases. Malignancy still holds poor prognosis as therapeutic options remain limited. Radiopharmaceutical and chemotherapy remains promising but no major breakthroughs have been achieved. Palliative care and lesion-based treatment remains the standard.

Keywords Pheochromocytoma • Paragangliomas • Secondary hypertension • Secondary diabetes mellitus

---

J.F. Robles • K. Pacak (✉)
Program in Reproductive and Adult Endocrinology, Eunice Kennedy Shriver National Institute of Child Health and Human Development, National Institute of Health, NIH Building 10, Center Drive, CRC, 1-East, Room 1-3140, MSC 1109, Bethesda, MD, USA
e-mail: karel@mail.nih.gov

L.B. Mercado-Asis
Section of Endocrinology and Metabolism, University of Santo Tomas Hospital, Manila, Philippines

C.A. Koch and G.P. Chrousos (eds.), *Endocrine Hypertension: Underlying Mechanisms and Therapy*, Contemporary Endocrinology, DOI 10.1007/978-1-60761-548-4_7,

Introduction

A pheochromocytoma is a rare catecholamine-producing tumor that can manifest as spells of hypertension accompanied by symptoms of sympathetic nervous system activation. Other patients remain asymptomatic and discovery of the tumor may be incidental. Diagnosis is challenging because there is no consistent clinical presentation. A significant number of patients remain misdiagnosed with potential fatal consequences.

As a physician, the task is to be able to consider these tumors in difficult cases of hypertension. Long-term complications related to cardiovascular effects from chronic exposure to high levels of catecholamines lead to significant morbidity. Early diagnosis and aggressive treatment can prevent this poor outcome.

Proving it is pheochromocytoma entails biochemical confirmation followed by accurate localization with imaging tests. Developments in the diagnosis of pheochromocytoma now favor the use of fractionated plasma metanephrines, while improvements in imaging studies now utilize combined PET and CT imaging to identify accurately the locations and reveal the extent of tumors. Identification of familial syndromes and gene mutations related to pheochromocytoma now emphasizes the important role of genetics in the detection of the disease especially among the young. Management requires adequate control of hypertension and its related symptoms with appropriate medications in preparation for definitive treatment, which is surgery.

Definitions

We define a pheochromocytoma as an intraadrenal paraganglioma and an extraadrenal pheochromocytoma as a sympathetic paraganglioma in the thorax, abdomen and pelvis, and other parts of the body [1]. These two have similar morphology and identical neuroendocrine phenotype and may sometimes share genetic predisposition [2]. In contrast, parasympathetic paragangliomas are tumors found in the head and neck.

Incidence

The prevalence among hypertensive patients is less than 0.1% [3, 4]. The Rochester epidemiology project reported an average annual incidence of 1 per 100,000 with half of the patients that were diagnosed during autopsy [5]. They can be found at any age group but the peak age is between 40 and 50 years old with almost equal male to female ratio [6]. Among adrenal incidentalomas up to 19% have been found to have pheochromocytoma [7].

Genetic Syndromes

Familial pheochromocytoma is associated with large, bilateral, multifocal, and extraadrenal tumors [8, 9]. Upto 27.4% were found to be hereditary in nature. The five most common genetic syndromes associated with pheochromocytoma are neurofibromatosis 1 (NF1), von Hippel-Lindau (VHL) syndrome, multiple endocrine neoplasia 2 (MEN2), and the paraganglioma syndromes (PGL1, PGL3, and PGL4). All of them are autosomal dominant.

Neurofibromatosis, with a defect in the NF1 gene, can present clinically with manifestations of multiple fibromas, café au lait spots and axillary skin freckling, and lisch nodules on the iris [10]. Pheochromocytoma is a minor feature occurring only in <5.5% [11]. They occur in the older age group as a single intraadrenal lesion that is usually benign [12, 13]. Since clinical diagnosis is straightforward, genetic testing is usually not carried out [8].

VHL syndrome results from a mutation in the VHL gene [14]. They are characterized by retinal and craniospinal hemangioblastomas, endolymphatic sac tumors, renal and pancreatic tumors or cyst, and broad ligament cystadenoma. Pheochromocytomas occur in 10–20% with a mean age of 30 years old [15]. They present as multiple intraadrenal tumors that secrete predominantly norepinephrine (NE) [16–18]. Long-term morbidity and mortality of patients with VHL syndrome are related to complications from complications of hemangioblastomas and metastatic renal cell carcinoma.

Multiple endocrine neoplasia (MEN) 2A and 2B have defects on the RET gene. Medullary thyroid cancer and pheochromocytomas are common to both syndromes. MEN2A has a predisposition to primary parathyroid hyperplasia while MEN2B may present with mucosal gangliomas. Approximately 50% of MEN 2 patients may have the related pheochromocytoma [8]. Age of onset is between 30 and 40 years old. They present with benign unilateral or bilateral lesions confined to the adrenal glands [19, 20]. In comparison to VHL-related pheochromocytomas, MEN2-related pheochromocytomas are more symptomatic and secrete more of epinephrine (EPI) [17]. Medullary thyroid cancer usually precedes the diagnosis of pheochromocytoma [21]. Early prophylactic thyroidectomy is recommended especially for MEN 2B [22, 23].

Succinate dehydrogenase (SDH)-related mitochondrial dysfunction leads to upregulation of hypoxic and angiogenic pathways that are believed to be involved in malignancy [24, 25]. Distinct clinical phenotypes have been identified with its subunits, SDHA with congenital Leigh syndrome, SDHB, SDHC, and SDHD with paraganglioma syndromes.

Paraganglioma syndrome 1 with SDHD mutation is closely related to head and neck paragangliomas, and then with multifocal tumors in the chest, abdomen, or pelvis [26]. Adrenal, head, and neck paragangliomas are always multiple but benign [26, 27]. Age-related penetrance is about 50% by the age of 30 years old [28]. Transmission is also autosomal dominant but may be masked by maternal imprinting resulting in only paternal transmission [29].

Paraganglioma syndrome 3 associated with SDHC mutation also manifest as head and neck tumors that are benign and seldom multifocal [30]. Its prevalence among head and neck paragangliomas is only 4%, but screening is recommended to identify the risk of inheritance. Clinical behavior appears to be similar to that of benign sporadic head and neck paragangliomas with a younger age presentation.

Paraganglioma syndrome 4 with SDHB mutation is the most significant. It is associated with paragangliomas of in head, neck, thorax, abdomen, and pelvis [27]. Frequency of mutation in pheochromocytoma patients is 7% [8]. They occur more commonly as extraadrenal tumors often multifocal [26]. Age-related penetrance is exhibited with a 50% risk of developing pheochromocytomas by the age of 30–35 years old [9]. The predominant biochemical secretion consists of NE or dopamine (DA) [31]. Carriers are known to have high risk of developing metastatic tumors with generally poorer prognosis [32–35]. Thus, in the presence of this mutation, management should be aggressive and prompt genetic testing of all first-degree relatives should be pursued to determine the presence of family-specific mutation [36].

Genetic Testing and Considerations

Selective genetic testing for genetic syndromes is recommended. Key considerations should include the presence of bilateral tumors that are more common to mutations of RET, VHL, and SDHB. These tumors may not occur at the same time, thus warrants close follow-up [37]. Pheochromocytomas associated with MEN2 always produce EPI while VHL-related pheochromocytomas secrete predominantly norepinephrine [17,18]. The presence of SDHB mutation should always be considered in metastatic pheochromocytoma since they have worse prognosis [34]. In general, patients with familial history for paragangliomas, multiple, extraadrenal tumors, or those presenting at young age are good candidates for genetic testing of pheochromocytoma [38].

Catecholamine Metabolism

The metabolism of catecholamines begins with tyrosine converted to 3,4-dihydroxyphenylalanine (DOPA) by the cystosolic enzyme tyrosine hydroxylase. This enzyme is found in the neurons of the central nervous system, sympathetic nerves, and chromaffin-producing cells [39]. This is the rate-limiting step of catecholamine synthesis that can be targeted by the pharmacologic agent metyrosine. Aromatic amino acid decarboxylase then catalyzes the conversion of DOPA to DA. The vesicular monoamine transporter (VMAT) is a membrane-embedded protein that transports monoamine neurotransmitter molecules into intraneuronal storage vesicles [40]. DA is transported into the storage vesicles where it is converter to NE by DA hydroxylase.

Phenylethanolamine *N*-methyltransferase (PNMT) is the enzyme responsible for conversion of norepinephrine to EPI [41]. It is largely restricted to the adrenal medulla but with detectable levels in the brain. EPI, NE, and DA are stored in the granules within chromaffin cells. EPI is derived mainly from the adrenal medulla while NE is produced from sympathetic nerves innervating the mesenteric organs, kidneys, and skeletal muscles [42]. Once released, NE acts on α1-adrenoceptors triggering vasoconstriction and hypertension. EPI acts on β2-adrenoceptors of the skeletal muscle vasculature causing vasodilation and hypotension [43].

The major pathway of metabolism of catecholamines occurs in the sympathetic neuronal cells involving the sequential action of monoamine oxidase (MAO) and aldose reductase on NE to form dihydroxyphenylglycol (DHPG). This by-product provides a biochemical index of NE turnover that increases with elevated levels of norepinephrine. Increments in NE concentrations can be estimated by simultaneous measurements of DHPG [44]. EPI is also metabolized to DHPG in the same manner. As DHPG diffuses to the extracellular fluid, it is metabolized by catechol-*O*-methyltransferase (COMT) to become methoxyhydroxyphenylglycol (MHPG). MHPG is converted in the liver by alcohol dehydrogenase to become the end product vanillylmandelic acid (VMA). DA is also acted upon by MAO and converted to dihydroxyphenylacetic acid (DOPAC). DOPAC is metabolized to homovanillic acid (HVA) becoming the end product of DA metabolism.

The alternate pathway begins with O-methylation of COMT of EPI, NE, and DA to their metabolites metanephrine, normetanephrine, and methoxytyramine, respectively [45]. This normally occurs in the extraneuronal tissues and adrenal chromaffin cells as a minor pathway but becomes the major pathway in pheochromocytoma cells. As metabolites of COMT, metanephrines reflect the actual levels of production of the chromaffin cells. Metanephrine and normetanephrine can be deaminated to form MHPG while methoxytyramine is converted directly to HVA. All catecholamines and their metabolites can be converted to sulfate-conjugated metabolites by sulfotransferase (SULT1A3) and are slowly removed through the urine [46].

Pheochromocytoma cells produce over 94% of the elevated plasma metanephrine and normetanephrine, which is derived from the metabolism of catecholamines it produces. This is done continuously and independently of any variations in catecholamine release [45].

Hypertension and Cardiovascular Consequences

The manifestations of pheochromocytoma represent periods of sudden release of catecholamines from the tumor. Hypertension is always accompanied by symptoms of catecholamines excess. A typical spell would begin with generalized pounding headache, palpitations, tachycardia, sweating, tremors, anxiety, and feeling of impending doom [47]. They usually occur weekly but can occur more often. Episodes last mostly within an hour often followed by generalized weakness and exhaustion. They may be precipitated by palpation of the tumor, postural changes, exertion, anxiety, trauma, pain, ingestion of foods or beverages containing tyramine (certain cheeses, beers, and wines), use of certain drugs (histamine, glucagon, tyramine, phenothiazine, metoclopramide, adrenocorticotropic hormone (ACTH)), intubation, induction of anesthesia, and operative manipulation [48].

Hypertension is a common presentation but its occurrence may be inconsistent. Half of the patients will have paroxysms while a third will present with persistent hypertension, and the rest can be normotensive [4]. EPI and NE have overlapping but

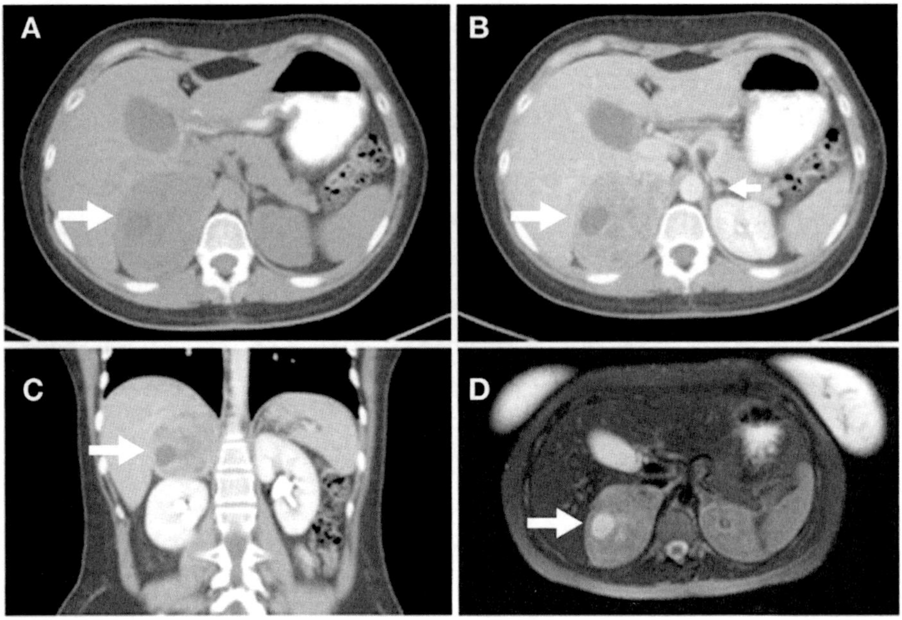

Fig. 7.1 A 23-year-old female who presented with severe left flank pain with normal blood pressure. Biochemical testing revealed elevated plasma and urine normetanephrine levels. Anatomic imaging showed the following results. (**a**) A large right suprarenal mass (*thick arrow*) measuring 8.5×6.3×7.2 cm. (**b**) The left adrenal gland is normal in size (*thin arrow*). (**c**) Axial images show the mass abutting the right lobe of the liver with heterogeneous enhancement on contrast. (**d**) T2-weighted MRI shows a heterogeneously enhancing right suprarenal mass. Patient had right adrenalectomy and the tumor was confirmed to be pheochromocytoma on pathology

distinct actions on the different groups of adrenoceptors [50]. NE causes α1-mediated vasoconstriction resulting in hypertension. EPI has a more potent effect on β2-adrenoceptors causing vasodilation resulting in hypotension. Both stimulate β1-adrenoceptors resulting in increased heart rate. EPI-secreting pheochromocytomas show episodic symptoms with signs of palpitations, lightheadedness, anxiety, and hyperglycemia. NE producing pheochromocytomas have more consistent symptoms of hypertension, sweating, and headache. DA predominant tumors usually present with normal blood pressure [50, 51] (Fig. 7.1) rarely with hypotension [52].

Desensitization of β-adrenoceptors can occur with prolonged stimulation of cells leading to diminished responsiveness of the cells to subsequent activation by catecholamines [53]. Other substances known to contribute to the clinical picture of pheochromocytoma include vasoactive intestinal peptide (VIP), ACTH, neuropeptide Y (NYP), atrial natriuretic peptide (ANP), growth hormone-releasing factor, somatostatin, parathyroid hormone-related peptide, calcitonin, and serotonin [54].

Sudden massive catecholamine release can cause severe vasoconstriction that can lead to severe cardiac dysrhythmias and pulmonary edema [55]. This can reflect on electrocardiography as prolonged QT interval and ST-T wave abnormalities mimicking coronary artery disease [56, 57]. Cardiomyopathy, acute myocarditis, cardiogenic shock, and sudden death are rare yet lethal complications that have been associated with pheochromocytoma [57–59]. Although the cause may be multifactorial and complex, injury to the myocardium from excess catecholamine plays a significant role. Pathologic examinations have revealed multifocal myocyte necrosis and replacement fibrosis with mixed inflammatory inflammation [60]. This can lead to intravascular hypovolemia and decreased cardiac output. The influence of catecholamines on vascular wall growth and thickening is believed to be the reason why there is a significant increase of intima-media thickness (IMT) in the common carotid artery of patients with pheochromocytoma [61].

Reversal of clinical manifestations and improvement in cardiac function were reported in several studies suggesting that early detection and intervention can prevent these fatal consequences [57–69, 62, 63].

Biochemical Evidence of Pheochromocytoma

Pheochromocytoma cells continuously metabolize catecholamines to metanephrines. Metanephrines reflect the actual levels of production of catecholamines in chromaffin cells. Subsequent studies have established that measurement of plasma or urine metanephrines for the diagnosis of pheochromocytoma was found to be superior to all other previous diagnostic tests [64–66]. Plasma metanephrines are measured in the free form while the urinary metanephrines are measured in the deconjugated form, both of which have advantages and disadvantages but with comparable results [66]. Measurement of plasma or urinary methoxytyramine may be done to detect DA-producing tumors [67]. Elevations of more than four times above the reference interval for both plasma and urine fractionated metanephrines are associated with almost 100% probability of having pheochromocytoma [64].

At present, liquid chromatography with tandem mass spectrometry (LC-MS/MS) is the ideal method for measuring plasma and urine fractionated metanephrines [68, 69]. This provides an effective method of purification with reduced interference from chromatographic contaminants such as medications. This method enables combined measurement of plasma NE, EPI, DA, and other metabolites such as DOPA, the precursor of catecholamines, and DOPAC, the deaminated metabolite of DA. While DHPG reflects the intraneuronal turnover of norepinephrine DOPA provides information on synthesis and transmission catecholamines. This enables comprehensive analysis of the dynamics of the patient's catecholamine system. Its limitation is primarily the cost and availability as only specialized centers are equipped to run these methods. High-pressure liquid chromatography (HPLC) remains the most common analytical method for biogenic amine quantitation. Its overall sensitivity and specificity is reported at 98 and 92%, respectively [70]. Enzyme-linked immunosorbent assay (ELISA) may also be used to determine the levels of metanephrines at sensitivity lower than liquid chromatography [71].

The phenotype of hormone secreted by the tumor can also provide information about the size and location of the tumor [72]. There is a strong positive relationship

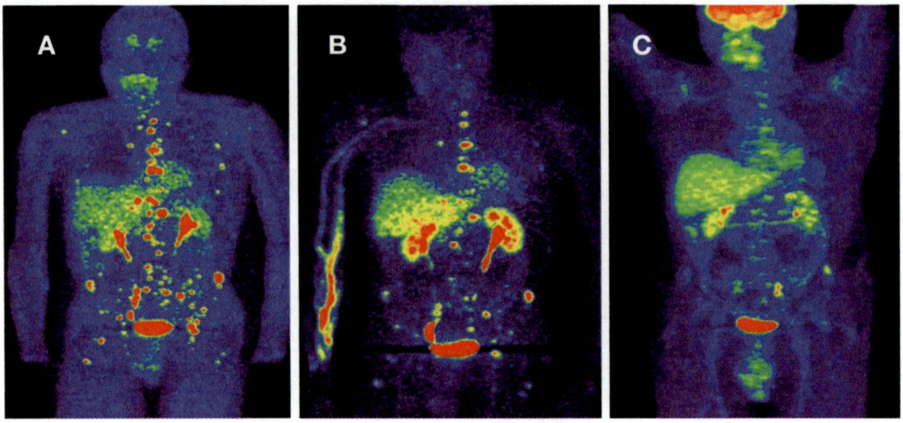

Fig. 7.2 A 24-year-old male presented with episodic hypertension. Several of his relatives were previously diagnosed with pheochromocytoma. Biochemical evaluation showed very high levels of plasma and urine normetanephrine. CT and MRI revealed a 3.6×2.6×2.8 cm retroperitoneal mass medial to the left kidney with multiple metastatic bone lesions. Functional imaging reveals the extent of metastatic disease using (**a**) FDA, (**b**) FDOPA, and (**c**) FDG PET imaging. Increased uptake of tracer is noted on the lumbar vertebrae, sacrum, and pelvis. The primary tumor was removed and the patient underwent chemotherapy. Genetic testing revealed that he had an SDHB mutation

between tumor diameter and summed plasma concentrations of free normetanephrine and metanephrine [72]. Adrenal tumors produce relatively high concentrations of plasma-free metanephrine compared to normetanephrine. Comparing sporadic and familial pheochromocytoma, biochemical parameters were found to be higher in sporadic than hereditary tumors [65]. Characteristic secretion patterns for syndromic pheochromocytomas reveal that MEN 2 patients secrete predominantly high metanephrines while VHL patients secrete more normetanephrine [18, 72] (Fig. 7.2).

Confounding Factors

Medications known to affect the results include phenoxybenzamine and tricyclic antidepressants, which are most frequently associated with false-positive results in plasma and urinary norepinephrine and normetanephrine. Selective α1-adrenoceptor blocking drugs, doxazosin, terazosin, and prazosin only increased urinary norepinephrine levels. β-Adrenoceptor blockers increase plasma metanephrine and urinary NE levels. Calcium channel blockers elevate plasma norepinephrine. Diuretics, angiotensin converting enzyme inhibitors, and angiotensin-1 receptor blockers have no influence on frequencies of false-positive biochemical results for any of the analytes [73].

Patient positioning at the time of blood extraction was found to affect the levels of plasma metanephrines. Upper reference limits of plasma-free metanephrines were higher in samples obtained from seated patients without preceding rest than from supine patients with preceding rest [74]. Catecholamine rich-diet only had substantial effects on plasma and urinary levels of free and deconjugated methoxytyramine [75].

An intravenous catheter should be inserted on the arm prior to letting the patient rest comfortable in the supine position for at least 20 min. Blood will be drawn from the catheter with the patient in supine position. Blood tests are best taken in the morning after an overnight fast.

Pharmacologic Test

The clonidine suppression test is utilized to distinguish between patients with pheochromocytoma and other causes of sympathetic activation [76]. Clonidine activates α2-adrenoceptors in the brain and sympathetic nervous system to suppress the release of NE. Baseline blood samples are taken for plasma normetanephrine followed by clonidine given at 0.3 mg/70 kg dose. Repeat plasma normetanephrine determination after 3 h should show a decrease in plasma normetanephrine of 40% from baseline values. Positive response consistent with pheochromocytoma is a lack of clonidine-induced suppression combined with a plasma normetanephrine concentration above the upper reference limit. Sensitivity of this test was reported at 96% with a specificity of 98–100% [73]. The use of glucagon stimulation test is no longer recommended because of the lack of sensitivity and risk for hypertensive complications. Glucagon-provoked increases in plasma catecholamines only revealed the presence of the tumor in less than 50% of affected patients [77].

Ancillary Laboratory Tests

The pro-hormone chromogranin A is also being utilized as an adjunct biochemical test in the diagnosis of pheochromocytoma [78–80]. It is secreted by a variety of peptide-producing endocrine neoplasms including pheochromocytoma, parathyroid adenoma, medullary thyroid cancer, carcinoids, oat-cell lung cancer, pancreatic islet-cell tumors, and aortic-body tumor [78]. Studies have established significant positive relationship between chromogranin A levels, tumor mass, and malignancy [81–83]. Serial measurements can be used to monitor treatment response.

Patients with pheochromocytomas may present with hyperglycemia because of α2-adrenergic inhibition of insulin release, EPI-induced inhibition of glucose uptake, adrenergic stimulation of hepatic glucose production, and α-adrenergic receptor desensitization. In young patients with hypertension and normal body weight, the presence of diabetes is a clinical clue to the diagnosis of pheochromocytoma [84, 85].

The main effect of the excess catecholamine secretion on lipid metabolism was increased lipolytic activity, lower serum triglyceride (TGL), and increased high density lipoprotein (HDL) cholesterol concentrations [86]. Treatment of pheochromocytoma with β-blockers may worsen the lipid profile of these patients by decreasing HDL and increasing TGL. In contrast, the selective α1-blocker increases HDL cholesterol and decreases TGL.

Patients suspected of having MEN 2 syndrome should be tested for intact parathyroid and serum calcium to rule out primary hyperparathyroidism. Serum calcitonin levels are elevated in patients with medullary thyroid cancer. Complete blood count may reveal transient leucocytosis during spells. Polycythemia from erythropoietin may be noted in VHL patients.

Most of the metabolic derangements noted during the diagnosis of pheochromocytoma are usually improved or reversed after the tumor is removed.

Tumor Localization Using Anatomical Imaging

Generally, imaging studies for pheochromocytoma follow biochemical diagnosis. This should be initiated if clinical evidence is strong and biochemical tests are positive. Patients with previous history of the tumors and hereditary predisposition are the exception [64]. Anatomical imaging is done to provide precise localization while functional imaging reveals nature, activity, and extent of the lesions. The CT and the MRI can detect tumors within the adrenal with a minimum size of 0.5–1 cm in diameter and extraadrenal lesions of at least 1–2 cm [87]. CT is fast and readily available in most medical centers. MRI has higher sensitivity, superior contrast resolution for extraadrenal lesions, and lacks ionizing radiation. It is the procedure of choice for children, pregnant women, and patients with allergies to contrast material.

Unenhanced CT provides density measurements of the lesions while succeeding delayed contrast studies quantify the washout characteristics and surrounding vascularity [88, 89]. The attenuation coefficient of lesions expressed as hounsfield units (HU) has been used to differentiate adrenal adenomas from tumors such as pheochromocytoma; values more than 10 HU supports the diagnosis of pheochromocytoma [90, 91]. Most sporadic pheochromocytomas are described as 2–3 cm in diameter with smaller lesion with homogenous appearance and larger lesions with inhomogenous appearance attributed to hemorrhage and necrosis [92]. On MRI, the T1-weighted sequences are equal to or higher than that of the liver, kidney, and muscle. T2-weighted MRI appearance is variable with smaller lesions appearing homogenous and larger lesions heterogeneous. Increasing heterogeneity correlated pathologically with increasing amounts of hemorrhage, necrosis, and fibrosis [93]. Pheochromocytomas enhance avidly with contrast and have a prolonged washout period. The addition of MR angiographic sequences is helpful in assessing the vascular supply of paragangliomas particularly in carotid body tumors [94]. In general, the majority of paragangliomas arise from the adrenal medulla. Of the 15% found outside of the adrenals, 46% are found in the renal hilum, 29% of the organ of Zuckerkandl, 10% of the thoracic paraspinal region, 10% in the bladder, and 2–4% of the head and neck region [95]. By order of significance, initial scan should be done on the abdomen and pelvis followed by the chest and neck.

Tumor Localization Using Functional Imaging

Functional imaging studies are done to prove that the tumor is pheochromocytoma and to reveal its extent. Radiolabeled ligands specific for catecholamine synthesis and metabolism as well as nonspecific ligands are utilized in nuclear imaging techniques to detect pheochromocytoma [96]. Metaiodobenzylguanidine (MIBG) is an analog of NE that is taken up by the human norepinephrine transporter system (hNET) into sympathomedullary cells and stored in the secretory granules via the VMAT [96]. MIBG has high affinity to hNET system but does not bind to adrenergic receptors nor metabolized [97]. ^{123}Iodine (^{123}I) is preferentially used over ^{131}iodine (^{131}I) as label because it allows better image quality, greater sensitivity, and reduced radiation exposure due to higher photon flow and shorter half-life [98]. Overall sensitivity in several series ranged between 75 and 89% [99, 100]. Sensitivity was consistently higher for adrenal and sporadic pheochromocytoma [100, 101].

Positron emission tomography (PET) imaging is a functional imaging technique based on detection of coincident photons originating from the annihilation of emitted positrons with electrons from surrounding tissues [102]. Biological substances labeled with positron emitters reveal lesions within minutes or hours after administration. It produces superior quality of images and subject patients to relatively low radiation exposure [97]. Combined anatomical and functional imaging has now been used to localize lesions with greater accuracy [102]. Complementing functional and anatomic imaging facilitates the distinction between pheochromocytoma and physiologic tracer accumulation in normal adrenal tissue [103].

Specific radioligands pass through the membrane hNET and target-specific steps in catecholamine metabolism. ^{11}C EPI and ^{11}C-hydroxyephedrine (^{11}C-HED) are NE analogs that were the first positron-emitting tracers for the sympathetic nervous system. ^{18}F-fluorodopamine (FDA) is an analog of DA that is taken in by both the plasma membrane and intracellular vesicular transporters in catecholamine secreting cells. Several studies have reported the utility of FDA imaging in the diagnosis pheochromocytoma [104–106]. It has comparable results with MIBG in detecting non-metastatic pheochromocytomas but higher sensitivity for metastatic lesions [107]. Established standard uptake values (SUV) for physiologic uptake of normal adrenal glands was <7.3 while pheochromocytoma-related uptake was >10.1 [103]. FDA results in lower radiation dose and faster procedure time. Its use is advocated for the evaluation of biochemically established adrenal, extraadrenal, and metastatic paragangliomas in localizing primary tumors and ruling out multifocal and metastatic lesions [108].

Nonspecific functional imaging labeled tracers utilize the amino acid transport system, glucose transporter, and somatostatin receptor. ^{18}Fluoro-L-dihydroxyphenylalanine (F-DOPA) is transported into the cell by the large amino acid transporter 2 (LAT2), then decarboxylated to ^{18}F-FDA, and then transported inside the vesicles through the VMAT. Pretreatment with carbidopa enhances the sensitivity of ^{18}F-DOPA for adrenal and extraadrenal paragangliomas by increasing the tumor to background ratio of tracer uptake [109]. This imaging was also found to be superior to MIBG scintigraphy with an overall sensitivity of 90% and specificity of 93% [110, 111]. ^{18}F-DOPA has the advantage of having little physiologic uptake in healthy adrenal tissues compared to previously imaging modalities [112]. Combining ^{18}F-DOPA with CT or MRI imaging improves sensitivity to 93–100% [110, 111]. Sensitivity of ^{18}F-DOPA for metastases associated with SDHB appears to be limited [109].

^{18}Fluoro-2-deoxy-D-glucose (FDG) PET scanning reflects excessive glucose uptake by the glucose transporter-1 (GLUT-1) among cancer cells related to a shift to anaerobic glycolysis known as the "Warburg effect" [113]. Uptake was reflective of inherent metastatic tendency and aggressive behavior [114]. Sensitivity was highest for SDHB metastatic lesions reaching 100%, a finding that is linked directly to the tumor biology of SDHB lesions [115]. False-positive results have been reported with areas with infection and inflammation [114].

Somatostatin receptor scintigraphy is used to detect the presence of somatostatin receptors types 1, 2a, and 3 in neuroendocrine tumors [116]. 111-Indium labeled octreotide is a radiolabeled somatostatin analog specific to somatostatin receptor 2 used for diagnosis and therapy for neuroendocrine tumors [117]. It can detect metastatic pheochromocytoma and head and neck paragangliomas with a sensitivity of 89% [118, 119]. Physiologic uptake is observed mainly in the kidneys [120]. Infection and inflammation are known to produce false-positive results [121].

In summary, the ^{18}F-FDA and ^{18}F-DOPA are the ideal imaging procedures to localize the primary tumor and rule out metastasis. The ^{18}F-DOPA is particularly useful in patients with head and neck paragangliomas [122]. ^{18}F-FDG is the best imaging procedure for SDHB-related pheochromocytoma. ^{123}I-MIBG and octreotide scan serves as an alternative imaging procedures that are also used to evaluate possible response to radiotherapy. Bone scintigraphy plays a role in staging of malignant pheochromocytoma especially with SDHB mutation [123] (Fig. 7.3).

Medical Treatment

Control of hypertension and accompanying symptoms are the immediate concerns that need to be addressed. The drug of choice is phenoxybenzamine, an irreversible, noncompetitive, α-adrenoceptor blocker. Its half-life is 24 h. Total daily dose of 1 mg/kg/day can be given in two to three divided doses and titrated accordingly. Initial dose can be started at 10 mg twice a day and increased in increments of 10–20 mg every 2–3 days [124]. Appropriate dosing can control paroxysms of hypertension and maintain BP at optimum level. Significant postural hypotension, reflex tachycardia, vomiting, and shock can be observed if the dose is too high.

Other α-blockers that can be used include prazosin given at 2–5 mg two to three times a day, Terazosin at 2–5 mg/day, and doxazosin at 2–8 mg/day. These are selective α1-adrenoceptor blockers that decrease total peripheral resistance and venous return. Severe hypotension may be observed after the first dose warranting it to be given at bedtime. Succeeding dose adjustments can be done more quickly with fewer side effects.

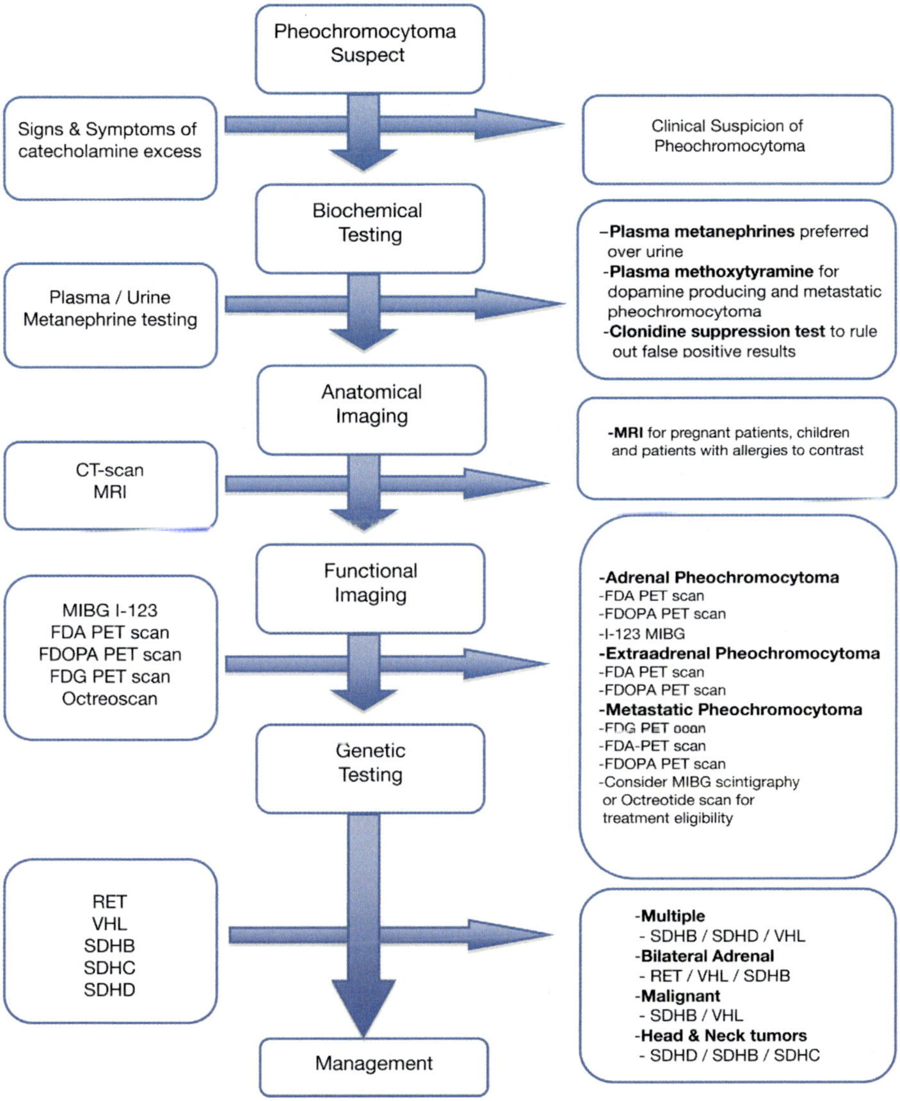

Fig. 7.3 Diagnostic approach to pheochromocytoma

β-Adrenoceptor blockers compliment the action of α-blockers in controlling hypertension. They also help control tachycardia brought about by catecholamine release or induced by α-adrenoceptor blockers. β1-selective blocker atenolol can be given at 12.5–25 mg two to three times a day or Metoprolol given at 25–50 mg three to four times a day. Alternatively, nonselective beta adrenoceptor blockers such as propanolol, timolol, nadolol, penbutolol, and sotalol can be used. Combined alpha and β-adrenoceptor blockers are not recommended because the fixed ratio favors beta blocking over alpha blocking effect. Emphasis is placed on starting after starting α-adrenoceptor blockers before β-adrenoceptor blockers because unopposed α-receptor activation can result to hypertensive crises [125].

Calcium channel blockers can be used as the primary antihypertensive drug in low-risk patients [124]. As an alternative, it can replace adrenoceptor blockers in case side effects cannot be tolerated or when hypotension is noted on intermittently hypertensive pheochromocytoma patients since they do not cause hypotension during normotensive period [126]. These drugs block the norepinephrine-mediated calcium influx into vascular muscle controlling hypertension and tachyarrhythmias. It can also be used as an additional medication for patients who remain hypertensive despite maximal adrenergic blocker medications [124]. Amlodipine can be given at 10–20 mg/day, Nicardipine at 60–90 mg/day, Nifedipine 30–90 mg/day, and Verapamil at 180–540 mg/day.

Alpha-methyl-L-tyrosine or metyrosine (Demser) inhibits tyroxine hydroxylase, the rate-limiting step of catecholamine biosynthesis. It depletes catecholamine stores and contributes in the control of hypertension particularly in patients with biochemically active tumors [127–128]. Treatment can be started with 250 mg every 8–12 h and titrated up to 1.5–2 g/day 1–3 weeks before the surgery [124]. Side effects include fatigue diarrhea, anxiety, depression, and cystalluria [129]. Central effects can be explained by the ability of metyrosine to cross the blood brain barrier. Symptoms can resolve when doses are lowered or discontinued.

Preoperative Management

Adrenergic blockade can be started 1–2 weeks prior to scheduled surgery to allow ample time to control hypertension, control the heart rate, and expand contracted volume. Phenoxybenzamine can be titrated daily according to blood pressure response. β-Blocker can be added after 3 days for tachycardic patients. Metyrosine and a calcium channel blocker can be added in patients with uncontrolled hypertension [124]. Last doses of phenoxybenzamine and metyrosine are given at midnight prior to operation.

High salt diet is given a few days after starting α-adrenoceptor blockers to help restore diminished blood volume. Fluid replacement is initiated 2 days prior to surgery and continued throughout the procedure to expand the intravascular volume and reduces the frequency and severity of postoperative hypotension. Hypotension and shock can result from diffuse vasodilation when the tumor is removed.

Surgical Management and Approach

Laparoscopic surgery is the procedure of choice for most pheochromocytomas and sympathetic paragangliomas. It is safe and effective since blood loss was significantly less, postoperative recovery time was shorter, and the procedure is less invasive [130–134]. Option to convert to open surgery should be considered in cases with unexpected difficulty in dissection, invasion, or adhesions [134–138]. Long-term

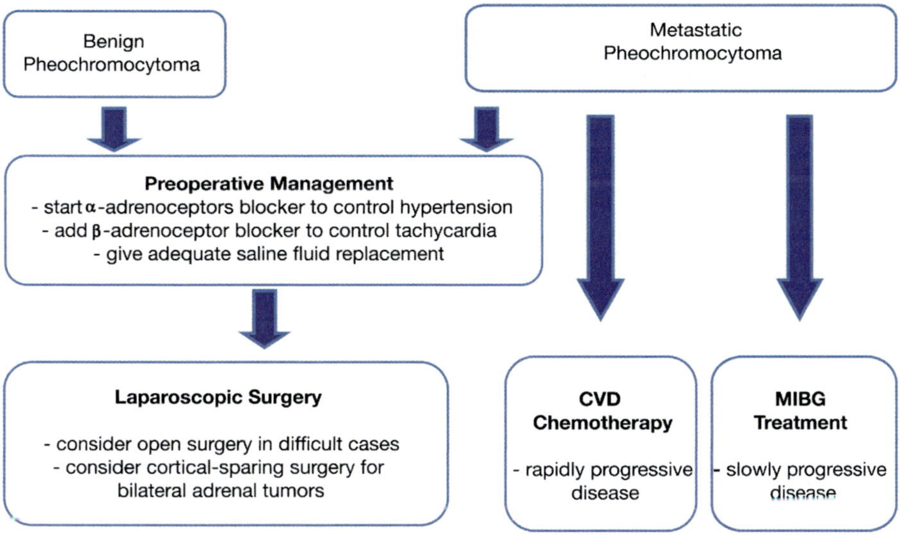

Fig. 7.4 Therapeutic approach to pheochromocytoma

follow-up of post-laparoscopic adrenalectomy patients confirmed favorable outcome beyond 3 years after the procedure [139]. Bilateral cortical sparing surgery should be considered for familial cancer syndromes with bilateral or multiple tumors to avoid the lifelong consequences of bilateral adrenalectomy [140, 141].

These tumors show enormous variability in cytology and histologic pattern that must be differentiated from other neuroendocrine tumors. Gross examination can reveal multiple and bilateral tumors that suggest familial disease. Malignancy is defined as the presence of metastases; local invasion alone is a poor predictor of metastases and the absence of apparent invasion does not preclude the development of metastases [142]. There is no histologic feature nor scoring system that can predict metastatic potential. Standardized pathologic reporting is advocated by the United States Association of Directors of Anatomic and Surgical pathology (ADSP) and the United Kingdom Royal College of Pathologist to include the list of potentially unfavorable findings that can help identify potentially malignant tumors. Immunohistochemical staining for Ki-67 on paraffin sections of monoclonal antibody MIB-1 has been correlated with malignancy but available data needs further support [138, 143] (Fig. 7.4).

Crisis Management

Considering the amount of hormones produced, it is likely that the stress of surgery can trigger the release of vast amounts of catecholamines resulting to uncontrolled hypertension and overall morbidity. Management requires the use of drugs that can be titrated with rapid action and short duration.

Sodium nitroprusside is a nonselective arterial and venous vasodilator that can be given as an infusion. It acts within 30 s and peaks within 2 min and loses its effect after 3 min. Hypertension can be controlled at doses between 0.5 and 5 μg/kg/min [144]. Doses >10 μg/kg/min for >10 min must be reduced or a second agent should be added because of risk of toxicity [145]. This is the first-line drug used to control intraoperative crisis.

Nicardipine is an intravenous dihydropyridine calcium channel blocker that can be utilized to prevent catecholamine-induced coronary vasospasm. Loading dose can be started at 1–2.5 mg for the first 2 min as bolus then maintained as an infusion at 5–15 mg/h [146].

Magnesium sulfate is beta agonist that acts as a vasodilator and antiarrhythmic. It can be used to control the manifestations of catecholamine excess by itself or in combination with other agents [147]. Loading dose of 1–2 g IV can be given, and then continued as IV infusion at 1–3 g/h.

Phentolamine is an intravenous competitive, nonselective α-adrenergic receptor antagonist, with a half-life of 19 min, and may be used as initial therapy for hypertensive crisis as an alternative if other medications are not available. A bolus of 5–15 mg can be given, and then infused at 12–120 mg/h.

Esmolol, a short acting selective β1-adrenergic adrenoceptor antagonist, can be used as adjuvant therapy for uncontrolled tachycardia. Loading dose of 500 μg/kg for 1 min then followed by an infusion at 50–300 μg/kg/min.

Hypotension can occur during surgery particularly after venous clamping and tumor isolation [148]. This can be managed by judicious administration of IV fluids or use of appropriate vasopressors. Phenylephrine can be given to cause α-adrenergic-mediated vasoconstriction without provoking catecholamine release. Alternatively, vasopressin may be used in small bolus doses and continued as infusion [149, 150].

Hypoglycemia can occur as a result of rebound release of insulin secretion after the removal of the tumor. This can be corrected with intravenous infusion of glucose [151]. Blood sugar should be monitored continuously since periods of hypoglycemia may persist for several days [152].

Operative outcome among patients with pheochromocytoma has vastly improved in recent years because of better perioperative management. Nonetheless, success is dependent on close monitoring and critical care by an expert multidisciplinary team.

Malignancy Implications and Management

Prevalence of malignancy has been reported to be between 5 and 26% [153]. SDHB mutation was found in 30–43% of malignant pheochromocytomas and paragangliomas [34, 35, 154]. The most common sites of metastases are the lymph nodes, bones, liver, and lungs. They can be present at the time of diagnosis or appear during recurrence. Overall, 5-year survival rate is between 40 and 74% [155, 156]. It is more common among extraadrenal pheochromocytomas [155, 157]. Malignant pheochromocytoma associated with SDHB mutation generally has a poorer prognosis [33, 154].

The signs and symptoms of catecholamine excess can be manifested in clinically functioning malignant pheochromocytoma [158]. DA can preferentially be secreted due to alterations of catecholamine synthesis in malignant pheochromocytoma cells [155]. Measurement of plasma-free methoxytyramine together with metanephrine and normetanephrine may be useful for identification of these tumors [155]. Markedly elevated chromogranin A levels correlate well with plasma metanephrines, size of tumor, and malignancy.

Anatomical imaging with both CT scan and MRI can identify metastatic and extraadrenal lesions above 1 cm in diameter [159]. Both imaging procedures are vital in the accurate localization of metastatic tumors. Functional imaging defines the extent of the disease and potential response to radiopharmaceuticals.

There is no effective cure for metastatic pheochromocytoma but surgery remains a viable option for tumor reduction if it is technically feasible [153]. Most treatments are palliative, directed at reducing the tumor burden, decreasing hormonal activity, and improving the quality of life [160].

Total adrenalectomy and resection of loco regional lymph node or complete excision of paragangliomas and removal of distant metastases are recommended [161]. Hepatic metastases can be treated with arterial embolization, chemoembolization, cryoembolization, radiofrequency ablation, or transcatheter arterial embolization in specialized centers [162, 164]. The risk increases with the size of the tumor but does not reliably predict malignancy in pheochromocytomas with local disease only [137].

I-131 MIBG therapy is useful only for slow to moderately progressive metastatic patients with lesions that take up this radionuclide. Cumulative results of I-131 MIBG treatment show partial tumor response of 25.3% and stable disease of 43.4% [165]. Higher MIBG doses have been associated with hematotoxicity. Response to somatostatin receptor therapy has failed to show significant improvement on biochemical and clinical response [126, 166]. Chemotherapy is considered among rapidly progressive metastatic disease as first-line treatment [167]. The most evaluated regimen uses Cyclophosphamide, Vincristine, and Dacarbazine (CVD) given for 2 days and cycled after 21 days. Toxicity was mild to moderate with remission period less than 2 years [167]. Recently, reported survival analysis of patients treated under this regimen did not reveal any significant improvement but provided effective palliation for patients with progressive and advanced pheochromocytoma.

Pheochromocytoma in the Young

The clinical presentation of pheochromocytoma in the young can be classified into two, a biochemically functioning tumor or an inactive incidental retroperitoneal mass [165]. Symptomatic tumors manifest similarly to adults with severe and sustained hypertension as the most striking symptom [168]. Biochemically inactive tumors can present as a mass that is often mistaken for the more common neuroblastoma [165]. Both tumors are derived from the neural crest cells and share the capability to secrete catecholamines but pheochromocytomas produce physiologically active hormones.

Most of the adrenal pheochromocytomas occur as unilateral lesions but a significant number present as bilateral lesions at the time of presentation or within a few years [168]. Up to 84% of multifocal tumors have genetic predisposition, with the most common defect is associated with VHL gene [36].

Biochemical confirmation of the tumor can be done with urine or plasma determination of metanephrine levels. The MRI is the preferred imaging modality for children. This can be complemented by functional information using ^{123}I-MIBG imaging, octreoscan, or PET scan using FDA or FDA for general evaluation and FDG for metastatic evaluation.

Preoperative therapy with phenoxybenzamine is given at 20–50 mg/day in two to three divided doses titrated to control hypertension [169]. Additional β-adrenergic blocker atenolol may be warranted in patients with uncontrolled hypertension, tachycardia, and dysrhythmias. This can be given at 20–60 mg daily in two to three doses. Metyrosine given at 250 mg/day two to four times a day can also be added to control adrenergic symptoms of the patient. Calcium channel blockers are alternative drugs that can be used to control hypertension. Volume replacement should be limited to 10 mL/kg/h because of the risk of catecholamine-induced pulmonary edema [170].

Laparoscopic surgery minimizes catecholamine-induced hemodynamic changes during surgery and overall perioperative morbidity [166, 171]. Adrenal sparing surgery should be considered because of the significant morbidity associated with the need for lifelong steroid replacement [166, 167]. Nonetheless, close follow-up is needed to check for possible recurrence. Malignancy is higher among young pheochromocytoma patients, a series reported an incidence of 47% [165]. Identified risk factors for the development of malignant tumors include a tumor size of >6 cm, extraadrenal lesion, and sporadic occurrence. Overall survival rate is favorable primarily because of early detection and aggressive intervention.

Summary

We discussed pheochromocytoma and extraadrenal paragangliomas as functional tumors of the neuroendocrine system. Both can secrete excessive amounts of catecholamines. Signs and symptoms are variable, but generally include hypertension.

Plasma or urine metanephrines are reliable biochemical tests that are sensitive to detect patients with biochemically active tumors. CT scan and MRI are anatomic imaging tests that remain vital for accurate preoperative assessment. Functional imaging can be diagnostic and therapeutic; it enables detection of tumor extent and assesses possible response to therapy.

Focus on genetic studies for familial predisposition for early detection is now at the forefront of research. Identification of SDHB mutations warrants aggressive treatment because of tumor propensity for metastasis with poor prognosis.

Surgery remains the cornerstone of treatment with potential cure for benign tumors and palliative management. Long-term follow-up is necessary to detect recurrence and metastasis. Malignancy still holds poor prognosis as therapeutic options remain limited. Radiopharmaceutical and chemotherapy remain promising but no major breakthrough has been achieved. Palliative care and lesion-based treatment remain the standard.

Acknowledgments This research was supported, in part, by the Intramural Research Program of the NIH, NICHD.

References

1. Delellis RA, Lloyd RV, Heitz PU, Eng C. Pathology and genetics of tumors of the endocrine organs. Lyon: IARC Press; 2004.
2. Tischler AS. Pheochromocytoma and extra-adrenal paraganglioma: updates. Arch Pathol Lab Med. 2008;132(8):1272–84.
3. Manger WM, Gifford RW. Pheochromocytoma. J Clin Hypertens (Greenwich). 2002;4(1): 62–72.
4. Bravo EL, Tagle R. Pheochromocytoma: state-of-the-art and future prospects. Endocr Rev. 2003;24(4):539–53.
5. Beard CM, Sheps SG, Kurland LT, Carney JA, Lie JT. Occurrence of pheochromocytoma in Rochester, Minnesota, 1950 through 1979. Mayo Clin Proc. 1983;58(12):802–4.
6. Ilias I, Pacak K. A clinical overview of pheochromocytomas/paragangliomas and carcinoid tumors. Nucl Med Biol. 2008;35 Suppl 1:S27–34.
7. Bin X, Qing Y, Linhui W, Li G, Yinghao S. Adrenal incidentalomas: experience from a retrospective study in a Chinese population. Urol Oncol. 2011;29(3):270–4.
8. Gimenez-Roqueplo AP, Lehnert H, Mannelli M, et al. Phaeochromocytoma, new genes and screening strategies. Clin Endocrinol (Oxf). 2006;65(6):699–705.
9. Amar L, Bertherat J, Baudin E, et al. Genetic testing in pheochromocytoma or functional paraganglioma. J Clin Oncol. 2005;23(34):8812–8.
10. Gutmann DH, Aylsworth A, Carey JC, et al. The diagnostic evaluation and multidisciplinary management of neurofibromatosis 1 and neurofibromatosis 2. JAMA. 1997;278(1):51–7.
11. Machens A, Brauckhoff M, Gimm O, Dralle H. Risk-oriented approach to hereditary adrenal pheochromocytoma. Ann N Y Acad Sci. 2006;1073:417–28.
12. Walther MM, Herring J, Enquist E, Keiser HR, Linehan WM. von Recklinghausen's disease and pheochromocytomas. J Urol. 1999;162(5):1582–6.
13. Bausch B, Borozdin W, Neumann HP. Clinical and genetic characteristics of patients with neurofibromatosis type 1 and pheochromocytoma. N Engl J Med. 2006;354(25):2729–31.
14. Glasker S, Neumann HPH, Koch CA, Vortmeyer AO. Von Hippel Lindau syndrome. Chapter 35 (Section editor: George P. Chrousos) in: Leslie De Groot, editor, online http://www.endotext.org/adrenal/adrenal35/adrenalframe35.htm.
15. Lonser RR, Glenn GM, Walther M, et al. von Hippel-Lindau disease. Lancet. 2003; 361(9374):2059–67.
16. Walther MM, Reiter R, Keiser HR, et al. Clinical and genetic characterization of pheochromocytoma in von Hippel-Lindau families: comparison with sporadic pheochromocytoma gives insight into natural history of pheochromocytoma. J Urol. 1999;162(3 Pt 1):659–64.
17. Eisenhofer G, Walther MM, Huynh TT, et al. Pheochromocytomas in von Hippel-Lindau syndrome and multiple endocrine neoplasia type 2 display distinct biochemical and clinical phenotypes. J Clin Endocrinol Metab. 2001;86(5):1999–2008.

18. Koch CA, Mauro D, Walther MM, et al. Pheochromocytoma in von Hippel-Lindau disease: distinct histopathologic phenotype compared to pheochromocytoma in multiple endocrine neoplasia type 2. Endocr Pathol. 2002;13(1):17–27.
19. Recasens M, Oriola J, Fernandez-Real JM, et al. Asymptomatic bilateral adrenal pheochromocytoma in a patient with a germline V804M mutation in the RET proto-oncogene. Clin Endocrinol (Oxf). 2007;67(1):29–33.
20. Gimm O, Koch CA, Januszewicz A, Opocher G, Neumann HP. The genetic basis of pheochromocytoma. Front Horm Res. 2004;31:45–60.
21. Bryant J, Farmer J, Kessler LJ, Townsend RR, Nathanson KL. Pheochromocytoma: the expanding genetic differential diagnosis. J Natl Cancer Inst. 2003;95(16):1196–204.
22. Brandi ML, Gagel RF, Angeli A, et al. Guidelines for diagnosis and therapy of MEN type 1 and type 2. J Clin Endocrinol Metab. 2001;86(12):5658–71.
23. Machens A, Niccoli-Sire P, Hoegel J, et al. Early malignant progression of hereditary medullary thyroid cancer. N Engl J Med. 2003;349(16):1517–25.
24. Gottlieb E, Tomlinson IP. Mitochondrial tumour suppressors: a genetic and biochemical update. Nat Rev Cancer. 2005;5(11):857–66.
25. Lee S, Nakamura E, Yang H, et al. Neuronal apoptosis linked to EglN3 prolyl hydroxylase and familial pheochromocytoma genes: developmental culling and cancer. Cancer Cell. 2005;8(2):155–67.
26. Neumann HP, Pawlu C, Peczkowska M, et al. Distinct clinical features of paraganglioma syndromes associated with SDHB and SDHD gene mutations. JAMA. 2004;292(8):943–51.
27. Benn DE, Gimenez-Roqueplo AP, Reilly JR, et al. Clinical presentation and penetrance of pheochromocytoma/paraganglioma syndromes. J Clin Endocrinol Metab. 2006;91(3):827–36.
28. Young Jr WF, Abboud AL. Editorial: paraganglioma–all in the family. J Clin Endocrinol Metab. 2006;91(3):790–2.
29. Baysal BE, Willett-Brozick JE, Lawrence EC, et al. Prevalence of SDHB, SDHC, and SDHD germline mutations in clinic patients with head and neck paragangliomas. J Med Genet. 2002;39(3):178–83.
30. Schiavi F, Boedeker CC, Bausch B, et al. Predictors and prevalence of paraganglioma syndrome associated with mutations of the SDHC gene. JAMA. 2005;294(16):2057–63.
31. Timmers HJ, Kozupa A, Eisenhofer G, et al. Clinical presentations, biochemical phenotypes, and genotype-phenotype correlations in patients with succinate dehydrogenase subunit B-associated pheochromocytomas and paragangliomas. J Clin Endocrinol Metab. 2007; 92(3):779–86.
32. Gimenez-Roqueplo AP, Favier J, Rustin P, et al. Functional consequences of a SDHB gene mutation in an apparently sporadic pheochromocytoma. J Clin Endocrinol Metab. 2002;87(10):4771–4.
33. Gimenez-Roqueplo AP, Favier J, Rustin P, et al. Mutations in the SDHB gene are associated with extra-adrenal and/or malignant phaeochromocytomas. Cancer Res. 2003;63(17):5615–21.
34. Amar L, Baudin E, Burnichon N, et al. Succinate dehydrogenase B gene mutations predict survival in patients with malignant pheochromocytomas or paragangliomas. J Clin Endocrinol Metab. 2007;92(10):3822–8.
35. Majumdar S, Friedrich CA, Koch CA, Megason GC, Fratkin JD, Moll GW. Compound heterozygous mutation with a novel splice donor region DN sequence variant in the succinate dehydrogenase subunit B gene in malignant paraganglioma. Pediatr Blood Cancer. 2010;54: 473–75.
36. Neumann HP, Bausch B, McWhinney SR, et al. Germ-line mutations in nonsyndromic pheochromocytoma. N Engl J Med. 2002;346(19):1459–66.
37. Neumann HP, Eng C. The approach to the patient with paraganglioma. J Clin Endocrinol Metab. 2009;94(8):2677–83.
38. Erlic Z, Neumann HP. When should genetic testing be obtained in a patient with phaeochromocytoma or paraganglioma? Clin Endocrinol (Oxf). 2009;70(3):354–7.
39. Eisenhofer G, Huynh TT, Hiroi M, Pacak K. Understanding catecholamine metabolism as a guide to the biochemical diagnosis of pheochromocytoma. Rev Endocr Metab Disord. 2001;2(3):297–311.

40. Edwards RH. The transport of neurotransmitters into synaptic vesicles. Curr Opin Neurobiol. 1992;2(5):586–94.
41. Cleary S, Brouwers FM, Eisenhofer G, et al. Expression of the noradrenaline transporter and phenylethanolamine N-methyltransferase in normal human adrenal gland and phaeochromocytoma. Cell Tissue Res. 2005;322(3):443–53.
42. Eisenhofer G, Rundquist B, Aneman A, et al. Regional release and removal of catecholamines and extraneuronal metabolism to metanephrines. J Clin Endocrinol Metab. 1995;80(10): 3009–17.
43. Kantorovich V, Eisenhofer G, Pacak K. Pheochromocytoma: an endocrine stress mimicking disorder. Ann N Y Acad Sci. 2008;1148:462–8.
44. Goldstein DS, Eisenhofer G, Stull R, Folio CJ, Keiser HR, Kopin IJ. Plasma dihydroxyphenylglycol and the intraneuronal disposition of norepinephrine in humans. J Clin Invest. 1988;81(1):213–20.
45. Eisenhofer G, Keiser H, Friberg P, et al. Plasma metanephrines are markers of pheochromocytoma produced by catechol-O-methyltransferase within tumors. J Clin Endocrinol Metab. 1998;83(6):2175–85.
46. Goldstein DS, Eisenhofer G, Kopin IJ. Sources and significance of plasma levels of catechols and their metabolites in humans. J Pharmacol Exp Ther. 2003;305(3):800–11.
47. Manger WM. The protean manifestations of pheochromocytoma. Horm Metab Res. 2009;41 (9):658–63.
48. Manger WM. Editorial. In search of pheochromocytomas. J Clin Endocrinol Metab. 2003; 88(9):4080–2.
49. Eisenhofer G, Kopin IJ, Goldstein DS. Catecholamine metabolism: a contemporary view with implications for physiology and medicine. Pharmacol Rev. 2004;56(3):331–49.
50. Ito Y, Fujimoto Y, Obara T. The role of epinephrine, norepinephrine, and dopamine in blood pressure disturbances in patients with pheochromocytoma. World J Surg. 1992;16(4): 759–63; discussion 763–4.
51. Bravo EL, Tarazi RC, Fouad FM, Textor SC, Gifford Jr RW, Vidt DG. Blood pressure regulation in pheochromocytoma. Hypertension. 1982;4(3 Pt 2):193–9.
52. Koch CA, Rodbard JS, Brouwers FM, Eisenhofer G, Pacak K. Hypotension in a woman with a metastatic dopamine-secreting carotid body tumor. Endocr Pract. 2003;9(4):310–4.
53. Tsujimoto G, Manger WM, Hoffman BB. Desensitization of beta-adrenergic receptors by pheochromocytoma. Endocrinology. 1984;114(4):1272–8.
54. Manger WM. An overview of pheochromocytoma: history, current concepts, vagaries, and diagnostic challenges. Ann N Y Acad Sci. 2006;1073:1–20.
55. Sode J, Getzen LC, Osborne DP. Cardiac arrhythmias and cardiomyopathy associated with pheochromocytomas. Report of three cases. Am J Surg. 1967;114(6):927–31.
56. Musuraca G, Imperadore F, Terraneo C, et al. Pheochromocytoma mimicking a non-ST elevation acute myocardial infarction. Cardiol J. 2009;16(4):355–7.
57. Menke-van der Houven van Oordt CW, Twickler TB, van Asperdt FG, Ackermans P, Timmers HJ, Hermus AR. Pheochromocytoma mimicking an acute myocardial infarction. Neth Heart J. 2007;15(7–8):248–51.
58. Attar MN, Moulik PK, Salem GD, Rose EL, Khaleeli AA. Phaeochromocytoma presenting as dilated cardiomyopathy. Int J Clin Pract. 2003;57(6):547–8.
59. Kelley SR, Goel TK, Smith JM. Pheochromocytoma presenting as acute severe congestive heart failure, dilated cardiomyopathy, and severe mitral valvular regurgitation: a case report and review of the literature. J Surg Educ. 2009;66(2):96–101.
60. Rosenbaum JS, Billingham ME, Ginsburg R, Tsujimoto G, Lurie KG, Hoffman BB. Cardiomyopathy in a rat model of pheochromocytoma. Morphological and functional alterations. Am J Cardiovasc Pathol. 1988;1(3):389–99.
61. Holaj R, Zelinka T, Wichterle D, et al. Increased carotid intima-media thickness in patients with pheochromocytoma in comparison to essential hypertension. J Hum Hypertens. 2009; 23(5):350–8.
62. Jang SY, Yang DH, Lee SH, et al. Recurrent catecholamine-induced cardiomyopathy in a patient with a pheochromocytoma. Korean Circ J. 2009;39(6):254–7.

63. Wu XM, Chen JJ, Wu CK, Lin LY, Tseng CD. Pheochromocytoma presenting as acute myocarditis with cardiogenic shock in two cases. Intern Med. 2008;47(24):2151–5.
64. Pacak K, Eisenhofer G, Ahlman H, et al. Pheochromocytoma: recommendations for clinical practice from the First International Symposium. October 2005. Nat Clin Pract Endocrinol Metab. 2007;3(2):92–102.
65. Lenders JW, Pacak K, Walther MM, et al. Biochemical diagnosis of pheochromocytoma: which test is best? JAMA. 2002;287(11):1427–34.
66. Grossman A, Pacak K, Sawka A, et al. Biochemical diagnosis and localization of pheochromocytoma: can we reach a consensus? Ann N Y Acad Sci. 2006;1073:332–47.
67. Eisenhofer G, Goldstein DS, Sullivan P, et al. Biochemical and clinical manifestations of dopamine-producing paragangliomas: utility of plasma methoxytyramine. J Clin Endocrinol Metab. 2005;90(4):2068–75.
68. Eisenhofer G, Goldstein D, Kopin I. Simultaneous liquid-chromatographic determination of plasma catecholamines and metabolites. Clin Chem. 2009;55(12):2223–4.
69. Perry CG, Sawka AM, Singh R, Thabane L, Bajnarek J, Young Jr WF. The diagnostic efficacy of urinary fractionated metanephrines measured by tandem mass spectrometry in detection of pheochromocytoma. Clin Endocrinol (Oxf). 2007;66(5):703–8.
70. Eisenhofer G, Siegert G, Kotzerke J, Bornstein SR, Pacak K. Current progress and future challenges in the biochemical diagnosis and treatment of pheochromocytomas and paragangliomas. Horm Metab Res. 2008;40(5):329–37.
71. Peaston RT, Graham KS, Chambers E, van der Molen JC, Ball S. Performance of plasma free metanephrines measured by liquid chromatography-tandem mass spectrometry in the diagnosis of pheochromocytoma. Clin Chim Acta. 2010;411(7–8):546–52.
72. Eisenhofer G, Lenders JW, Goldstein DS, et al. Pheochromocytoma catecholamine phenotypes and prediction of tumor size and location by use of plasma free metanephrines. Clin Chem. 2005;51(4):735–44.
73. Eisenhofer G, Goldstein DS, Walther MM, et al. Biochemical diagnosis of pheochromocytoma: how to distinguish true- from false-positive test results. J Clin Endocrinol Metab. 2003;88(6):2656–66.
74. Lenders JW, Willemsen JJ, Eisenhofer G, et al. Is supine rest necessary before blood sampling for plasma metanephrines? Clin Chem. 2007;53(2):352–4.
75. de Jong WH, Eisenhofer G, Post WJ, Muskiet FA, de Vries EG, Kema IP. Dietary influences on plasma and urinary metanephrines: implications for diagnosis of catecholamine-producing tumors. J Clin Endocrinol Metab. 2009;94(8):2841–9.
76. Bravo EL, Tarazi RC, Fouad FM, Vidt DG, Gifford Jr RW. Clonidine-suppression test: a useful aid in the diagnosis of pheochromocytoma. N Engl J Med. 1981;305(11):623–6.
77. Lenders JW, Pacak K, Huynh TT, et al. Low sensitivity of glucagon provocative testing for diagnosis of pheochromocytoma. J Clin Endocrinol Metab. 2010;95(1):238–45.
78. Grossrubatscher E, Dalino P, Vignati F, et al. The role of chromogranin A in the management of patients with phaeochromocytoma. Clin Endocrinol (Oxf). 2006;65(3):287–93.
79. Bilek R, Safarik L, Ciprova V, Vlcek P, Lisa L. Chromogranin A, a member of neuroendocrine secretory proteins as a selective marker for laboratory diagnosis of pheochromocytoma. Physiol Res. 2008;57 Suppl 1:S171–9.
80. Miehle K, Kratzsch J, Lenders JW, Kluge R, Paschke R, Koch CA. Adrenal incidentaloma diagnosed as pheochromocytoma by plasma chromogranin A and plasma metanephrines. J Endocrinol Invest. 2005;28(11):1040–2.
81. Giovanella L, Squin N, Ghelfo A, Ceriani L. Chromogranin A immunoradiometric assay in diagnosis of pheochromocytoma: comparison with plasma metanephrines and 123I-MIBG scan. Q J Nucl Med Mol Imaging. 2006;50(4):344–7.
82. d'Herbomez M, Forzy G, Bauters C, et al. An analysis of the biochemical diagnosis of 66 pheochromocytomas. Eur J Endocrinol. 2007;156(5):569–75.
83. Rao F, Keiser HR, O'Connor DT. Malignant pheochromocytoma. Chromaffin granule transmitters and response to treatment. Hypertension. 2000;36(6):1045–52.
84. La Batide-Alanore A, Chatellier G, Plouin PF. Diabetes as a marker of pheochromocytoma in hypertensive patients. J Hypertens. 2003;21(9):1703–7.

85. East HE, Subauste JS, Gandhi A, Koch CA. 10 things you need to know about secondary causes of diabetes mellitus. J Miss State Med Assoc. 2012;in press.
86. Winocour PH, Masud T, Clark F, Cooper BG, Laker MF, Alberti KG. Lipid and lipoprotein metabolism in familial combined hyperlipidaemia during treatment of sporadic phaeochromocytoma: a case study. Postgrad Med J. 1992;68(799):371–5.
87. Zapanti E, Ilias I. Pheochromocytoma: physiopathologic implications and diagnostic evaluation. Ann N Y Acad Sci. 2006;1088:346–60.
88. Lockhart ME, Smith JK, Kenney PJ. Imaging of adrenal masses. Eur J Radiol. 2002;41(2): 95–112.
89. Heinz-Peer G, Memarsadeghi M, Niederle B. Imaging of adrenal masses. Curr Opin Urol. 2007;17(1):32–8.
90. Korobkin M, Brodeur FJ, Yutzy GG, et al. Differentiation of adrenal adenomas from nonadenomas using CT attenuation values. AJR Am J Roentgenol. 1996;166(3):531–6.
91. Hamrahian AH, Ioachimescu AG, Remer EM, et al. Clinical utility of noncontrast computed tomography attenuation value (hounsfield units) to differentiate adrenal adenomas/hyperplasias from nonadenomas: Cleveland Clinic experience. J Clin Endocrinol Metab. 2005; 90(2):871–7.
92. Mayo-Smith WW, Boland GW, Noto RB, Lee M. From the RSNA refresher courses—State-of-the-art adrenal imaging. Radiographics. 2001;21(4):995–1012.
93. Jacques AE, Sahdev A, Sandrasagara M, et al. Adrenal phaeochromocytoma: correlation of MRI appearances with histology and function. Eur Radiol. 2008;18(12):2885–92.
94. Sahdev A, Sohaib A, Monson JP, Grossman AB, Chew SL, Reznek RH. CT and MR imaging of unusual locations of extra-adrenal paragangliomas (pheochromocytomas). Eur Radiol. 2005;15(1):85–92.
95. Whalen RK, Althausen AF, Daniels GH. Extra-adrenal pheochromocytoma. J Urol. 1992; 147(1):1–10.
96. Shulkin BL, Ilias I, Sisson JC, Pacak K. Current trends in functional imaging of pheochromocytomas and paragangliomas. Ann N Y Acad Sci. 2006;1073:374–82.
97. Ilias I, Shulkin B, Pacak K. New functional imaging modalities for chromaffin tumors, neuroblastomas and ganglioneuromas. Trends Endocrinol Metab. 2005;16(2):66–72.
98. Brink I, Hoegerle S, Klisch J, Bley TA. Imaging of pheochromocytoma and paraganglioma. Fam Cancer. 2005;4(1):61–8.
99. Wiseman GA, Pacak K, O'Dorisio MS, et al. Usefulness of 123I-MIBG scintigraphy in the evaluation of patients with known or suspected primary or metastatic pheochromocytoma or paraganglioma: results from a prospective multicenter trial. J Nucl Med. 2009;50(9): 1448–54.
100. Bhatia KS, Ismail MM, Sahdev A, et al. 123I-metaiodobenzylguanidine (MIBG) scintigraphy for the detection of adrenal and extra-adrenal phaeochromocytomas: CT and MRI correlation. Clin Endocrinol (Oxf). 2008;69(2):181–8.
101. Taieb D, Sebag F, Hubbard JG, Mundler O, Henry JF, Conte-Devolx B. Does iodine-131 meta-iodobenzylguanidine (MIBG) scintigraphy have an impact on the management of sporadic and familial phaeochromocytoma? Clin Endocrinol (Oxf). 2004;61(1):102–8.
102. Lonsdale MN, Beyer T. Dual-modality PET/CT instrumentation-today and tomorrow. Eur J Radiol. 2010;73(3):452–60.
103. Timmers HJ, Carrasquillo JA, Whatley M, et al. Usefulness of standardized uptake values for distinguishing adrenal glands with pheochromocytoma from normal adrenal glands by use of 6-18F-fluorodopamine PET. J Nucl Med. 2007;48(12):1940–4.
104. Pacak K, Eisenhofer G, Carrasquillo JA, Chen CC, Li ST, Goldstein DS. 6-[18F]fluorodopamine positron emission tomographic (PET) scanning for diagnostic localization of pheochromocytoma. Hypertension. 2001;38(1):6–8.
105. Ilias I, Yu J, Carrasquillo JA, et al. Superiority of 6-[18F]-fluorodopamine positron emission tomography versus [131I]-metaiodobenzylguanidine scintigraphy in the localization of metastatic pheochromocytoma. J Clin Endocrinol Metab. 2003;88(9):4083–7.
106. Kaji P, Carrasquillo JA, Linehan WM, et al. The role of 6-[18F]fluorodopamine positron emission tomography in the localization of adrenal pheochromocytoma associated with von Hippel-Lindau syndrome. Eur J Endocrinol. 2007;156(4):483–7.

107. Timmers HJ, Eisenhofer G, Carrasquillo JA, et al. Use of 6-[18F]-fluorodopamine positron emission tomography (PET) as first-line investigation for the diagnosis and localization of non-metastatic and metastatic phaeochromocytoma (PHEO). Clin Endocrinol (Oxf). 2009;71(1):11–7.
108. Havekes B, King K, Lai EW, Romijn JA, Corssmit EP, Pacak K. New imaging approaches to phaeochromocytomas and paragangliomas. Clin Endocrinol (Oxf). 2009;72(2):137–45.
109. Timmers HJ, Hadi M, Carrasquillo JA, et al. The effects of carbidopa on uptake of 6-18F-Fluoro-L-DOPA in PET of pheochromocytoma and extraadrenal abdominal paraganglioma. J Nucl Med. 2007;48(10):1599–606.
110. Fiebrich HB, Brouwers AH, Kerstens MN, et al. 6-[F-18]Fluoro-L-dihydroxyphenylalanine positron emission tomography is superior to conventional imaging with (123) I-metaiodobenzylguanidine scintigraphy, computer tomography, and magnetic resonance imaging in localizing tumors causing catecholamine excess. J Clin Endocrinol Metab. 2009;94(10):3922–30.
111. Luster M, Karges W, Zeich K, et al. Clinical value of 18F-fluorodihydroxyphenylalanine positron emission tomography/computed tomography (18F-DOPA PET/CT) for detecting pheochromocytoma. Eur J Nucl Med Mol Imaging. 2010;37(3):484–93.
112. Hoegerle S, Altehoefer C, Ghanem N, et al. Whole-body 18F dopa PET for detection of gastrointestinal carcinoid tumors. Radiology. 2001;220(2):373–80.
113. Warburg O, Wind F, Negelein E. The metabolism of tumors in the body. J Gen Physiol. 1927;8(6):519–30.
114. Belhocine T, Spaepen K, Dusart M, et al. 18FDG PET in oncology: the best and the worst (Review). Int J Oncol. 2006;28(5):1249–61.
115. Timmers HJ, Kozupa A, Chen CC, et al. Superiority of fluorodeoxyglucose positron emission tomography to other functional imaging techniques in the evaluation of metastatic SDHB-associated pheochromocytoma and paraganglioma. J Clin Oncol. 2007;25(16):2262–9.
116. Mundschenk J, Unger N, Schulz S, Hollt V, Steinke R, Lehnert H. Somatostatin receptor subtypes in human pheochromocytoma: subcellular expression pattern and functional relevance for octreotide scintigraphy. J Clin Endocrinol Metab. 2003;88(11):5150–7.
117. McCarthy KE, Woltering EA, Anthony LB. In situ radiotherapy with 111In-pentetreotide. State of the art and perspectives. Q J Nucl Med. 2000;44(1):88–95.
118. Ilias I, Chen CC, Carrasquillo JA, et al. Comparison of 6-18F-fluorodopamine PET with 123I-metaiodobenzylguanidine and 111in-pentetreotide scintigraphy in localization of non-metastatic and metastatic pheochromocytoma. J Nucl Med. 2008;49(10):1613–9.
119. Koopmans KP, Jager PL, Kema IP, Kerstens MN, Albers F, Dullaart RP. 111In-octreotide is superior to 123I-metaiodobenzylguanidine for scintigraphic detection of head and neck paragangliomas. J Nucl Med. 2008;49(8):1232–7.
120. de Jong M, Breeman WA, Bakker WH, et al. Comparison of (111)In-labeled somatostatin analogues for tumor scintigraphy and radionuclide therapy. Cancer Res. 1998;58(3):437–41.
121. Vanhagen PM, Krenning EP, Reubi JC, et al. Somatostatin analogue scintigraphy in granulomatous diseases. Eur J Nucl Med. 1994;21(6):497–502.
122. King K, Chen CC, Alexopoulos DK, Whatkey MA, Reynolds JC, Patronas N, et al. Functional imaging of SDHx-related head and neck paragangliomas: Comparison of ^{18}F-fluorodihydroxyphenylalanine, ^{18}Ffluorodopamine, ^{18}F-fluoro-2-deoxy-D-glucose PET, ^{123}I-metaiodobenzylguanidine scintigraphy, and ^{111}In-pentetreotide scintigraphy. J Clin Endocrinol Metab. 2011;96(9):2779–85.
123. Zelinka T, Timmers HJ, Kozupa A, et al. Role of positron emission tomography and bone scintigraphy in the evaluation of bone involvement in metastatic pheochromocytoma and paraganglioma: specific implications for succinate dehydrogenase enzyme subunit B gene mutations. Endocr Relat Cancer. 2008;15(1):311–23.
124. Pacak K. Preoperative management of the pheochromocytoma patient. J Clin Endocrinol Metab. 2007;92(11):4069–79.
125. Sibal L, Jovanovic A, Agarwal SC, et al. Phaeochromocytomas presenting as acute crises after beta blockade therapy. Clin Endocrinol (Oxf). 2006;65(2):186–90.
126. Bravo EL. Pheochromocytoma. Cardiol Rev. 2002;10(1):44–50.

127. Steinsapir J, Carr AA, Prisant LM, Bransome Jr ED. Metyrosine and pheochromocytoma. Arch Intern Med. 1997;157(8):901–6.
128. Perry RR, Keiser HR, Norton JA, et al. Surgical management of pheochromocytoma with the use of metyrosine. Ann Surg. 1990;212(5):621–8.
129. van der Horst-Schrivers AN, Kerstens MN, Wolffenbuttel BH. Preoperative pharmacological management of phaeochromocytoma. Neth J Med. 2006;64(8):290–5.
130. Mellon MJ, Sundaram CP. Laparoscopic adrenalectomy for pheochromocytoma versus other surgical indications. JSLS. 2008;12(4):380–4.
131. Humphrey R, Gray D, Pautler S, Davies W. Laparoscopic compared with open adrenalectomy for resection of pheochromocytoma: a review of 47 cases. Can J Surg. 2008;51(4):276–80.
132. Meyer-Rochow GY, Soon PS, Delbridge LW, et al. Outcomes of minimally invasive surgery for phaeochromocytoma. ANZ J Surg. 2009;79(5):367–70.
133. Ippolito G, Palazzo FF, Sebag F, Thakur A, Cherenko M, Henry JF. Safety of laparoscopic adrenalectomy in patients with large pheochromocytomas: a single institution review. World J Surg. 2008;32(5):840–44; discussion 845–46.
134. Jaroszewski DE, Tessier DJ, Schlinkert RT, et al. Laparoscopic adrenalectomy for pheochromocytoma. Mayo Clin Proc. 2003;78(12):1501–4.
135. Kasahara T, Nishiyama T, Takahashi K. Laparoscopic adrenalectomy for pheochromocytoma: evaluation of experience and strategy at a single institute. BJU Int. 2009;103(2):218–22.
136. Dimas S, Roukounakis N, Kafetzis I, et al. Feasibility of laparoscopic adrenalectomy for large pheochromocytomas. JSLS. 2007;11(1):30–3.
137. Shen WT, Sturgeon C, Clark OH, Duh QY, Kebebew E. Should pheochromocytoma size influence surgical approach? A comparison of 90 malignant and 60 benign pheochromocytomas. Surgery. 2004;136(6):1129–37.
138. Singer J, Koch CA, Kassahun W, Lamesch P, Eisenhofer G, Kluge R, et al. A patient with a large recurrent pheochromocytoma demonstrating the pitfalls of diagnosis. Nat Rev Endocrinol. 2011;7(12):749–55.
139. Castilho LN, Simoes FA, Santos AM, Rodrigues TM, dos Santos CA Jr. Pheochromocytoma: a long-term follow-up of 24 patients undergoing laparoscopic adrenalectomy. Int Braz J Urol. 2009;35(1):24–31; discussion 32–5.
140. Petri BJ, van Eijck CH, de Herder WW, Wagner A, de Krijger RR. Phaeochromocytomas and sympathetic paragangliomas. Br J Surg. 2009;96(12):1381–92.
141. Asari R, Scheuba C, Kaczirek K, Niederle B. Estimated risk of pheochromocytoma recurrence after adrenal-sparing surgery in patients with multiple endocrine neoplasia type 2A. Arch Surg. 2006;141(12):1199–205; discussion 1205.
142. Tischler AS, Kimura N, McNicol AM. Pathology of pheochromocytoma and extra-adrenal paraganglioma. Ann N Y Acad Sci. 2006;1073:557–70.
143. Kimura N, Watanabe T, Noshiro T, Shizawa S, Miura Y. Histological grading of adrenal and extra-adrenal pheochromocytomas and relationship to prognosis: a clinicopathological analysis of 116 adrenal pheochromocytomas and 30 extra-adrenal sympathetic paragangliomas including 38 malignant tumors. Endocr Pathol Spring. 2005;16(1):23–32.
144. Reisin E, Huth MM, Nguyen BP, Weed SG, Gonzalez FM. Intravenous fenoldopam versus sodium nitroprusside in patients with severe hypertension. Hypertension. 1990;15(2 Suppl): I59–62.
145. Friederich JA, Butterworth JFt. Sodium nitroprusside: twenty years and counting. Anesth Analg. 1995;81(1):152–62.
146. Joris JL, Hamoir EE, Hartstein GM, et al. Hemodynamic changes and catecholamine release during laparoscopic adrenalectomy for pheochromocytoma. Anesth Analg. 1999;88(1):16–21.
147. James MF, Cronje L. Pheochromocytoma crisis: the use of magnesium sulfate. Anesth Analg. 2004;99(3):680–6; table of contents.
148. Shupak RC. Difficult anesthetic management during pheochromocytoma surgery. J Clin Anesth. 1999;11(3):247–50.
149. Augoustides JG, Abrams M, Berkowitz D, Fraker D. Vasopressin for hemodynamic rescue in catecholamine-resistant vasoplegic shock after resection of massive pheochromocytoma. Anesthesiology. 2004;101(4):1022–4.

150. Deutsch E, Tobias JD. Vasopressin to treat hypotension after pheochromocytoma resection in an eleven-year-old boy. J Cardiothorac Vasc Anesth. 2006;20(3):394–6.
151. Akiba M, Kodama T, Ito Y, Obara T, Fujimoto Y. Hypoglycemia induced by excessive rebound secretion of insulin after removal of pheochromocytoma. World J Surg. 1990;14(3):317–24.
152. Jude EB, Sridhar CB. Prolonged hypoglycaemia following surgical removal of phaeochromocytoma. Postgrad Med J. 2000;76(891):39–40.
153. Eisenhofer G, Bornstein SR, Brouwers FM, et al. Malignant pheochromocytoma: current status and initiatives for future progress. Endocr Relat Cancer. 2004;11(3):423–36.
154. Brouwers FM, Eisenhofer G, Tao JJ, et al. High frequency of SDHB germline mutations in patients with malignant catecholamine-producing paragangliomas: implications for genetic testing. J Clin Endocrinol Metab. 2006;91(11):4505–9.
155. John H, Ziegler WH, Hauri D, Jaeger P. Pheochromocytomas: can malignant potential be predicted? Urology. 1999;53(4):679–83.
156. Fitzgerald PA, Goldsby RE, Huberty JP, et al. Malignant pheochromocytomas and paragangliomas: a phase II study of therapy with high-dose 131I-metaiodobenzylguanidine (131I-MIBG). Ann N Y Acad Sci. 2006;1073:465–90.
157. Amar L, Servais A, Gimenez-Roqueplo AP, Zinzindohoue F, Chatellier G, Plouin PF. Year of diagnosis, features at presentation, and risk of recurrence in patients with pheochromocytoma or secreting paraganglioma. J Clin Endocrinol Metab. 2005;90(4):2110–6.
158. Goldstein RE, O'Neill JA Jr., Holcomb GW, III, et al. Clinical experience over 48 years with pheochromocytoma. Ann Surg. 1999;229(6):755–64; discussion 764–6.
159. Ilias I, Pacak K. Current approaches and recommended algorithm for the diagnostic localization of pheochromocytoma. J Clin Endocrinol Metab. 2004;89(2):479–91.
160. Chrisoulidou A, Kaltsas G, Ilias I, Grossman AB. The diagnosis and management of malignant phaeochromocytoma and paraganglioma. Endocr Relat Cancer. 2007;14(3):569–85.
161. Brauckhoff M, Gimm O, Dralle H. Preoperative and surgical therapy in sporadic and familial pheochromocytoma. Front Horm Res. 2004;31:121–44.
162. Kebebew E, Duh QY. Benign and malignant pheochromocytoma: diagnosis, treatment, and follow-Up. Surg Oncol Clin N Am. 1998;7(4):765–89.
163. Pacak K, Linehan WM, Eisenhofer G, Walther MM, Goldstein DS. Recent advances in genetics, diagnosis, localization, and treatment of pheochromocytoma. Ann Intern Med. 2001;134(4):315–29.
164. Takahashi K, Ashizawa N, Minami T, et al. Malignant pheochromocytoma with multiple hepatic metastases treated by chemotherapy and transcatheter arterial embolization. Intern Med. 1999;38(4):349–54.
165. Pham TH, Moir C, Thompson GB, et al. Pheochromocytoma and paraganglioma in children: a review of medical and surgical management at a tertiary care center. Pediatrics. 2006; 118(3):1109–17.
166. Walther MM. New therapeutic and surgical approaches for sporadic and hereditary pheochromocytoma. Ann N Y Acad Sci. 2002;970:41–53.
167. Brunt LM, Lairmore TC, Doherty GM, Quasebarth MA, DeBenedetti M, Moley JF. Adrenalectomy for familial pheochromocytoma in the laparoscopic era. Ann Surg. 2002; 235(5):713–20; discussion 720–1.
168. Barontini M, Levin G, Sanso G. Characteristics of pheochromocytoma in a 4- to 20-year-old population. Ann N Y Acad Sci. 2006;1073:30–7.
169. Ein SH, Pullerits J, Creighton R, Balfe JW. Pediatric pheochromocytoma. A 36-year review. Pediatr Surg Int. 1997;12(8):595–8.
170. Turner MC, Lieberman E, DeQuattro V. The perioperative management of pheochromocytoma in children. Clin Pediatr (Phila). 1992;31(10):583–9.
171. Vargas HI, Kavoussi LR, Bartlett DL, et al. Laparoscopic adrenalectomy: a new standard of care. Urology. 1997;49(5):673–8.

Part II
Other Potential Causes of Endocrine Hypertension

Chapter 8
Hypertension in Growth Hormone Excess and Deficiency

Daniel H.P. Towie and George R. Merriam

Abstract Cardiovascular and cerebrovascular morbidity and mortality are increased in both acromegaly and adult growth hormone deficiency (GHD), and a significant portion of this elevated risk can be attributed to hypertension. Despite taking into account the effects of derangement of other pituitary hormones that often accompany these conditions and of treatments used for acromegaly or GHD, much appears attributable to the direct and indirect effects of abnormal levels of GH or IGF-I themselves. The hypothesized mechanisms for hypertension have been the subjects of much more study in acromegaly than in GHD; but at present there is no clear consensus on the most important abnormalities underlying hypertension in either condition, nor even on its prevalence, with a wide range of estimates from less than 20% to more than 70% in acromegaly, and 25–30% in GHD. The divergent results arise from differences in the techniques used to measure blood pressure and also the rates of hypertension in the background populations. Mechanisms postulated to underlie hypertension in acromegaly include expansion of plasma volume, direct renal effects, changes in vascular compliance, increased sympathetic tone, and indirect effects due to insulin resistance and to sleep apnea. Hypothesized mechanisms in GHD include endothelial dysfunction and increased vascular stiffness; but several other factors, such as increased sympathetic tone, paradoxically overlap with factors thought to play a role in acromegaly as well. This overlap may signify a U-shaped curve for the effects of GH and IGF-I on blood pressure regulation, with optimum effects within the normal range, but data are currently insufficient to demonstrate this with any certainty. Perhaps the strongest evidence linking acromegaly with abnormal BP is resolution or improvement of hypertension with successful treatment of GH excess.

D.H.P. Towie
Bristol Royal Infirmary, University of Bristol Faculty of Medicine, Bristol, UK

G.R. Merriam (✉)
Department of Medicine, Division of Metabolism, Endocrinology and Nutrition,
University of Washington School of Medicine, VA Puget Sound Health Care System,
9600 Veterans Drive SW, Tacoma, WA 98493, USA
e-mail: merriam@uw.edu

C.A. Koch and G.P. Chrousos (eds.), *Endocrine Hypertension: Underlying Mechanisms and Therapy*, Contemporary Endocrinology, DOI 10.1007/978-1-60761-548-4_8,

Keywords Acromegaly • Aldosterone • Angiotensin • Blood pressure • Cardiovascular disease • Catecholamines • Cerebrovascular disease • Endothelial reactivity • Growth hormone • Growth hormone deficiency • Hypertension • Insulin-like growth factor-I • Nitrogen oxides • Renin • Risk factors • Sympathetic nervous system • Vasodilatation

Introduction

The coordinated actions of many hormones are needed to support normal growth, including thyroid hormone, sex steroids, and cortisol, and those effects continue in adult life. Perhaps because of its name and earlier scarcity, little attention was paid until relatively recently to the effects of growth hormone (GH) once statural until growth has ceased; and yet it also continues to play an important role in adult life as a partitioning hormone, stimulating bone and cardiac and skeletal muscle and reducing fat, particularly intra-abdominal fat. GH stimulates retention of sodium and body water. Hypertension in patients with GH excess—gigantism and acromegaly—is common and not unexpected. However, there is a doubling of cardiovascular mortality and an excess of hypertension in growth hormone deficiency (GHD) as well. Therefore, in recent years, blood pressure dysregulation in GH excess and deficiency has become a major research focus. This chapter briefly discusses effects of GH on blood pressure in normal physiology and the prevalence and pathophysiology of hypertension in both acromegaly and GHD.

GH/IGF-I and Blood Pressure in Normal Populations

Several studies suggest a relationship between circulating insulin-like growth factor-I (IGF-I) levels and blood pressure (BP) within the general population; however little literature exists linking GH and BP variability. Evidence in this area appears to be conflicting; however it might be of relative importance if IGF-I levels in the apparently normal range were to be associated with changes in blood pressure as this could lead to possible future antihypertensive therapeutic targets.

In 2008 Colao's group carried out a study in 404 subjects with no history of pituitary or cardiovascular disease. Heavy smokers and alcohol drinkers were excluded. In this population, 27% had mild or severe hypertension. The IGF-I standard deviation score (SDS) was negatively correlated with systolic and diastolic blood pressure (DBP), and a negative IGF-I SDS predicted hypertension in their population. Lower levels of IGF-I, after adjustment for age, were associated with hypertension, and this was shown to be independent of glucose tolerance—a potential confounding factor [1].

Using 715 subjects from the Västerbotten Intervention Project cohort in Sweden, Hunt and colleagues conducted a cross-sectional analysis of the relationship between

IGF-I, IGF binding proteins (IGFBPs), and a number of cardiovascular risk factors, including blood pressure [2]. They found that DBP correlated negatively with IGF-I levels but that the association with systolic blood pressure (SBP) was nonsignificant. They subdivided the subjects into quartiles of IGF-I and found an inverse proportionality between hypertension and IGF-I quartile—subjects with higher levels of IGF-I having less hypertension—however this lost significance when it was adjusted for BMI. This indicates that the association may be weak or that BMI influences both IGF-I levels and blood pressure independently. When the hypertensive section of the cohort was examined, however, they found a significantly lower mean IGF-I compared with the non-hypertensive subgroup even after adjusting for BMI and IGFBP-3. A weakness highlighted by the authors is that 94 of their cohort were receiving antihypertensive therapy, making it impossible to know their "natural" blood pressure. This likely influenced results; however we cannot know in what way as no post hoc analysis was done. Furthermore, they comment that higher insulin levels in hypertensive subjects may explain the lower IGF-I titers, and thus the correlation may be indirect.

Another group used a different Swedish random sample of 392 subjects between the ages of 25 and 64 years. Although initially their results showed an inverse correlation between IGF-I and SBP, and also DBP in women, when adjusted for age these results became statistically nonsignificant [3].

These papers indicate a possible link between BP and IGF-I outside the context of extremes of the GH/IGF-I axis but are not indicative of causality. Their findings are in line with those from other cohorts, including one comprising patients with type 1 diabetes mellitus (T1DM); within this population of 246 Caucasians with T1DM, they found lower IGF-I levels were strongly associated with systolic hypertension and diastolic hypertension in women. These results remained significant when adjusted for age, sex, and age at diagnosis of T1DM. Furthermore lower levels of free serum IGF-I were associated with more diabetic neuropathy, nephropathy, and retinopathy [4]. The authors cite evidence that in T1DM, inflammatory cytokines activate suppressor of cytokine signaling (socs) genes that reduce GH activity by a post-receptor mechanism, leading to lower serum IGF-I.

A number of studies have found no significant association between IGF-I and hypertension. One such study of young black and white men comprised cross-sectional and prospective longitudinal analyses of their cohort at 2, 7, and 10 years [5]. Some age-adjusted inverse associations between BP and IGF-I were seen in black males at 10 years, but these lost significance after adjustment for other confounding covariables (body mass index, physical activity score, alcohol intake, and cigarettes/day).

Other groups have found contradictory results, with increased IGF-I in hypertensive patients as opposed to healthy controls, with highest levels in hypertensive patients with left ventricular hypertrophy [6, 7].

Given the relative weakness of evidence linking both excess and inadequacy of the GH/IGF-I axis with hypertension, it is unsurprising that it is weaker still when looking at the more subtle differences in IGF-I within the normal range, in populations not known to have significantly deranged neuroendocrine systems. This lack of clarity may reflect inability of studies to detect the association, or the absence of association, or the number of confounding variables. It is of note that little investigation of GH itself has been performed in the context of the normal population. IGF-I is often used in the clinical setting as a proxy marker of diurnal GH secretion because its levels remain more stable in the blood. It is especially important when considering so-called normal populations to remember that IGF-I can also be affected by other factors, particularly carbohydrate metabolism and insulin secretion. In the settings of acromegaly and GHD we can be sure that GH/IGF-I levels are congruously high and low respectively and can hypothesize that they may be causing the observed changes to blood pressure. However, when looking at "normal" populations we cannot know whether high-normal IGF-I levels truly reflect high GH levels, which hormone is associated with blood pressure changes and, indeed whether there is a causal relationship.

Acromegaly

Acromegaly is a state of abnormally increased GH action, usually due to a GH-secreting pituitary adenoma. While it most often occurs in middle age, when it begins in childhood before epiphyseal closure it can lead to abnormally increased stature, or "gigantism." Even when it sets in after linear growth has ceased, major sequelae of acromegaly include cardiovascular, respiratory, metabolic, musculoskeletal, and neoplastic complications. The effects of acromegaly within the cardiovascular system are particularly important as it appears that these may be the main contributors to patients' elevated mortality [8]. While the effects of acromegaly on the heart itself are well defined and extensively investigated, hypertension in acromegaly—although long recognized—has garnered less interest.

Cardiomyopathy is common in acromegaly—particularly if duration of disease is long, when cardiomegaly is found in up to 90% of patients at postmortem [9]. This concentric biventricular hypertrophy without enlargement of the chambers develops independently of hypertension and other risk factors, in response to elevated circulating GH/IGF-I. However, concomitant hypertension has been shown to be an independent risk factor for cardiac pathology (75% vs. 37.2% in uncomplicated acromegaly) [10]. Before regular success with treatment was achieved, cardiovascular events were the leading cause of mortality [8]. More recent evidence suggests that mortality is still higher than the general population and that apart from the degree of elevation of GH/IGF-I, the presence of hypertension is one of the strongest predictors of mortality [11, 12]. Acromegaly-associated hypertension is also reportedly resistant to normal antihypertensive treatment [13].

Despite the importance of hypertension to the prognosis of acromegalic patients, there remains a lack of consensus over the association between acromegaly and hypertension, its prevalence and whether it is reversible; there is also little understanding of the pathogenesis of hypertension in this condition.

Clinical Evidence of Hypertension in Acromegaly

Estimated Prevalence

Before attempting to qualify the relationship between BP and excess activity in the GH/IGF-I axis, the association requires quantification.

There are numerous series that estimate the prevalence of high blood pressure (HBP) within acromegalic populations. The results, however, vary widely—from 17.5 to 57% in larger series [14] and even more widely in smaller samples [15] (see Table 8.1).

Table 8.1 Prevalence of hypertension in acromegaly: summary of the literature

References	No. cases	Prevalence (%)	Measurement	Criteria for hypertension (mmHg)
Nabarro [123]	256	30.5	Clinical	Not known
Rodrigues et al. [24]	34	26	Clinical	160/95
Kraatz et al. [23]	158	31.6	Clinical	160/95
Kraatz et al. [23] recalculated		50.6		140/90
Molitch [124]	639	23	Clinical	Not known
Ezzat et al. [64]	500	51	Clinical	140/90
Ohtsuka et al. [25]	64	37.5	Clinical	160/95
Ohtsuka et al. [25] recalculated		57.8		140/90
Lopez-Velasco et al. [125]	39	33.3	Clinical	140/90
Minniti et al. [17]	40	42.5	Clinical	140/90
Minniti et al. [17]	40	17.5	ABPM	136/84
Terzolo et al. [21]	16	31.2	ABPM	136/84
Colao et al. [10, 39]	130	35.4	Clinical	DBP 90
Fukuda et al. [126]	65	38	Clinical	Not known
Jaffrain-Rea et al. [18]	68	51.5	Clinical	140/90
	68	47	ABPM	135/85
Otsuki et al. [127]	21	57	Clinical	140/90
Pietrobelli et al. [19]	25	56	Clinical	140/90
	25	40	ABPM	136/84
Weiss et al. [128]	55	38.2	Clinical	Not known
Jaffrain-Rai et al. [20]	31	45.1	Clinical	140/90
	31	35.5	ABPM	136/84
Vitale et al. [14]	200	46	Clinical	140/90
Damjanovic et al. [41]	23	39	Clinical	Not known
Mestron et al. [129]	1,036	39.1	Medical records	Medical records
Colao et al. [26] (elderly pts)	57	82	Clinical	140/90
Colao et al. [13, 34]	89	57.3	Clinical	140/90
Sucunza et al. [27]	60	37.7	Clinical	Not known
Ciresi et al. [15]	12	66.7	Clinical	140/90
Melnichenko et al. [31]	232	80.2	Clinical	Not known
Colao et al. [29]	45	46.7	Clinical	90 DBP

Redrawn and updated from Vitale et al. [14], including criteria required for diagnosis of hypertension and prevalence recalculated where possible using modern definitions

ABPM = 24-h ambulatory blood pressure monitoring

Clinical = manual sphygmomanometer

Worldwide prevalence of hypertension in the general population, although difficult to estimate accurately, was thought to be 26.4% and rising in 2000 [16]. Comparison of these figures therefore casts aspersions as to whether acromegaly and hypertension are related, particularly whether they are associated in all patient groups. The wide variation among estimates for the frequency of hypertension may reflect different methods of assessing BP, different definitions of hypertension, the use of small samples, specific differences between populations being studied where control groups are not used, or confounding factors such as concomitant use of antihypertensives.

Some authors have argued that the method of BP measurement plays a key role in the divergent estimates. Minniti and colleagues [17] compared the prevalence of hypertension as diagnosed with a manual sphygmomanometer, following an accepted protocol (42.5%), with results from ambulatory BP measurement (ABPM, 17.5%) taken at regular intervals in acromegalic subjects. They found that only 40% of patients found to be hypertensive by clinical assessment were confirmed as hypertensive with ABPM. They then questioned whether hypertension in acromegaly had been overestimated in previous studies. Subsequent studies, however, that made measurements using both clinical and ABPM techniques have reported both less discrepancy between the techniques and a higher prevalence of hypertension using ABPM [18–21]. In addition to this, the difference that Minniti et al. found may represent mainly the "white coat" hypertension phenomenon that has been found by others to be associated with the development of frank hypertension [22]. Furthermore, the evidence that hypertension is an independent and strong predictor of mortality in acromegalic patients [11, 12] was formulated from clinical assessment of BP, so the prevalences calculated using similar methods are likely to hold significance. Estimates of hypertension's prevalence remain diverse regardless of method used to assess BP. This suggests other factors are contributing to the results' heterogeneity.

One other possible cause of the variability in results is the use of different reference ranges and definitions for hypertension. Most of the papers that provide a prevalence of hypertension used a criterion of >140 mmHg systolic and/or >90 mmHg diastolic BP. Some papers did not report their criteria, although in papers published since 2000 it may be fair to assume that a similar definition was used. Some used only a diastolic BP >90 mmHg as a criterion and some older papers used the prior threshold of >160 mmHg systolic over >95 mmHg diastolic [23–25]. By today's standards this would underestimate prevalence. Two of these papers define BP >140/90 mmHg but <160/95 mmHg as "borderline hypertension," and patients in this category would have been classified as hypertensive in the other studies. If these patients are added to the prevalence figures, the prevalence of 31.6% in Kraatz and colleagues' 1990 paper [23] becomes 50.6%. In Ohtsuka et al.'s study [25], the prevalence of 37.5% becomes 57.8%. Although this reduces the range of the results somewhat, it is still substantial. This residual variability may be due to the relatively small samples size in most studies, a result of the relative infrequency of acromegaly. Lastly, given the many factors that predispose to hypertension, it is likely that the different study populations had differing mixes of family history, race, diet, or other variables. This is particularly relevant in studies where control groups from the same population were not used.

Prevalence Compared to Control Populations

Some of the studies have included internal comparison groups, which allow a better estimation of the association between acromegaly and hypertension. One group compared the frequency of hypertension between a retrospective series of 158 acromegalic subjects and a large, local epidemiological study [23], only finding a raised prevalence of hypertension in female patients. Hypertension was found in 19.6% of acromegalics. However, when the figures were recalculated using modern definitions, hypertension is considerably more common in both sexes, with 50.6% of patients being hypertensive vs. 32.9% in the comparison population. A Japanese group found that the prevalence of hypertension was higher in a retrospective cohort of 64 acromegalics (37.5%) than in the local population (20–25%) [25]. They found that 75% of patients with acromegaly classified as hypertensive (using the old definition) had a family history of hypertension compared to 25.9% of normotensive acromegalics. This effect may have been diluted when hypertension is defined by modern standards as only 23.1% of their "borderline hypertensive" acromegalics had a positive family history. However, since a family history of hypertension increases the risk of hypertension in non-acromegalics as well, this may be a confounder rather than a specific effect.

A larger subsequent study used 200 cases and controls matched for age, sex, body mass index, and lifestyle factors and found hypertension in 46% of acromegalic cases and 25% ($p<0.0001$) of controls [14]; cases had significantly higher diastolic and systolic BPs. In contrast to some other studies, gender did not influence the acromegaly-hypertension association; they also found that a family history of hypertension was more common in controls than patients, in contrast with Kraatz et al. [23]. Hypertension was positively correlated with age in both groups, although it occurred 10 years earlier in cases than in controls. The strength of this study lies in its relatively large size and the use of controls matched for factors that could otherwise confound the results (the prevalence also agrees with worldwide estimates [16]); however, there is no mention of blinding of investigators which may be a weakness.

One study looked at hypertension in a cohort of 57 patients who were diagnosed with acromegaly when older than 60, comparing them with gender and age-matched controls [26]. They found that 82% of the patients, whereas only 67% of controls were hypertensive. Mean systolic and diastolic BPs were significantly higher in cases. The authors note that many of the acromegalic patients are being treated unsuccessfully for hypertension. This may imply that hypertension associated with acromegaly is relatively refractory to treatment.

Two studies have compared controls with a mix of acromegalic patients—treatment naïve, and those receiving or who recently received unsuccessful treatment of their acromegaly. Sucunza et al. found that 37.7% of acromegalic patients ($n=19$) were hypertensive compared with only 15% of controls ($n=105$) [27]. Ciresi's group also did a small study of acromegaly patients mostly receiving therapy, 12 of whom were not responding completely. They compared the 12 with active acromegaly against 21 controls and found hypertension in 66.7% of cases and 0% of controls [15]. These papers do corroborate the evidence from other stronger studies;

however, they are both small and contained many patients receiving acromegaly treatment, a potentially confounding attribute as a search of the literature shows that somatostatin analogues (SSA), a mainstay of medical therapy for acromegaly, may themselves increase BP [28].

Thus, despite the wide range of prevalence findings, the association between acromegaly and hypertension appears to have a strong base of evidence. The best evidence comes from the Naples group's case–control study of 400 subjects [14]; their result that 46% of patients with acromegaly are hypertensive by clinical assessment (compared with 25% of controls) also falls around the mean of the other studies' results. This does not, however, provide evidence of a causal relationship.

Resolution of Hypertension with Treatment of Acromegaly?

One observation that would provide a stronger argument for causality is if treatment of acromegaly reduces or resolves hypertension. The evidence surrounding this is mixed, with some studies finding a reduction in BP while others showing no effect. There may also be differences between the different methods of treatment—medical vs. surgical.

The best study to address this question may be that of Colao et al. from 2008 [13]. They retrospectively selected 105 treatment-naïve acromegalic patients, all receiving therapy for hypertension. Hypertension was successfully controlled in only 14% of patients; the remainder continue to be hypertensive despite therapy. Subjects received a variety of treatments, which normalized GH and IGF-I levels in 72%. In this group both systolic and diastolic mean BP fell by 13.1% and 11.4% respectively ($p<0.0001$), independent of treatment method. The reduction in BP was not statistically significant in patients whose acromegaly therapy was unsuccessful. This study of hypertensives found that basal systolic and diastolic BPs were correlated with GH and IGF-I levels. Furthermore, there was a significant correlation between the percentage reduction in GH/IGF-I levels and the percentage reduction in systolic and diastolic BPs.

Their findings of both a degree of dose–response relationship between GH/IGF-I levels and BP, and a significant reduction in BP and uncontrolled hypertension when acromegaly is controlled represent the strongest evidence yet that acromegaly does cause hypertension. Limitations of the study include the exclusion of hypertensive patients who were not receiving antihypertensives and the lack of blinding. These may have biased results, however, the overwhelming strengths of this study designed—unlike others—specifically to detect a change in BP with acromegaly treatment lend considerable weight to the argument that acromegaly causes a potentially reversible hypertension. The subsequent year the same group produced a study looking at patients (some of whom have also been included in the previous study after shorter follow-up) who received only SSA treatment for 5 years (excluding patients who were initially or subsequently managed surgically) [29]. They observed a reduction in hypertension greater than 50% ($p=0.027$). This reduction retained significance when patients were analyzed by sex or type of SSA.

One study of 31 patients (11 hypertensives) who underwent successful surgery for acromegaly measured pre- and post-operative BP clinically and using ABPM. They found significant reductions in systolic and diastolic BPs by clinical measurement [20]. With ABPM they found that 24 h, daytime and nighttime systolic pressures fell significantly; however, corresponding diastolic changes were nonsignificant.

These papers provide focused data about whether treatment of acromegaly improves the associated hypertension by removing confounding diluent effects in other papers of small initial numbers of hypertensive patients and patients who do not respond adequately to treatment. Another paper by Delaroudis and colleagues [30] found a significant reduction in BP in 18 patients on SSAs that achieved only partial control of their GH/IGF-I levels. A Russian group recently presented data on a sample of 232 acromegalic patients, 80.2% of whom were hypertensive. They report a normalization of BP in patients whose acromegaly began before age 45, but not in others [31]. Other groups have found a link between age and cardiovascular comorbidities in acromegaly. A phenomenon also recognized in acromegalic cardiomyopathy [32], duration of disease, is likely to play a role in this. A Dutch study looking at comorbidities of patients in long-term remission from acromegaly found that compared to epidemiological data, only patients aged 50–70 were significantly more hypertensive than controls [33]. Some groups looking at whether remission of acromegaly results in resolution of hypertension have found less or no association. It should be mentioned that few of these studies focus on hypertension as a primary outcome; most are looking at changes in other conditions, usually cardiomyopathy.

Colao et al. published another study in 2008 looking at improvement in cardiovascular morbidity by different successful acromegaly treatments: surgery vs. SSAs [34]. In this case only diastolic BP decreased significantly, but with both treatment approaches. Overall, there was a nonsignificant trend to a reduction in the number of hypertensives with both treatments. This may not have reached statistical significance because the analysis subdivided hypertension into stages 1 and 2 and patients were divided by treatment, meaning small samples. A significant reduction in diastolic BP alone was also found in another paper when GH/IGF-I levels were normalized [35]. Another study found that patients in remission after surgical treatment of acromegaly had significantly lower diastolic BP than those whose surgery had failed, but hypertension prevalence and systolic BP were not significantly different [36].

A 2007 meta-analysis of 18 papers (none were randomized control trials) which examined the effect of SSAs on the heart in acromegaly found no significant effect on hypertension [37]. However, hypertension was not one of the inclusion criteria, meaning certain papers were ignored including more recent studies that used the best designs for detecting changes in hypertension. Another reason that the meta-analysis may have failed to detect a significant difference is that many of the studies were done before the currently accepted definition of remission of acromegaly. The mean level of post-treatment GH after an oral glucose tolerance test (OGTT) was 7.6 μg/L—today an accepted level for remission is <1 μg/L [38]. This incomplete remission of acromegaly may have meant that changes in BP were insignificant;

however, another group have found significant changes with partial control of acromegaly (although mean nadir GH was lower at 2.35 μg/L) [30]. Other potential explanations include that the possibility that follow-up was not sufficiently long to see resolution of hypertension, possible effects of different age demographics, that heterogeneity influenced results or that low numbers of hypertensives meant that mean BP changes were small when diluted with non-hypertensive patients.

Apart from this meta-analysis, papers from other groups found no significant reduction in BP or hypertension. One series including 15 patients (4 hypertensives) [39] found no significant reduction. Two reasonably sized (43 and 61 patient) studies compared those with successful remission of acromegaly with those with partial remission and with controls; neither found any difference in BP or hypertension [40, 41]. One study of 10 patients treated with a subcutaneous SSA (octreotide) found a significant increase in mean 24 h and nighttime systolic and diastolic BPs with ABPM [28]. They hypothesize that this may be due either to vasoconstrictive effects of octreotide on the splanchnic vasculature, increasing systemic circulating volume, or because ABPM provides a better assessment of hypertension than clinical measurements. It seems possible that SSAs produce this effect only transiently, and if other studies measure BP clinically at another time to treatment this effect might be missed. Perhaps only ABPM, with its long-term measurements would detect this change.

The combination of these findings presents a mixed picture. Methodologically, the strongest studies do find a reduction in BP. However, we cannot ignore evidence from the meta-analysis and other studies that found no change. Despite having flaws in their design for detecting change in BP (most not having been designed with this aim) they demonstrate that BP reduction with treatment of acromegaly may only happen in certain patients or settings, with certain treatments, or that changes are small. More studies are required, including the use of ABPM and larger cohorts looking for changes in BP in both hypertensives and normotensives. Samples need to be large so that data can be analyzed for those whose treatment is successful and for those who remain acromegalic.

The Nature of Acromegaly-Associated Hypertension

A very small number of groups have attempted to elucidate the nature of the BP change that occurs in acromegaly. As seen above some have found that hypertension is predominantly diastolic or systolic, however there is also evidence from studies using ABPM about BP patterns in acromegaly, particularly loss of the normal circadian fall in nocturnal BP or "non-dipping." Non-dipping has been found to be independently associated with significant cardiovascular morbidity [42]; two population studies have estimated its prevalence in a cohort of Swedish men (6.2%) [43] and in normotensive non-diabetic Finnish subjects (18.8%) [44]. Jaffrain-Rai and colleagues found that 44.1% of 68 acromegalic patients were non-dippers [18]. They analyzed to look for interaction with the glucose tolerance of patients—since diabetes mellitus is independently associated with non-dipping—but no such interaction existed. They do highlight the important fact that lack of nocturnal fall in BP may be confounded by the coexistence of sleep apnea—this could cause nocturnal hypertension and is found in acromegaly. Another study ($n=25$) found a high prevalence of non-dipping in both normotensive patients (40%) and hypertensive patients with acromegaly (60%), and that non-dipping was associated with higher GH levels [19]. These agreed with a previous smaller paper [21] but contradict findings of Minniti et al. who found only one of seven hypertensive acromegalic patients were non-dippers [17]. The latter paper also found a very large difference between the prevalence of hypertension when using clinical measurements or ABPM (as mentioned above) so the population may have been atypical. Another group have presented data showing similarly high levels of non-dipping (57%) in acromegalics regardless of whether hypertensive or not [45]. The only evidence where controls were used is from a small study that found non-dipping was more common in acromegalics (62%) vs. controls (12%, $p<0.01$) [21]. In summary, it appears that the non-dipping profile may be associated with acromegaly, beyond that expected for the hypertension and impaired glucose tolerance seen in the condition. Whether this effect is mediated by concomitant obstructive sleep apnea remains to be clarified.

Conclusions

Evidence from case series and case–control studies suggest strongly that acromegaly is associated with elevated BP. The prevalence remains unclear, with estimates ranging from 17.5% to over 80%, however most studies, particularly larger ones designed to look at hypertension in acromegaly find it to be between approximately 40 and 60%, and higher than in matched controls. Acromegaly may also cause the non-dipping nocturnal BP pattern.

As mentioned above, hypertension is of significance in acromegaly because of its negative impact on acromegalic cardiomyopathy and as a predictor of mortality. It appears that treatment of acromegaly can lead to an improvement of hypertension; however, there is not sufficient evidence about effects of management of hypertension on mortality in acromegaly. It also remains to be clarified whether the effects are directly from GH/IGF-I excess or indirectly e.g. from obstructive sleep apnea; there does not seem to be a consistent correlation between either GH/IGF-I levels or duration of disease and degree of hypertension [20], pointing to a complex association.

Possible Mechanisms for Hypertension in Acromegaly

Expansion of Plasma Volume

There is quite extensive evidence to suggest that acromegaly is associated with an augmentation of the body's fluid volumes. In a cross-sectional study, one group found that average extracellular water was 6 L greater for 16 acromegalic patients than for 18 controls ($p<0.01$) [46], these results were in agreement with findings from a larger population [47]. There is also a good body of evidence that these expansions in body water resolve with both surgical and medical treatment, reviewed in detail elsewhere [48, 49].

Plasma volume and extracellular water are closely related to the body's exchangeable pool of sodium. The finding that this pool of sodium is increased in acromegalics [47, 50], including in hypertensive patients [25] lends support to this theory. The cause of this change in plasma volume and exchangeable sodium pool is not clear; however the association is consistent, so it is likely that this is at least one of the pro-hypertensive changes in acromegaly.

Direct Effect by GH or IGF-I

It has been suggested that hypertension and this expansion of plasma volume in acromegaly may also be induced indirectly via a number of pathways, including direct actions of GH and/or IGF-I on the kidney. Indeed, both GH and IGF-I receptors are expressed in the kidney [51] which has led to investigation of this as a possible link.

Direct action of GH was first suggested as early as the 1960s [52]. The majority of subsequent evidence comes mainly from animal models, non-acromegalic subjects, and from effects on channels outside the kidney as a proxy for renal activity (comprehensively reviewed elsewhere [48]). A number of studies have looked at activity of the sodium-potassium pump (Na^+/K^+ATPase) in other tissues, with contradictory conclusions about it being up-regulated [53] or down-regulated [54] in acromegaly. Given this inconsistency in the literature, the paucity of human trials and difficulty in distinguishing activity attributable to GH or IGF-I we cannot be sure of a GH-mediated effect.

GH can cause an increase in the glomerular filtration rate (GFR) of normal subjects [55] and a raised GFR is seen in acromegalic patients [50, 56]. However, this is also seen with administration of IGF-I, which suppresses GH secretion, in normal subjects; so IGF-I may be the direct mediator [57]. The direction of causality between increased plasma volume and increased GFR also remains to be defined.

Renin-Angiotensin-Aldosterone System and Brain Natriuretic Peptide

The renin-angiotensin-aldosterone (RAA) system and brain natriuretic peptide (BNP) have both been implicated as possible indirect mechanisms of hypertension in acromegaly. However, some of the results have subsequently been found to be irreproducible. One group produced a paper thoroughly examining this integrated endocrine axis [58]. They found that there was no significant difference between active and remitted acromegalic subjects for plasma renin activity, aldosterone levels, plasma atrial natriuretic peptide (ANP) or amount of natriuresis, nor was there a significant change in BNP levels after treatment of acromegalic subjects. Limitations

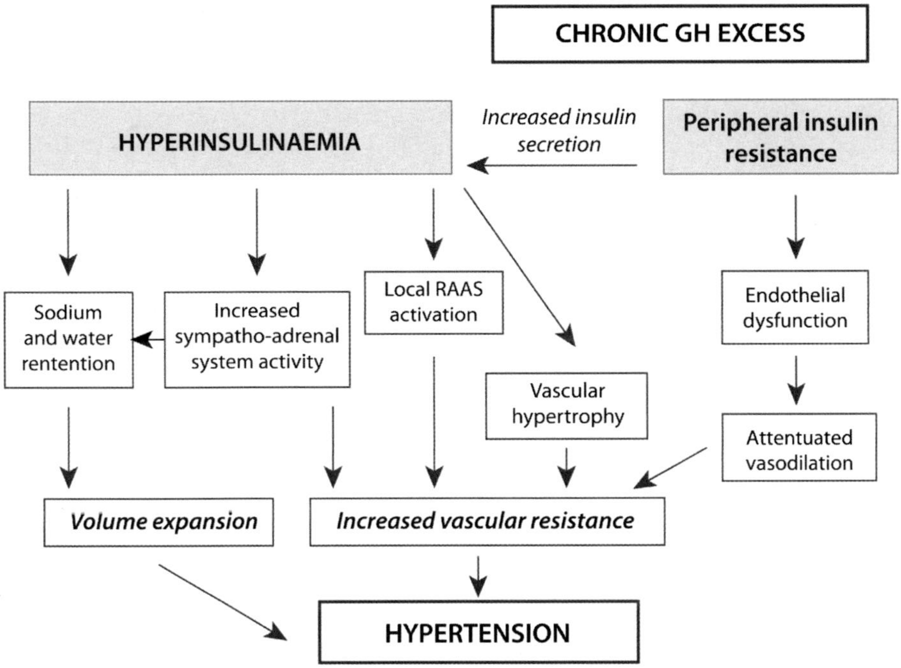

Fig. 8.1 Summary of proposed mechanisms of insulin-mediated hypertension in acromegaly. Reprinted with permission: Bondanelli et al. [76]

of the study include the fact that none of the patients had significant hypertension (all <160/90 mmHg) so we cannot be sure these changes do not occur in hypertensives, although plasma volume was significantly increased in active patients. Also, their definition of remission was less strict than today's so it is possible that treatment of acromegaly was incomplete. Furthermore, some have criticized the accuracy of the early ANP/BNP assays [52, 59]. This paper does, however, provide evidence that BNP and the RAA system may not be the key mediators of acromegaly-associated hypertension, which is supported by other groups' findings concerning the RAA system [23, 60, 61]. Many do, however, believe it is implicated somehow in acromegaly [62] and since it seems to be important in BP changes when GH is given to controls [63], further investigation is warranted.

Insulin-Mediated Mechanisms

A common feature of acromegaly is insulin resistance and resultant hyperinsulinemia [64]. Some have proposed that insulin causes hypertension through a number of mechanisms, as outlined in Fig. 8.1. Many groups have found that hypertension is more prevalent among acromegalic patients with impaired glucose tolerance or diabetes than those without [10, 18, 65, 66], although others' findings disagree [64] and some found the association only between abnormalities of carbohydrate metabolism and non-dipping profiles [19]. It is also not clear whether there is confounding; impaired carbohydrate metabolism and hypertension may commonly coexist, because they are both found in severe acromegaly or certain patient subgroups. However, one group found no interaction between hypertension or carbohydrate metabolism and either GH or IGF-I levels [18].

Evidence from non-acromegalic patients does provide a number of putative links. Insulin is known to have its own role in sodium homeostasis, causing increased tubular reabsorption [67], and is thought to cause an increase in sympathetic nervous system activity, activation of the RAA, and vascular effects [67, 68]. There is, however, a dearth of evidence from acromegalic patients and we are therefore unsure of the role of insulin in this association.

Sympathetic Activity

Increased sympathetic tone in acromegaly has been suggested as the cause of hypertension and while some have found raised plasma catecholamines in active acromegaly vs. controls [69, 70] (possibly because acromegalic patients were older than controls in Rozenberg et al. [69]), most have found urinary and plasma levels to be normal [71–74]. Bondanelli and colleagues found normal plasma catecholamine levels, but an absence of their normal nocturnal drop in acromegalic patients, which returned after surgical treatment of acromegaly [75]. This may have relevance to the non-dipping BP profile, but may also be related to obstructive sleep apnea. Once again, there is insufficient evidence to convincingly confirm or refute sympatho-adrenomedullary hyperactivity as being of major importance in acromegaly-associated hypertension. The issue is further confused by the fact that insulin resistance, sleep apnea, and expansion of plasma volume may all cause abnormal autonomic outflow [76]. Increased sympathetic activity may, therefore, be a side product of these conditions, the intermediate link between them and hypertension, or completely unrelated.

Cardiovascular Effects

Patients with acromegaly have been observed to have a hyperkinetic heart with increased output and cardiac index [77, 78]. Coupled with evidence of dysfunctional regulation of systemic vascular resistance, the possibility of this as a cause of hypertension in acromegaly has been raised. Although systemic vascular resistance is thought to be reduced in uncomplicated acromegaly, it appears that cardiac output may be distributed abnormally peripherally as measurements of brachial artery hemodynamics revealed increased local resistance compared with controls [79]. Others have found impaired endothelium-dependent vasodilation in the upper limb that may explain this [80]. Endothelium-dependent structural changes in vessels have also been reported, with increased intima-media thickness (IMT) in active acromegalics compared with healthy controls and inactive patients [81], although when patients were matched with controls for vascular risk factors there was no significant difference [82]. Increased IMT can be a result of hypertension, impaired glucose tolerance, and other cardiovascular risk factors [77]. Increased IMT can also be a primary change to cause hypertension [83]. The discovery of increased IMT in normotensive acromegalic patients [84] suggests that this change may contribute to hypertension; however it is unclear whether this is a direct effect of GH/IGF-I or an indirect effect of impaired glucose tolerance. It appears that vascular dysfunction and structural change may be present in acromegaly and may contribute to hypertension; however, further studies are required to clarify this.

Sleep Apnea Syndrome

As mentioned previously, one possible intermediate link between acromegaly and hypertension is sleep apnea syndrome (SAS). SAS is seen commonly in acromegaly—estimates range from 20 to 80% [85]—and hypertension is associated with SAS in 40–60% in the general population [86]. Despite this, there is little recognition of this in the literature concerning acromegaly and hypertension and very few papers investigate SAS as a potential confounding comorbidity. One study mentions that the severity of SAS was greater in hypertensive acromegalics than normotensives [87]. The proposed pathophysiology of hypertension in SAS is shown in Fig. 8.2, and includes alterations in sympathetic activity and endothelial dysfunction as discussed above. It also includes reduced nitric oxide (NO) production, which has been

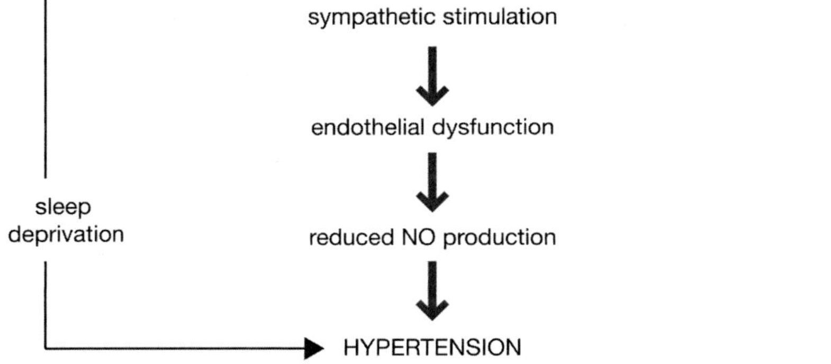

Fig. 8.2 Proposed mechanism of development of hypertension in sleep apnea. Reprinted with permission: Fatti et al. [86]

detected by one group [88]. SAS of course is not limited to acromegalics; in non-acromegalic patients with SAS, GH secretion and IGF-I levels have been reported to be reduced, perhaps because of elevated cortisol due to the hypoxemia and resultant frequent near-awakening (for review see [89]).

Conclusion: Acromegaly

These represent some of the major mechanistic theories concerning the association between acromegaly and hypertension. Hypertension is probably, as in the general population, a product of numerous factors in acromegaly. The evidence reviewed above shows some of these possible factors individually and the overlap between them. Future research must consider these several issues in an integrated fashion.

Growth Hormone Deficiency

Introduction

Hypopituitarism without growth hormone replacement is known to be associated with cardiovascular disease and premature mortality. In the context of deficiency of numerous other hormones which affect the cardiovascular system and the potential for under- or over-replacement of these hormones, it is difficult to study the effects of GH on BP in isolation. In addition, BP is one interconnected cardiovascular variable along with other factors such as lipid profiles, body composition, fat distribution, and cardiac function—all of which have been shown to vary with GH deficiency and replacement [90–92]. GH replacement has been shown to improve some cardiovascular morbidity and cardiovascular risk in patients with hypopituitarism [93, 94]. In this section the epidemiological relationship will be discussed and the response of BP to GH replacement as well as some proposed mechanisms to explain any association.

Hypertension in GHD Patients

A number of studies have looked at the increased cardiovascular risk profile in hypopituitary patients. Older studies have looked at patients who were adequately replaced for all other pituitary hormones but not GH. Rosen et al. looked at a group of such patients in comparison with a local cohort, the World Health Organization's MONICA study population of cardiovascular disease. They found a significantly increased prevalence of treated hypertension in the GHD patients but no absolute difference in BP. This difference was neither explained by increased diabetes mellitus nor smoking rates (actually higher in controls). One major possible interfering factor is that patients in the study may have more medical attention and therefore have been more likely to have hypertension detected and treated. However, if this had been the case one might expect the absolute BP values to have differed [95].

The largest study of adult-onset GHD is one of 926 Spanish patients with untreated GHD of different causes, as compared with a separately studied population of nearly 30,000 normal Spanish subjects. They found a prevalence of hypertension (as defined by use of antihypertensive medication or SBP >140 mmHg and DBP >90 mmHg) to be 22.6 and 21.7% among male and female GHD patients respectively, which is higher than the 14.8% found in the reference population [96].

Examining congenital syndromes of isolated GH absence or ineffectivity may exclude the possible interference from excess or under-replacement of other pituitary hormones. Barreto-Filho and colleagues examined a homogenous population of 16 patients with familial isolated GH deficiency secondary to a non-functional growth hormone-releasing hormone receptor (GHRH-R). Compared with a matched control group SBP alone was significantly higher. They also found a blunted ability of the cardiovascular system to respond to orthostatic stress (increased drop in SBP and reduced rise in DBP vs. controls) [97]. The authors make a comparison with another study's population possessing a different null-mutation in the GHRH-R; in this study they found asymptomatic hypotension. The blood pressure values were likely inaccurate due to use of an inappropriately large cuff on the patients, however, this was considered not sufficient to explain the considerable hypotension and when they remeasured certain subjects' BP using a pediatric cuff, patients were still found to be hypotensive [98]. Isolated systolic hypotension has also been reported [91]. Interestingly, a literature search reveals no evidence of changes in blood pressure in patients with GH resistance (Laron syndrome), in whom Laron states that "resting blood pressure is within normal limits" [99].

Large studies of GHD patients seem to confirm an adverse BP profile; however, there are no reports of extreme differences and the evidence is more mixed concerning BP in congenital syndromes of isolated GHD.

Resolution of Hypertension in GHD with Treatment

As in acromegaly, where there is doubt about the validity of the association of GHD and hypertension it is useful to look at the effect that GH replacement therapy has on blood pressure and rates of hypertension. A number of studies have examined this.

Of the studies looking at the treatment of GHD, there are several that have found a decrease in DBP but not SBP. A meta-analysis of the literature performed in 2004 including only double-blind, randomized control trials included ten trials that reported monitoring of BP. They showed no significant change in SBP but a significant decrease in DBP (−1.8 mmHg). The overall meta-analysis included 27 other trials and the authors note that most of these would have included some monitoring of

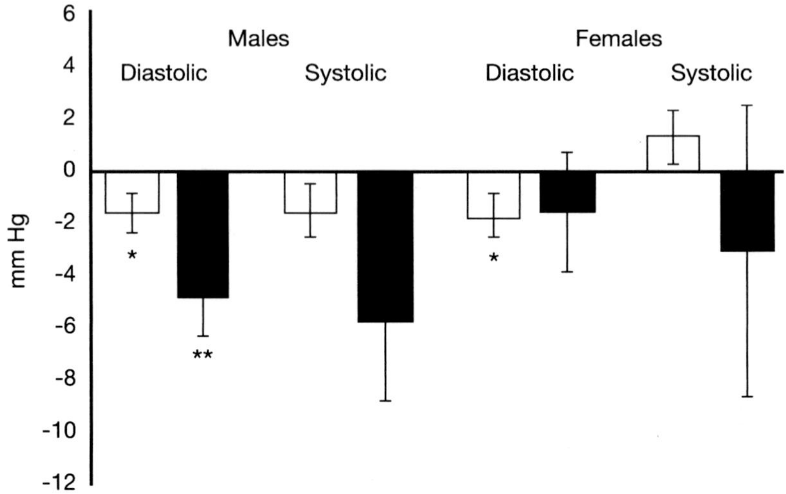

Fig. 8.3 Changes in diastolic and systolic blood pressure after 6 months of GH replacement in adult GH deficient patients younger (*open bars*) and older (*black bars*) than age 65. $^{*}p<0.05$; $^{**}p<0.01$. Reprinted with permission: Monson et al. [104]

BP (possibly for safety). They concluded that the other trials probably did not find any significant change in BP with GH treatment; this may have introduced bias but the data are interesting as they use only trials with rigorous design [90]. Another small study from 1994 found an isolated reduction in DBP (79 to 72 $p<0.05$) in the 10 patients they studied in their placebo, double blinded 6-month cross-over study [100]. Fideleff and colleagues' findings were similar from a group of mixed adult-onset and congenital GHD as compared to controls. They found a significant decrease in DBP alone over 4 years of GH treatment (–4 mmHg, $p<0.035$) which did not vary depending on age of onset of GHD [101]. Another group looked at the effect of 7 years of GH replacement and found a significant reduction in resting DBP vs. controls but a small increase in SBP. Increased SBP was also seen in the control population so this was attributed to age-related changes [102].

The KIMS database (Kabi International Metabolism Study, now called the Pfizer International Metabolic Database) is a pharmacovigilence study monitoring patients receiving GH replacement. There are no control groups but the study benefits from being large (over 1,000 patients) and from long follow-up. One group's baseline analysis found that using a target blood pressure of <130/85 mmHg, 26% of patients were hypertensive, including 15% that were on antihypertensive medications. The authors considered this to be an "adverse profile," although there was no control group for comparison. Over 2 years' follow-up there was no change in mean BP values; however, there was a small reduction in the number of patients exceeding the target BP of 130/85 mmHg from 26 to 23% ($p=0.01$) [103].

Another analysis of the KIMS database looked at the effect of at least 6 months GH replacement in hypopituitary patients over the age of 65 as compared with patients under 65 years old. In patients under 65 and male patients over 65 there was a trend to reduce DBP but this change was nonsignificant in females over 65 (Fig. 8.3).

They state their own previous findings from the KIMS data that show reductions in BP with GH replacement to be correlated with baseline BP; they feel this would explain their findings of a trend to reduce SBP only in older patients, given that BP was positively correlated with age [104].

Another group's paper examined similar parameters in children (mean age 9.3 years) at baseline and 2 years follow-up after GH treatment vs. matched controls [105]. They found no difference at baseline or change in SBP or DBP with treatment, which would fit with Monson et al.'s findings [104]. A confounding factor may be that childrens' blood pressure is recognized to rise as they get older.

Recently, a meta-analysis of 11 studies examining the effects of GH replacement in an older GHD population (over 60 years old) found no overall significant BP change in the five studies that included data on BP. One study found no change, one a transient fall in BP, and three found reduced DBP only [106]. They also found no effect of GH on cardiac structure or function. As mentioned above, others have found a reduction in BP with GH replacement; however, there is a strong body of evidence to suggest that cardiac function improves with GH treatment [26]. This suggests that either elderly peoples' cardiovascular systems are less able to respond to GH than younger individuals' or that the study was not sufficiently powered to detect the changes in BP and cardiac function found in other studies.

Some studies have found a reduction in both diastolic and SBPs with GH treatment. Abdu et al. found a significant drop in both measures of BP after 6 and 12 months follow-up. When taken in context with improvement in lipid profiles, body fat distribution and proxy measurements of endothelial dysfunction, these amounted to a reduction in absolute and relative risk of coronary artery disease as calculated by the Framingham risk equation [107].

Measurements of blood pressure have been made using alternative methods. Smith et al. used calculated central aortic pressures by assessment of the peripheral pulse waveforms in GHD patients and controls before and after 6 months of GH or placebo administration [108]. These data were included in the meta-analysis by Maison et al. [90]. At baseline they found nonsignificant trends of increased BP in the GHD patients over controls. After 6 months treatment recipients of GH had a significantly lower SBP and DBP in calculations of aortic pressures as compared with placebo-treated patients, however, similar trends were not significant for measurements at the brachial artery. They also showed significant reductions in markers of endothelial dysfunction (a risk factor for atherogenesis) with GH and attribute improvements found in central BP to reduced arterial wall stiffness [108].

Ahmad and colleagues used ABPM to assess BP and circadian rhythms in BP [94]. They found a significant drop in both SBP and DBP in their 22 patients after 12 months GH treatment. There was no evidence of absence of the normal circadian BP variation before or after GH treatment—a factor known to be associated with cardiovascular disease as discussed above. However, others have found increased rates of systolic non-dipping in untreated GHD [109]. Conversely, Moller et al. found no significant change in 24 h ABPM between those treated with GH or placebo in their younger group of GHD patients [110].

This is not the only study to find no significant difference in BP with GH replacement particularly over shorter time-frames [110–113]. As mentioned above, a number of studies within the meta-analysis of Maison et al. may also not have found an effect.

One early study reported an increased SBP in response to 6 months' GH replacement in 24 subjects [114]. A recent analysis of another large adult GHD pharmacovigilance study, Lilly's Global Hypopituitary Control and Complications Study (HypoCCS), looked at 346 GHD patients before and after 3 years' treatment with GH [115]. Surprisingly, they found a significant increase in hypertension (on antihypertensives or BP >130/85 mmHg) after GH replacement. This is a long follow-up time with a large population and may represent longer-term changes to BP with GH treatment. However, it may also be explained by the aging of the population—important in this study given the long follow-up, as well as the effect that being in a study population might have on prescription of antihypertensive medication which would increase the number qualifying as hypertensive. Furthermore, the baseline numbers of patients found to be hypertensive was very high (59.8%). The 346 cases were selected from a population of 7,895 patients and were the only ones to have full records of the five variables measured (BP, triglycerides, fasting glucose, high-density lipoprotein cholesterol, and waist circumference) at baseline and 3 years follow-up. This equates to 4% of the total cohort and it is possible that these patients had more comprehensive records because their health was worse than other patients who did not have a complete record. This might also explain the high level of hypertension in the cohort.

Contradictory results make it difficult to say with any certainty about the effect of GH replacement in GHD but the strongest evidence comes from Maison et al.'s meta-analysis because of the quality of the included trials. Its findings are also supported by a number of other studies; however, it may be that effects are different according to age group studied.

Possible Mechanisms

Given the sometimes contradictory results concerning BP, GHD and GH replacement, this area has received little direct scrutiny in the literature on other cardiovascular effects of GHD. As such, there is a lack of strong evidence on possible mechanisms of GHD-induced hypertension.

One explanation offered by a number of authors, including Ahmad et al., suggests that the problems arise from abnormal vascular reactivity or endothelial dysfunction. Citing evidence that GH's effects on the cardiovascular system are mediated by IGF-I and that IGF-I can cause vasodilatation via a nitric oxide (NO)-dependent mechanism (reviewed elsewhere [116]), they propose this as a mechanism [94]. Treatment of GHD over 12 months in a randomized placebo-control trial showed increased NO formation and a 30% fall in peripheral arterial resistance. There was no fall in BP but this may have been negated by the increase in cardiac output seen [117]. Others have found a reduction in total peripheral resistance to accompany a fall in diastolic BP [100]. Capaldo and colleagues found that in young GHD sufferers, vascular dysfunction was found even in the absence of severe diabetes mellitus, hypertension, and hypercholesterolemia—all of which are associated with GHD—suggesting that this might be the primary change [118]. This dysregulation of the vascular system was not found in treated GHD patients, who had similar responses to controls. They hypothesize that the reason for vascular dysfunction in GHD is the absence of the GH/IGF-I vasodilator effect which is probably mediated by NO (reduced endothelial production and reduced smooth muscle cell sensitivity).

Abdu et al. agree with some of the hypotheses raised by Ahmad et al. concerning NO production. However, they feel that GH replacement's effect on hypertension is not in itself as significant as the overall improvement in endothelial function and vascular regulation. They give this more importance as it is reflected in an improvement in a number of cardiovascular risk factors, including hypertension, by redressing the imbalance of vasoactive substances [107].

As mentioned above, Smith et al. examined endothelial dysfunction and large artery stiffness and found that this was increased in GHD patients and reversible with GH replacement. Stiffening of the vasculature is known to increase central blood pressure, something they demonstrated in GHD patients [108]. Evidence regarding arterial stiffening in non-GHD patients shows that this can be caused by hypertension, but may also exacerbate hypertension in a bi-directional manner [119].

Some have suggested stimulation of the renin-angiotensin-aldosterone system (RAS) as the effect of GH that may reduce blood pressure in GH replacement. An increase in sodium retention with involvement of the RAS has been shown after 6 months GH replacement [120]. Others have found no change in the RAS but fluid retention due to suppression of BNP, although this was only over 15 days of GH treatment in non-GHD subjects [113]. Others have found 7 days of GH replacement in GHD patients to cause fluid retention, not due to RAS or ANP changes, but rather to renal tubular effects [112].

A role for increased sympathetic nervous system output has also been hypothesized. Patients with GHD had significantly higher muscle sympathetic nerve activity than controls, their DBP was also elevated and DBP correlated positively with sympathetic activity in patients but not controls [121].

Lastly, Egecioglu and colleagues studied GH receptor knock out (KO) mice and found lower SBP than their wild-type equivalents [122]. The KO mice were found to have more NO bioavailability, which the group posed as a possible explanation. There was no difference in aldosterone levels although renin was raised in KO mice. This may be in accord with some groups' findings of hypotension in populations with genetic syndromes of GH resistance [98]. It is possible that other physiological systems are compensating during early development, which is not possible in adult-onset GHD.

Conclusion: GH Deficiency

Evidence on hypertension in GHD is far sparser and the association far less clear than that in acromegaly. From large population studies it appears that hypertension is a feature of the GHD syndrome, although it is unclear whether there are differences between adult and childhood-onset GHD. Whether GH replacement therapy in these patients leads to a reduction in blood pressure also remains uncertain. Treatment of GHD causes widespread changes in body composition, lipids, cardiac and vascular function, and as such it is hard to isolate effects on BP. Furthermore, little direct study has been done on BP in this setting. It may be, however, that focusing on BP in this way is not relevant to mortality and morbidity. It has been shown that replacement of GH reduces the excess cardiovascular mortality associated with untreated GHD [93]. Perhaps the focus of investigation should therefore be on the effects of GH replacement on the vascular system as a whole, with BP as one important aspect of that given its known importance as a cardiovascular risk factor.

General Conclusions

Summarizing the above discussions, the evidence that hypertension is a feature in acromegaly is persuasive, a fact found to be important because of the impact on cardiac function and morphology and, subsequently, life expectancy. Estimates of its prevalence are variable but it may be 40–60%. Diurnal BP rhythms may also be negatively affected. It appears that hypertension usually resolves or at least improves with treatment of acromegaly; however, whether this is accompanied by a reduction in mortality remains to be clarified, as do the pathways by which GH excess causes hypertension.

In GHD, we can be less sure, but it appears that hypertension may also be increased in this syndrome. Further direct study would be required to clarify this and whether hypertension resolves with treatment of GHD. There is no evidence to suggest that hypertension is independently associated with increased mortality in GHD; thus it may be that research should be focused on cardiovascular function as a whole, including blood pressure, rather than BP in isolation.

In the normal population the association among GH, IGF-I, and blood pressure is very uncertain, with contradictory results. This may be the area that merits most attention in future research, as the possibility for improving public health may be significant. The effect on blood pressure of administration of low doses of GH to hypertensives with lower levels of IGF-I would be of great interest.

Looking at these seemingly contradictory findings it is hard to describe a simple role for GH in hypertension—currently the evidence is not available. What is certain is that GH both in excess and deficiency is associated with worse cardiovascular outcomes, potentially in a U-shaped relationship. Less certain, but possibly more important is the question over GH's role in hypertensive patients without gross derangement of their GH or IGF-I levels, as this may offer a small chance to help many people worldwide.

Acknowledgment We gratefully acknowledge the assistance of Ms. Monica Kletke in the preparation of this chapter.

References

1. Colao A, Di Somma C, Cascella T, et al. Relationships between serum IGF1 levels, blood pressure, and glucose tolerance: an observational, exploratory study in 404 subjects. Eur J Endocrinol. 2008;159(4):389–97.
2. Hunt KJ, Lukanova A, Rinaldi S, et al. A potential inverse association between insulin-like growth factor I and hypertension in a cross-sectional study. Ann Epidemiol. 2006; 16(7):563–71.
3. Landin-Wllhelmsen K, Wllhelmsen L, Lappast G, et al. Serum insulin-like growth factor I in a random population sample of men and women: relation to age, sex, smoking habits, coffee consumption and physical activity, blood pressure and concentrations of plasma lipids, fibrinogen, parathyroid hormone and osteocalcin. Clin Endocrinol. 1994;41(3):351–7.
4. Capoluongo E, Pitocco D, Lulli P, et al. Inverse correlation between serum free IGF-I and IGFBP-3 levels and blood pressure in patients affected with type 1 diabetes. Cytokine. 2006;34(5–6):303–11.
5. Colangelo LA, Liu K, Gapstur SM. Insulin-like growth factor-1, insulin-like growth factor binding protein-3, and cardiovascular disease risk factors in young black men and white men: the CARDIA Male Hormone Study. Am J Epidemiol. 2004;160(8):750–7.
6. Andronico G, Mangano MT, Nardi E, et al. Insulin-like growth factor 1 and sodium-lithium countertransport in essential hypertension and in hypertensive left ventricular hypertrophy. J Hypertens. 1993;11(10):1097–101.
7. Díez J, Laviades C. Insulin-like growth factor-1 and cardiac mass in essential hypertension: comparative effects of captopril, lisinopril and quinapril. J Hypertens Suppl. 1994;12(4): S31–6.
8. Courville C, Mason VR. The heart in acromegaly. Arch Intern Med. 1938;61(5):704–13.
9. Lie JT. Pathology of the heart in acromegaly: anatomic findings in 27 autopsied patients. Am Heart J. 1980;100(1):41–52.
10. Colao A, Baldelli R, Marzullo P, et al. Systemic hypertension and impaired glucose tolerance are independently correlated to the severity of the acromegalic cardiomyopathy. J Clin Endocrinol Metab. 2000;85(1):193–9.
11. Holdaway IM, Rajasoorya RC, Gamble GD. Factors influencing mortality in acromegaly. J Clin Endocrinol Metab. 2004;89(2):667–74.
12. Melmed S. Clinical perspective. Acromegaly and cancer: not a problem? J Clin Endocrinol Metab. 2001;86(7):2929–34.
13. Colao A, Terzolo M, Bondanelli M, et al. GH and IGF-I excess control contributes to blood pressure control: results of an observational, retrospective, multicentre study in 105 hypertensive acromegalic patients on hypertensive treatment. Clin Endocrinol. 2008;69(4):613–20.
14. Vitale G, Pivonello R, Auriemma RS, et al. Hypertension in acromegaly and in the normal population: prevalence and determinants. Clin Endocrinol. 2005;63(4):470–6.
15. Ciresi A, Amato MC, Vetro C, et al. Adrenal morphology and function in acromegalic patients in relation to disease activity. Endocrine. 2009;36(2):346–54.
16. Kearney PM, Whelton M, Reynolds K, et al. Global burden of hypertension: analysis of worldwide data. Lancet. 2005;365(9455):217–23.
17. Minniti G, Moroni C, Jaffrain-Rea ML, et al. Prevalence of hypertension in acromegalic patients: clinical measurement versus 24-hour ambulatory blood pressure monitoring. Clin Endocrinol. 1998;48(2):149–52.
18. Jaffrain-Rea M, Moroni C, Baldelli R, et al. Relationship between blood pressure and glucose tolerance in acromegaly. Clin Endocrinol. 2001;54(2):189–95.
19. Pietrobelli DJ, Akopian M, Olivieri AO, et al. Altered circadian blood pressure profile in patients with active acromegaly. Relationship with left ventricular mass and hormonal values. J Hum Hypertens. 2001;15(9):601–5.
20. Jaffrain-Rea M, Minniti G, Moroni C, et al. Impact of successful transsphenoidal surgery on cardiovascular risk factors in acromegaly. Eur J Endocrinol. 2003;148(2):193–201.

21. Terzolo M, Matrella C, Boccuzzi A, et al. Twenty-four hour profile of blood pressure in patients with acromegaly. Correlation with demographic, clinical and hormonal features. J Endocrinol Invest. 1999;22(1):48–54.
22. Obara T, Ohkubo T, Imai Y. Long-term risk in subjects with white-coat hypertension. Hypertension. 2009;54(5):e133.
23. Kraatz C, Benker G, Weber F, et al. Acromegaly and hypertension: Prevalence and relationship to the renin-angiotensin-aldosterone system. J Mol Med. 1990;68(12):583–7.
24. Rodrigues EA, Caruana MP, Lahiri A, et al. Subclinical cardiac dysfunction in acromegaly: evidence for a specific disease of heart muscle. Br Heart J. 1989;62(3):185–94.
25. Ohtsuka H, Komiya I, Aizawa T, Yamada T. Hypertension in acromegaly: hereditary hypertensive factor produces hypertension by enhancing IGF-I production. Endocr J. 1995;42(6): 781–7.
26. Colao A, Pivonello R, Spinelli L, et al. A retrospective analysis on biochemical parameters, cardiovascular risk and cardiomyopathy in elderly acromegalic patients. J Endocrinol Invest. 2007;30(6):497–506.
27. Sucunza N, Barahona MJ, Resmini E, et al. Gender dimorphism in body composition abnormalities in acromegaly: males are more affected than females. Eur J Endocrinol. 2008; 159(6):773–9.
28. Fallo F, Barzon L, Boscaro M, Casiglia E, Sonino N. Effect of octreotide on 24-h blood pressure profile in acromegaly. Am J Hypertens. 1998;11(5):591–6.
29. Colao A, Auriemma RS, Galdiero M, Lombardi G, Pivonello R. Effects of initial therapy for five years with somatostatin analogs for acromegaly on growth hormone and insulin-like growth factor-I levels, tumor shrinkage, and cardiovascular disease: A prospective study. J Clin Endocrinol Metab. 2009;94(10):3746–56.
30. Delaroudis SP, Efstathiadou ZA, Koukoulis GN, et al. Amelioration of cardiovascular risk factors with partial biochemical control of acromegaly. Clin Endocrinol. 2008;69(2): 279–84.
31. Melnichenko G, Syirkin A, Pronin V, et al. Prevalence and peculiarity of arterial hypertension treatment in acromegaly patients; 2009. Available at: http://www.endocrine-abstracts.org/ea/0020/ea0020P293.htm. Accessed 21 Jan 2010.
32. Colao A, Marzullo P, Cuocolo A, et al. Reversal of acromegalic cardiomyopathy in young but not in middle-aged patients after 12 months of treatment with the depot long-acting somatostatin analogue octreotide. Clin Endocrinol. 2003;58(2):169–76.
33. Biermasz NR, Pereira AM, Smit JWA, Romijn JA, Roelfsema F. Morbidity after long-term remission for acromegaly: persisting joint-related complaints cause reduced quality of life. J Clin Endocrinol Metab. 2005;90(5):2731–9.
34. Colao A, Pivonello R, Galderisi M, et al. Impact of treating acromegaly first with surgery or somatostatin analogs on cardiomyopathy. J Clin Endocrinol Metab. 2008;93(7):2639–46.
35. Colao A, Pivonello R, Auriemma RS, et al. Efficacy of 12-month treatment with the GH receptor antagonist pegvisomant in patients with acromegaly resistant to long-term, high-dose somatostatin analog treatment: effect on IGF-I levels, tumor mass, hypertension and glucose tolerance. Eur J Endocrinol. 2006;154(3):467–77.
36. Serri O, Beauregard C, Hardy J. Long-term biochemical status and disease-related morbidity in 53 postoperative patients with acromegaly. J Clin Endocrinol Metab. 2004;89(2):658–61.
37. Maison P, Tropeano A, Macquin-Mavier I, Giustina A, Chanson P. Impact of somatostatin analogs on the heart in acromegaly: A metaanalysis. J Clin Endocrinol Metab. 2007; 92(5):1743–7.
38. Giustina A, Barkan A, Casanueva FF, et al. Criteria for cure of acromegaly: a consensus statement. J Clin Endocrinol Metab. 2000;85(2):526–9.
39. Colao A, Marzullo P, Ferone D, et al. Cardiovascular effects of depot long-acting somatostatin analog sandostatin LAR in acromegaly. J Clin Endocrinol Metab. 2000;85(9):3132–40.
40. Puder JJ, Nilavar S, Post KD, Freda PU. Relationship between disease-related morbidity and biochemical markers of activity in patients with acromegaly. J Clin Endocrinol Metab. 2005;90(4):1972–8.

41. Damjanovic SS, et al. Clinical indicators of biochemical remission in acromegaly: does incomplete disease control always mean therapeutic failure? Clin Endocrinol (Oxf). 2005;62(4):410–7.
42. Cuspidi C, Macca G, Sampieri L, et al. Target organ damage and non-dipping pattern defined by two sessions of ambulatory blood pressure monitoring in recently diagnosed essential hypertensive patients. J Hypertens. 2001;19(9):1539–45.
43. Bjorklund K, Lind L, Andren B, Lithell H. The majority of nondipping men do not have increased cardiovascular risk: a population-based study. J Hypertens. 2002;20(8):1501–6.
44. Vasunta RL, Kesaniemi YA, Ukkola O. Plasma adiponectin concentration is associated with ambulatory daytime systolic blood pressure but not with the dipping status. J Hum Hypertens. 2009. Available at: http://dx.doi.org/10.1038/jhh.2009.98. Accessed 8 Feb 2010.
45. Paisley A, Roberts M, Heagerty A, Trainer P. 24-hour ambulatory blood pressure monitoring (ABPM) in patients with acromegaly and the value of clinic blood pressure measurements. Available at: http://www.endocrine-abstracts.org/ea/0007/ea0007P127.htm. Accessed 5 Feb 2010.
46. Gibney J, Wolthers T, Burt MG, et al. Protein metabolism in acromegaly: differential effects of short- and long-term treatment. J Clin Endocrinol Metab. 2007;92(4):1479–84.
47. Bengtsson B-Å, Brummer RM, Eden S, Bosaeus I. Body composition in acromegaly. Clin Endocrinol. 1989;30(2):121–30.
48. Møller J. Effects of growth hormone on fluid homeostasis. Clinical and experimental aspects. Growth Horm IGF Res. 2003;13(2–3):55–74.
49. Katznelson L. Alterations in body composition in acromegaly. Pituitary. 2009;12(2):136–42.
50. Ikkos D, Luft R, Sjögren B. Body water and sodium in patients with acromegaly. J Clin Invest. 1954;33(7):989–94.
51. Hammerman MR, Miller SB. Renal cellular biology of growth hormone and insulin-like growth factor I. Pediatr Nephrol. 1991;5(4):505–8.
52. Biglieri EG, Watlington CO, Forsham PH. Sodium retention with human growth hormone and its subfractions. J Clin Endocrinol Metab. 1961;21(4):361–70.
53. Ng LL, Evans DJ. Leucocyte sodium transport in acromegaly. Clin Endocrinol (Oxf). 1987;26(4):471–80.
54. Salomon F, Cuneo RC, Hesp R, et al. Basal metabolic rate in adults with growth hormone deficiency and in patients with acromegaly: relationship with lean body mass, plasma insulin level and leucocyte sodium pump activity. Clin Sci. 1992;83(3):325–30.
55. Christiansen JS, Gammelgaard J, Ørskov H, et al. Kidney function and size in normal subjects before and during growth hormone administration for one week. Eur J Clin Invest. 1981;11(6):487–90.
56. Falkheden T, Sjogren B. Extracellular fluid volume and renal function in pituitary insufficiency and acromegaly. Acta Endocrinol. 1964;46(1):80–8.
57. Guler HP, Schmid C, Zapf J, Froesch ER. Effects of recombinant insulin-like growth factor I on insulin secretion and renal function in normal human subjects. Proc Natl Acad Sci USA. 1989;86(8):2868–72.
58. Deray G, Chanson P, Maistre G, et al. Atrial natriuretic factor in patients with acromegaly. Eur J Clin Pharmacol. 1990;38(5):409–13.
59. Hall C, Rouleau JL, Moyè L, et al. N-terminal proatrial natriuretic factor. An independent predictor of long-term prognosis after myocardial infarction. Circulation. 1994;89(5):1934–42.
60. McKnight JA, McCance DR, Hadden DR, et al. Basal and saline-stimulated levels of plasma atrial natriuretic factor in acromegaly. Clin Endocrinol (Oxf). 1989;31(4):431–8.
61. Cain JP, Williams GH, Dluhy RG. Plasma renin activity and aldosterone secretion in patients with acromegaly. J Clin Endocrinol Metab. 1972;34(1):73–81.
62. Mulatero P, Veglio F, Maffei P, et al. CYP11B2–344T/C Gene polymorphism and blood pressure in patients with acromegaly. J Clin Endocrinol Metab. 2006;91(12):5008–12.
63. Moller J, Moller N, Frandsen E, et al. Blockade of the renin-angiotensin-aldosterone system prevents growth hormone-induced fluid retention in humans. Am J Physiol Endocrinol Metab. 1997;272(5):E803–8.

64. Ezzat S, Forster MJ, Berchtold P, et al. Acromegaly. Clinical and biochemical features in 500 patients. Medicine (Baltimore). 1994;73(5):233–40.
65. Ikeda T, Terasawa H, Ishimura M, et al. Correlation between blood pressure and plasma insulin in acromegaly. J Intern Med. 1993;234(1):61–3.
66. Słowińska-Srzednicka J, Zgliczyński S, Soszyński P, Zgliczyński W, Jeske W. High blood pressure and hyperinsulinaemia in acromegaly and in obesity. Clin Exp Hypertens A. 1989;11(3):407–25.
67. DeFronzo RA. The effect of insulin on renal sodium metabolism. Diabetologia. 1981;21(3): 165–71.
68. Reaven GM, Lithell H, Landsberg L. Hypertension and associated metabolic abnormalities—the role of insulin resistance and the sympathoadrenal system. N Engl J Med. 1996;334(6):374–82.
69. Rozenberg I, Manchon P, Sabetier C, Hazard J, Lhoste F. Effects of thyrotrophin-releasing hormone on plasma catecholamine levels in acromegalics. Acta Endocrinol. 1985; 109(1):19–24.
70. Rio G, Velardo A, Mascadri C, et al. Baseline and stimulated catecholamine secretion in normotensive patients with active acromegaly: acute effects of continuous octreotide infusion. Eur J Endocrinol. 2000;142(2):179–86.
71. Cryer PE. Plasma norepinephrine and epinephrine in acromegaly. J Clin Endocrinol Metab. 1975;41(3):542–5.
72. Loon GRV. Abnormal plasma catecholamine responses in acromegalics. J Clin Endocrinol Metab. 1979;48(5):784–9.
73. Moore TJ, Thein-Wai W, Dluhy RG, et al. Abnormal adrenal and vascular responses to angiotensin II and an angiotensin antagonist in acromegaly. J Clin Endocrinol Metab. 1980;51(2): 215–22.
74. Capaldo B, Lembo G, Rendina V, et al. Muscle sympathetic nerve activity in patients with acromegaly. J Clin Endocrinol Metab. 2000;85(9):3203–7.
75. Bondanelli M, Ambrosio MR, Franceschetti P, et al. Diurnal rhythm of plasma catecholamines in acromegaly. J Clin Endocrinol Metab. 1999;84(7):2458–67.
76. Bondanelli M, Ambrosio MR, degli Uberti EC. Pathogenesis and prevalence of hypertension in acromegaly. Pituitary. 2001;4(4):239–49.
77. Clayton RN. Cardiovascular function in acromegaly. Endocr Rev. 2003;24(3):272–7.
78. Thuesen L, Christensen SE, Weeke J, Orskov H, Henningsen P. A hyperkinetic heart in uncomplicated active acromegaly. Explanation of hypertension in acromegalic patients? Acta Med Scand. 1988;223(4):337–43.
79. Chanson P, Megnien JL, del Pino M, et al. Decreased regional blood flow in patients with acromegaly. Clin Endocrinol (Oxf). 1998;49(6):725–31.
80. Maison P, Demolis P, Young J, et al. Vascular reactivity in acromegalic patients: preliminary evidence for regional endothelial dysfunction and increased sympathetic vasoconstriction. Clin Endocrinol. 2000;53(4):445–51.
81. Colao A, Spiezia S, Cerbone G, et al. Increased arterial intima-media thickness by B-M mode echo Doppler ultrasonography in acromegaly. Clin Endocrinol (Oxf). 2001;54(4):515–24.
82. Brevetti G, Marzullo P, Silvestro A, et al. Early vascular alterations in acromegaly. J Clin Endocrinol Metab. 2002;87(7):3174–9.
83. Folkow B. Physiological aspects of primary hypertension. Physiol Rev. 1982;62(2):347–504.
84. Colao A, Marzullo P, Lombardi G. Effect of a six-month treatment with lanreotide on cardiovascular risk factors and arterial intima-media thickness in patients with acromegaly. Eur J Endocrinol. 2002;146(3):303–9.
85. Colao A, Ferone D, Marzullo P, Lombardi G. Systemic complications of acromegaly: epidemiology, pathogenesis, and management. Endocr Rev. 2004;25(1):102–52.
86. Fatti LM, Scacchi M, Pincelli AI, Lavezzi E, Cavagnini F. Prevalence and pathogenesis of sleep apnea and lung disease in acromegaly. Pituitary. 2001;4(4):259–62.
87. van Haute FRB, Taboada GF, Correa LL, et al. Prevalence of sleep apnea and metabolic abnormalities in patients with acromegaly and analysis of cephalometric parameters by magnetic resonance imaging. Eur J Endocrinol. 2008;158(4):459–65.

88. Ronconi V, Giacchetti G, Mariniello B, et al. Reduced nitric oxide levels in acromegaly: cardiovascular implications. Blood Press. 2005;14(4):227–32.
89. Lanfranco F, Motta G, Minetto MA, Baldi M, Balbo M, Ghigo E, Arvat E, Maccario M. Neuroendocrine alterations in obese patients with sleep apnea syndrome. Int J Endocrinol. 2010;article 474518:11.
90. Maison P, Griffin S, Nicoue-Beglah M, et al. Impact of growth hormone (GH) treatment on cardiovascular risk factors in GH-deficient adults: a metaanalysis of blinded, randomized, placebo-controlled trials. J Clin Endocrinol Metab. 2004;89(5):2192–9.
91. Cittadini A, Cuocolo A, Merola B, et al. Impaired cardiac performance in GH-deficient adults and its improvement after GH replacement. Am J Physiol. 1994;267(2 Pt 1):E219–25.
92. McCallum RW, Petrie JR, Dominiczak AF, Connell JMC. Growth hormone deficiency and vascular risk. Clin Endocrinol. 2002;57(1):11–24.
93. Svensson J, Bengtsson B-Å, Rosen T, Oden A, Johannsson G. Malignant disease and cardiovascular morbidity in hypopituitary adults with or without growth hormone replacement therapy. J Clin Endocrinol Metab. 2004;89(7):3306–12.
94. Ahmad AM, Hopkins MT, Weston PJ, Fraser WD, Vora JP. Effects of GH replacement on 24-h ambulatory blood pressure and its circadian rhythm in adult GH deficiency. Clin Endocrinol. 2002;56(4):431–7.
95. Rosen T, Eden S, Larson G, Wilhelmsen L, Bengtsson B. Cardiovascular risk factors in adult patients with growth hormone deficiency. Acta Endocrinol. 1993;129(3):195–200.
96. Sanmarti A, Lucas A, Hawkins F, Webb S, Ulied A. Observational study in adult hypopituitary patients with untreated growth hormone deficiency (ODA study). Socio-economic impact and health status. Collaborative ODA (observational GH deficiency in adults) group. Eur J Endocrinol. 1999;141(5):481–9.
97. Barreto-Filho JAS, Alcantara MRS, Salvatori R, et al. Familial isolated growth hormone deficiency is associated with increased systolic blood pressure, central obesity, and dyslipidemia. J Clin Endocrinol Metab. 2002;87(5):2018–23.
98. Maheshwari HG, Silverman BL, Dupuis J, Baumann G. Phenotype and genetic analysis of a syndrome caused by an inactivating mutation in the growth hormone-releasing hormone receptor: Dwarfism of Sindh. J Clin Endocrinol Metab. 1998;83(11):4065–74.
99. Laron Z. Laron syndrome (primary growth hormone resistance or insensitivity): the personal experience 1958–2003. J Clin Endocrinol Metab. 2004;89(3):1031–44.
100. Caidahl K, Edén S, Bengtsson BA. Cardiovascular and renal effects of growth hormone. Clin Endocrinol (Oxf). 1994;40(3):393–400.
101. Fideleff HL, Boquete HR, Stalldecker G, Giaccio AV, Sobrado PGV. Comparative results of a 4-year study on cardiovascular parameters, lipid metabolism, body composition and bone mass between untreated and treated adult growth hormone deficient patients. Growth Horm IGF Res. 2008;18(4):318–24.
102. Chrisoulidou A, Beshyah SA, Rutherford O, et al. Effects of 7 years of growth hormone replacement therapy in hypopituitary adults. J Clin Endocrinol Metab. 2000;85(10):3762–9.
103. Abs R, Feldt-Rasmussen U, Mattsson AF, et al. Determinants of cardiovascular risk in 2589 hypopituitary GH-deficient adults–a KIMS database analysis. Eur J Endocrinol. 2006; 155(1):79–90.
104. Monson JP, Abs R, Bengtsson B-Å, et al. Growth hormone deficiency and replacement in elderly hypopituitary adults. KIMS Study Group and the KIMS International Board, Pharmacia and Upjohn International Metabolic Database. Clin Endocrinol (Oxf). 2000; 53(3):281–9.
105. Salerno M, Esposito V, Farina V, et al. Improvement of cardiac performance and cardiovascular risk factors in children with GH deficiency after two years of GH replacement therapy: an observational, open, prospective, case–control study. J Clin Endocrinol Metab. 2006;91(4):1288–95.
106. Kokshoorn N, Biermasz NR, Roelfsema F, et al. Growth hormone replacement therapy in elderly growth hormone deficient patients: a systematic review. Eur J Endocrinol. 2011; 164(5):657–65.

107. Abdu TAM, Elhadd TA, Buch H, et al. Recombinant GH replacement in hypopituitary adults improves endothelial cell function and reduces calculated absolute and relative coronary risk. Clin Endocrinol. 2004;61(3):387–93.
108. Smith JC, Evans LM, Wilkinson I, et al. Effects of GH replacement on endothelial function and large-artery stiffness in GH-deficient adults: a randomized, double-blind, placebo-controlled study. Clin Endocrinol. 2002;56(4):493–501.
109. Krzyzanowska K, Schnack C, Mittermayer F, et al. High prevalence of abnormal circadian blood pressure regulation and impaired glucose tolerance in adults with hypopituitarism. Exp Clin Endocrinol Diabetes. 2005;113(8):430–4.
110. Moller J, Fisker S, Rosenfalck A, et al. Long-term effects of growth hormone (GH) on body fluid distribution in GH deficient adults: a four months double blind placebo controlled trial. Eur J Endocrinol. 1999;140(1):11–6.
111. Saccà L, Cittadini A, Fazio S. Growth hormone and the heart. Endocr Rev. 1994;15(5):555–73.
112. Hoffman D, Crampton L, Sernia C, Nguyen T, Ho K. Short-term growth hormone (GH) treatment of GH-deficient adults increases body sodium and extracellular water, but not blood pressure. J Clin Endocrinol Metab. 1996;81(3):1123–8.
113. Møller J, Jørgensen JO, Møller N, et al. Expansion of extracellular volume and suppression of atrial natriuretic peptide after growth hormone administration in normal man. J Clin Endocrinol Metab. 1991;72(4):768–72.
114. Salomon F, Cuneo RC, Hesp R, Sönksen PH. The effects of treatment with recombinant human growth hormone on body composition and metabolism in adults with growth hormone deficiency. N Engl J Med. 1989;321(26):1797–803.
115. Attanasio AF, Mo D, Erfurth EM, et al. Prevalence of metabolic syndrome in adult hypopituitary growth hormone (GH)-deficient patients before and after GH replacement. J Clin Endocrinol Metab. 2010;95(1):74–81.
116. Böger RH. Nitric oxide and the mediation of the hemodynamic effects of growth hormone in humans. J Endocrinol Invest. 1999;22(5 Suppl):75–81.
117. Böger RH, Skamira C, Bode-Böger SM, et al. Nitric oxide may mediate the hemodynamic effects of recombinant growth hormone in patients with acquired growth hormone deficiency. A double-blind, placebo-controlled study. J Clin Invest. 1996;98(12):2706–13.
118. Capaldo B, Guardasole V, Pardo F, et al. Abnormal vascular reactivity in growth hormone deficiency. Circulation. 2001;103(4):520–4.
119. Franklin SS. Arterial stiffness and hypertension: a two-way street? Hypertension. 2005; 45(3):349–51.
120. Cuneo RC, Salomon F, Wilmshurst P, et al. Cardiovascular effects of growth hormone treatment in growth-hormone-deficient adults: stimulation of the renin-aldosterone system. Clin Sci. 1991;81(5):587–92.
121. Sverrisdottir YB, Elam M, Herlitz H, Bengtsson B-Å, Johannsson G. Intense sympathetic nerve activity in adults with hypopituitarism and untreated growth hormone deficiency. J Clin Endocrinol Metab. 1998;83(6):1881–5.
122. Egecioglu E, Andersson IJ, Bollano E, et al. Growth hormone receptor deficiency in mice results in reduced systolic blood pressure and plasma renin, increased aortic eNOS expression, and altered cardiovascular structure and function. Am J Physiol Endocrinol Metab. 2007;292(5):E1418–25.
123. Nabarro JDN. Acromegaly. Clin Endocrinol (Oxf). 1987;26:481–512.
124. Molitch ME. Clinical manifestations of acromegaly. Endocrinol Metab Clinics N Am. 1992;21:597–614.
125. Lopez-Velasco R, et al. Cardiac involvement in acromegaly: specific myocardiopathy or consequence of systemic hypertension? J Clin Endocrinol Metab. 1997;82:1047–53.
126. Fukuda I, Hizuka N, Murakami Y, Itoh E, Yasumoto K, Sata A, et al. Clinical features and therapeutic outcomes of 65 patients with acromegaly at Tokyo Women's Medical University. Internal Medicine. 2001;40:987–92.
127. Otsuki M, et al. Characterization of premature atherosclerosis of carotid arteries in acromegalic patients. Clin Endocrinol (Oxf). 54:791–96.

128. Weiss V, et al. Prevalence of the sleep apnea syndrome in acromegaly population. J Endocrinol Invest. 2001;23:515–19.
129. Mestron A, Webb SM, Astorga R, Benito P, Catala M, Gaztambide S, et al. Epidemiology, clinical characteristics, outcome, morbidity and mortality in acromegaly based on the Spanish Acromegaly Registry (Registro Espanol de Acromegalia, REA). Eur J Endocrinol. 2004; 151(4):439–46.

Chapter 9
Primary Hyperparathyroidism and Hypertension

Angela L. Carrelli and Shonni J. Silverberg

Abstract Although an association between primary hyperparathyroidism and hypertension has been reported in the literature for decades, the nature of this association has been fraught with controversy. There is wide variability in the reported prevalence of hypertension in primary hyperparathyroidism and conflicting data on whether surgical cure of primary hyperparathyroidism reverses hypertension. This chapter reviews the possible link between these two conditions, explores the potential mechanisms of this association, and evaluates whether hypertension is reversible with surgical cure of primary hyperparathyroidism. We conclude that the link between hypertension and primary hyperparathyroidism remains unclear and the data regarding reversibility with surgical cure unconvincing. Review of available data provides no reason to reconsider the conclusions of the recent International Guidelines for Surgery in Asymptomatic Primary Hyperparathyroidism, which do not include hypertension as an indication for surgery.

Keywords Primary hyperparathyroidism • Hypertension • Calcium • Parathyroid hormone

Introduction

Primary hyperparathyroidism is defined as hypercalcemia in the presence of elevated or inappropriately normal parathyroid hormone (PTH) levels. Although an association between primary hyperparathyroidism and hypertension has been reported in

A.L. Carrelli • S.J. Silverberg (✉)
Department of Medicine, Division of Endocrinology, College of Physicians and Surgeons, Columbia University, New York, NY, USA
e-mail: sjs5@columbia.edu

C.A. Koch and G.P. Chrousos (eds.), *Endocrine Hypertension: Underlying Mechanisms and Therapy*, Contemporary Endocrinology, DOI 10.1007/978-1-60761-548-4_9,

the literature for decades, the nature of this association has been fraught with controversy [1]. There is wide variability in the reported prevalence of hypertension in primary hyperparathyroidism and conflicting data on whether surgical cure of primary hyperparathyroidism reverses hypertension. This chapter will review the possible link between hypertension and primary hyperparathyroidism, explore the potential mechanisms of this association, and evaluate whether hypertension is reversible with surgical cure of primary hyperparathyroidism. We will begin with an abbreviated discussion of primary hyperparathyroidism itself: its typical presentation, evaluation, and treatment.

Clinical Presentation of Primary Hyperparathyroidism

Primary hyperparathyroidism has a reported incidence of up to 1 in 500 to 1 in 1,000, making it a relatively common endocrine disorder [2, 3]. Hypercalcemia is its biochemical hallmark. Primary hyperparathyroidism is the most common cause of hypercalcemia in the outpatient setting and, when combined with malignancy, is responsible for 90% of all cases of hypercalcemia. Primary hyperparathyroidism most often presents in the sixth decade of life and occurs more commonly in women than men with a 3:1 ratio.

The clinical picture of primary hyperparathyroidism has changed markedly over the past 50 years. The initial descriptions of classical primary hyperparathyroidism depicted a disease of "stones, bones, groans, and moans" with prominent skeletal and renal complications. The associated bone disease, osteitis fibrosa cystica, was characterized radiographically by brown tumors of the long bones, bone cysts, subperiosteal bone resorption of the distal phalanges, a "salt and pepper" appearance of the skull on X-ray due to erosions, and tapering of the distal clavicles [2]. Nephrolithiasis was also often associated with classical primary hyperparathyroidism, with an incidence of 33% in the 1960s. However, this phenotype of primary hyperparathyroidism is now rarely seen in Western countries. With the advent of multichannel screening tests in the early 1970s, primary hyperparathyroidism shifted from a disease that presented with classic symptoms to an asymptomatic disease found on screening blood tests. Today, less than 5% of patients in the United States with primary hyperparathyroidism have overt bone disease due to hyperparathyroidism and only 15–20% have associated nephrolithiasis [2]. In addition, it is estimated that three-quarters of patients with the disease in the United States do not have any clear symptoms [3].

In 80% of cases, primary hyperparathyroidism is due to a single parathyroid adenoma, while multiple parathyroid adenomas are reported in 2–4% of cases. Approximately 10–15% of patients with primary hyperparathyroidism have involvement of all four parathyroid glands, occasionally in association with a familial syndrome such as multiple endocrine neoplasia (MEN) type 1 or 2A.

Evaluation of Primary Hyperparathyroidism

The diagnosis of primary hyperparathyroidism is most commonly made upon evaluation of an asymptomatic elevation in serum calcium. The history and physical exam often do not provide additional clues to the diagnosis. The hallmark of the disease is the biochemical finding of hypercalcemia with an elevated PTH level. However, a PTH level that is in the mid to upper range of normal in the presence of hypercalcemia is also indicative of the disorder, because in nonparathyroid-mediated hypercalcemia PTH levels are suppressed. In addition, laboratory tests often reveal low-normal phosphorus levels, due to the phosphaturic effect of PTH. Forty percent of patients with primary hyperparathyroidism have hypercalciuria [3]. Because of the effect of PTH on conversion of 25-hydroxyvitamin D to 1,25-dihydroxyvitamin D, 1,25-dihydroxyvitamin D levels tend to be in the upper range of normal and levels are actually elevated in one-third of patients with primary hyperparathyroidism. However, most patients with primary hyperparathyroidism have 25-hydroxyvitamin D levels below 30 ng/mL, the cut-point for vitamin D sufficiency. As a result, the most recent International Workshop on the Management of Asymptomatic Primary Hyperparathyroidism recommended measurement of 25-hydroxyvitamin D levels in all patients and consideration of vitamin D supplementation if 25-hydroxyvitamin D levels are less than 20 ng/mL [4]. This International Workshop also recognized a phenotype of primary hyperparathyroidism in which PTH levels are elevated but serum calcium levels are normal (normocalcemic primary hyperparathyroidism). Causes of secondary hyperparathyroidism must be ruled out in order to make this diagnosis.

Although osteitis fibrosa cystica is no longer common, the skeleton remains an important target organ of the disease. While plain films of the bone do not yield much information, bone densitometry shows preferential bone loss at cortical sites due to the actions of PTH on bone, as reflected by lower bone mineral density at the distal one-third of the radius. Bone density at the more cancellous lumbar spine tends to be well preserved and readings at the hip tend to be intermediate between those at the spine and forearm [3]. The information from bone mineral densitometry is also important for establishing a treatment plan as this data is included in the clinical management guidelines, which will be addressed in the next section.

Renal ultrasound and spiral computed tomography are the preferred imaging modalities to detect renal stones when nephrolithiasis is suspected. Patients with renal stones are considered to have symptomatic primary hyperparathyroidism, which has important implications for clinical management.

Treatment of Primary Hyperparathyroidism

Primary hyperparathyroidism can be cured by removing the affected gland(s). All patients with symptoms of primary hyperparathyroidism, including fractures or kidney stones, are advised to have surgery. There is ongoing discussion regarding

Table 9.1 Current guidelines for surgery in asymptomatic primary hyperparathyroidism

Measurement	Surgery recommended in all who meet the following guideline
Age	<50 years old
Bone mineral density	*T*-score <–2.5 at any site and/or prior fragility fracture
Creatinine clearance (calculated)	<60 mL/min
Serum calcium	>1 mg/dL above the upper limit of normal

Adapted from Bilezikian et al. [5]

the management of asymptomatic primary hyperparathyroidism, in which patients have no specific symptoms or signs attributable to elevated calcium or PTH. Over the past two decades, the guidelines for management of patients with asymptomatic primary hyperparathyroidism have evolved. The most recent guidelines from the Third International Workshop on the Management of Asymptomatic Primary Hyperparathyroidism were released in the beginning of 2009 (see Table 9.1) [5]. The 2002 guidelines included 24 h urinary excretion >400 mg/day as an indication for surgery, but because of evidence that hypercalciuria itself does not correlate to risk of nephrolithiasis, this is no longer part of the guidelines. The presence of hypertension is not considered an indication for parathyroidectomy.

Localization studies to identify possible parathyroid adenomas are not necessary for the diagnosis of primary hyperparathyroidism, but are often done to assist with a planned surgery. The most commonly used localization studies are sestamibi scans and cervical ultrasound [6]. Improvement in such preoperative localization techniques, and the development of rapid intraoperative PTH assays have contributed to a shift from conventional four gland parathyroid exploration to minimally invasive parathyroidectomy procedures [6]. Minimally invasive parathyroidectomy procedures have estimated cure rates of 95–98%, with complication rates of 1–3% in initial explorations [6].

Cardiovascular Manifestations of Primary Hyperparathyroidism

The cardiovascular manifestations of primary hyperparathyroidism are a frequently discussed and evolving topic. Studies on the cardiovascular manifestations of the disorder have assessed a variety of endpoints, including cardiovascular mortality, hypertension, coronary artery disease, presence and extent of valvular and myocardial calcifications, left ventricular hypertrophy, cardiac conduction system disease, and carotid plaque [7–16]. Much of the discrepant data in the literature can be reconciled by the wide variations in disease severity studied. Reports on cohorts with symptomatic disease and marked hypercalcemia cannot be compared with those on populations in whom there are minimal calcium and PTH elevations in the absence of overt symptomatology.

While a full discussion of the cardiovascular manifestations of primary hyperparathyroidism is beyond the scope of this chapter, a brief review of the evolution of cardiovascular mortality is instructive, as it demonstrates the change in disease presentation and manifestation over time. Increased cardiovascular mortality is well described in patients with severe and moderately severe primary hyperparathyroidism [17–19]. The increase in mortality was reported to decrease with time following parathyroidectomy [19, 20].

Mortality is not clearly increased in patients with mild hyperparathyroidism. Analysis of 1,052 patients who underwent surgical treatment for primary hyperparathyroidism (median preoperative calcium 11.2 mg/dL) found no increase in mortality compared to the general population after a median follow-up of 12 years [21]. Indeed, the only population-based study from the United States did not find an increase in cardiovascular mortality in a mildly hypercalcemic cohort (relative risk: 0.6) [22]. A report by Nilsson et al. may explain the shift in mortality rates over time. Their study of over 10,000 Swedish patients treated for primary hyperparathyroidism between 1958 through 1997 found increased mortality in the overall cohort compared to the normal population. However, there was no increase in mortality in the subgroup of patients operated on in more recent years (1985–1997) [7]. One possible explanation for this observation is that the patients seen more recently had lower serum calcium levels. Another study suggesting that the decline in mortality may be associated with a decline in disease severity finds improved survival in cases from recent years when patients had lower preoperative serum calcium levels [20]. Only one population-based study in patients with mild untreated primary hyperparathyroidism reported an increased risk of mortality [23]. However, criteria for the diagnosis of primary hyperparathyroidism in this study raise the possibility that patients with other disorders may have been included in this cohort, making it difficult to interpret these findings. In summary, while increased mortality was seen in more severe primary hyperparathyroidism, the majority of existing studies do not demonstrate strong evidence for increased cardiovascular mortality in milder disease. This change may be due to the decline in calcium levels, although other factors, such as advances in treatment for cardiovascular disease, may also be responsible [15].

Hypertension

Hypertension is often seen in patients with primary hyperparathyroidism. The reported prevalence of hypertension in primary hyperparathyroidism varies widely among different studies, ranging from around 20 to 80% [8, 24–28]. There has been significant debate regarding the nature of this association as well as the impact of surgical cure. To further explore this relationship, we will focus on potential mechanisms linking hypertension and primary hyperparathyroidism and review the current data on the reversibility of hypertension with surgical cure of primary hyperparathyroidism. If surgical cure were shown to improve hypertension, this would have important implications for management of the parathyroid disease.

Mechanisms of Hypertension in Primary Hyperparathyroidism

Multiple mechanisms have been proposed to explain the possible link between hyperparathyroidism and hypertension. Several hypotheses attribute the association to one or both of the cardinal biochemical abnormalities seen in primary hyperparathyroidism, the elevations in serum calcium and PTH levels. Other theories link hypertension to associated findings, such as renal insufficiency, hypomagnesemia, and PTH effects on the renin-aldosterone system.

Hypercalcemia has been proposed to underlie the association between hypertension and primary hyperparathyroidism. Suggestive data comes from several studies in nonhyperparathyroid subjects. In one, the acute hypercalcemia resulting from an infusion of calcium in healthy volunteers resulted in increased systolic blood pressure [29]. In this study, hypercalcemia led to a dose-dependent impairment in endothelial vasodilatory function, suggesting that alterations in vasodilatory response could explain the resultant rise in blood pressure. Alternatively, calcium may be related to hypertension via its role in vascular smooth muscle cells contraction [30]. Similar results linking calcium infusion and rise in blood pressure were seen in another study investigating calcium infusion in both normotensive and hypertensive subjects [31]. This study also showed the rise in blood pressure could be prevented by administration of a calcium channel blocker. In primary hyperparathyroidism, a study of ambulatory blood pressure in 53 patients, of whom 47% were hypertensive, found that 24 h and daytime diastolic blood pressure values were significantly associated with serum ionized calcium in the hypertensive patients [8]. No associations were found between the blood pressure measurements and PTH. However, even if calcium is important in this association, data suggest that this relationship is likely to be complex. For example, when acute hypercalcemia was induced in patients with undetectable PTH levels (due to postoperative hypoparathyroidism) no rise in blood pressure was seen, while a euparathyroid control group did have a significant rise in systolic blood pressure. This suggests a possible role for PTH as a mediator of this relationship [32].

Similarly, data on a possible role for PTH in the association of primary hyperparathyroidism with hypertension is not straightforward. PTH causes dose-dependent transient vasodilation while chronic continuous infusion of PTH in normotensive subjects results in hypercalcemia and hypertension [33, 34]. PTH may be indirectly involved in the mechanism causing hypertension via stimulation of renin as discussed below, or more directly via a prostimulatory effect (mediated by calcium or by PTH activation of the renal 1-alpha hydroxylase enzyme) or prosclerotic effect on vascular smooth muscle cells [35, 36]. Population-based studies also suggest a link between PTH and hypertension in nonhyperparathyroid subjects. For example, a study of 1,205 older men and women found a positive association between blood pressure and serum PTH levels [37]. It is not clear whether this could be mediated by another factor, and whether those with higher PTH levels might have secondary hyperparathyroidism and an alternate reason for both PTH elevation and increased blood pressure. Thus in primary hyperparathyroidism data on the association of blood pressure with either PTH or calcium are conflicting, with studies suggesting one or the other may be responsible, and others revealing no relationship between PTH or calcium and blood pressure [38].

Impaired renal function has also been implicated as the possible link between primary hyperparathyroidism and hypertension. A review of 115 patients with primary hyperparathyroidism found that 54.8% were hypertensive. The patients with both primary hyperparathyroidism and hypertension had significantly higher serum urea and creatinine than the patients with primary hyperparathyroidism who were normotensive [39]. In addition, serum urea was associated with systolic blood pressure among all patients with primary hyperparathyroidism, while no correlations were found between blood pressure and either calcium or PTH. A similar association between renal dysfunction and hypertension in primary hyperparathyroidism has been reported in other studies, but it remains unclear if renal dysfunction is caused by hypertension in these patients, or if it is the underlying link between hypertension and primary hyperparathyroidism [40]. Additionally, renal dysfunction is not a consistent finding in studies investigating these associations [26, 38]. The study of 194 patients with primary hyperparathyroidism in which calcium and PTH did not correlate to blood pressure, found no difference in renal function between those with and without hypertension [38].

Another hypothesis regarding the cause of hypertension in patients with primary hyperparathyroidism proposes a potential role for hypomagnesemia in this association [41, 42]. Both experimental and epidemiologic data have suggested a link between hypomagnesemia and cardiovascular pathology, including hypertension [43, 44]. Hypomagnesemia leads to increased intracellular calcium levels, which may alter vascular smooth muscle contraction. In addition, magnesium efflux itself may be linked to calcium signaling pathways [44]. In an experiment on isolated coronary arteries, removal of magnesium from the surrounding organ chamber solution was associated with impaired endothelium-dependent vasodilation. This effect was reversed by replacement of magnesium [45]. This relationship has also been shown in human studies in vivo. In a study involving healthy young adults, infusion of intra-arterial magnesium increased endothelium-dependent vasodilation, although there was no change in systemic blood pressure [46].

The possible role of hypomagnesemia in mediating hypertension in the setting of hypercalcemia was first reported in studies using animal models. In a study involving hypercalcemic dogs, lowering magnesium levels was associated with increased peripheral resistance [42]. Primary hyperparathyroidism may cause hypomagnesemia because hypercalcemia results in decreased renal magnesium reabsorption. There is epidemiologic data that may support this theory. A retrospective study of 89 patients with primary hyperparathyroidism who underwent parathyroidectomy found no difference between the hypertensive ($N=43$) and normotensive ($N=46$) patients in terms of calcium, creatinine clearance, or phosphorus levels. However, the hypertensive patients had significantly lower mean serum magnesium levels [41]. Other than this limited observational data, it remains unclear whether hypomagnesemia actually plays a role in an association between hypertension and primary hyperparathyroidism.

The renin-stimulating ability of PTH, which is thought to be mediated through the inhibition of calcium influx, has also been mentioned as the possible link between primary hyperparathyroidism and hypertension [47]. PTH stimulates renin release in the proglomerular arterioles of rat kidneys [47, 48]. However, most studies investigating the role of the renin-aldosterone system in patients with primary hyperparathyroidism involved only very small groups of patients, and many were done over 30 years ago. In one of the earliest studies, 4 of 7 patients with primary hyperparathyroidism had elevated plasma renin activity (PRA) and hypertension, which both normalized following parathyroidectomy [49]. However, in another study in which patients with primary hyperparathyroidism and hypertension with elevated baseline PRA were given saralasin, an angiotensin inhibitor, no effect on blood pressure was found [50]. Similarly negative results were found in another small study (N=11) [51]. Studies examining changes in the renin-angiotensin-aldosterone system pre- and post-parathyroidectomy also have conflicting results. In a study of 16 normotensive patients with primary hyperparathyroidism, basal PRA and stimulated PRA and aldosterone levels were shown to be elevated. Although these levels normalized following parathyroidectomy, there was no clinically significant change in blood pressure [52]. Another study found no difference in PRA and aldosterone levels between patients with primary hyperparathyroidism and those with essential hypertension or normotensive controls [53]. The same study found no change in PRA, aldosterone levels, or blood pressure 1 and 6 months post-parathyroidectomy. Finally, among 34 patients with primary hyperparathyroidism, the PRA and aldosterone levels were higher in the patients with hypertension (10 patients) compared to the levels in patients who were normotensive [54]. Additionally, in 8 of 10 of the patients with primary hyperparathyroidism and hypertension, the renin and aldosterone levels normalized, as did their blood pressure, following parathyroidectomy. With such contradictory results and underpowered studies, no firm support currently exists for the association between the renin-aldosterone system and hypertension in primary hyperparathyroidism.

Multiple Endocrine Neoplasia

While there remains considerable controversy regarding the presence of a true association between hypertension and primary hyperparathyroidism in sporadic disease, the same is not true for patients with primary hyperparathyroidism in the setting of MEN. Hypertension in this subgroup of patients can be caused by the presence of an MEN-related pheochromocytoma. The most common clinical sign of pheochromocytomas is hypertension, which is seen in 85–90% of cases [55].

Hyperparathyroidism is a feature seen in both MEN type 1 and 2A. MEN1 is a hereditary syndrome associated with hyperparathyroidism, pituitary adenomas, and pancreatic islet cell tumors. Primary hyperparathyroidism is the most common and often the first feature of MEN1 and there is almost 100% penetrance by age 50 [56]. Another common feature of MEN1 is the presence of entero-pancreatic islet tumors, which occur in 30–75% of MEN1 patients, and include gastrinomas in 40% of MEN1 patients [56]. The Zollinger-Ellison syndrome (ZES) features a gastrinoma, recurrent peptic ulcers, and elevated gastrin levels [57]. When primary hyperparathyroidism and ZES are simultaneously present, the hypercalcemia may worsen ZES because it increases gastrin secretion and also decreases responsiveness to antisecretory agents [56, 58]. Parathyroidectomy improves ZES by normalizing calcium levels, leading to decreased gastrin production. Pheochromocytomas are usually not present in MEN1, but there are case reports of some families having MEN1-related pheochromocytomas, which may then present with hypertension [55]. However, pheochromocytomas are a more common feature in MEN type 2A, which is an autosomal dominant genetic syndrome characterized by the presence of hyperparathyroidism, medullary thyroid cancer, and pheochromocytoma [59]. Primary hyperparathyroidism is seen in 15–20% of patients with MEN2A, while approximately 50% develop pheochromocytomas. Overall, the clinical features of primary hyperparathyroidism in MEN2A are similar to as in sporadic cases. Interestingly, among MEN2 patients with pheochromocytomas, only about 50% have associated hypertension [55]. In addition, in these patients the hypertension is more often paroxysmal and not sustained.

The presence of a pheochromocytoma in patients with MEN-related primary hyperparathyroidism likely explains the link between primary hyperparathyroidism and hypertension in this subgroup. Hypertension in these cases is often attributable to catecholamine excess from the pheochromocytoma and would be expected to resolve following pheochromocytoma resection. After successful removal of a pheochromocytoma, only 25% of patients have persistent hypertension, which is then probably due to coexistent essential hypertension [55]. Unlike the link between improvement in ZES and treatment of primary hyperparathyroidism, there are no data to suggest that parathyroidectomy affects hypertension related to an underlying pheochromocytoma in MEN patients. The subject of hypertension and pheochromocytoma will be covered in much greater detail elsewhere, in Chap. 10.

Reversibility of Hypertension by Parathyroidectomy

If a direct link exists between primary hyperparathyroidism and hypertension, successful parathyroidectomy with resultant cure would be expected to reverse the elevated blood pressure. In several older studies from the 1970s and 1980s, hypertension was reported to improve following parathyroidectomy in up to half of all hypertensive patients [26, 27, 40]. However, in these studies, mean serum calcium levels were markedly higher than we see today, as high as 12.75 mg/dL [40]. Even in older studies with higher mean serum calcium levels, improvement in hypertension following parathyroidectomy was not always seen. For example, in a retrospective review from 1982 (preoperative calcium level 11.7 mg/dL), hypertension reversed in only 2 of the 15 patients following surgery [25].

Furthermore, some observational studies raised the possibility that hypertension could actually worsen following surgery [60, 61]. Fifteen year follow-up of a cohort enrolled in 1969 found higher systolic blood pressure, and a greater rise in blood pressure over time, in the patients who underwent parathyroidectomy as compared to those with persistent untreated hyperparathyroidism, although the number of

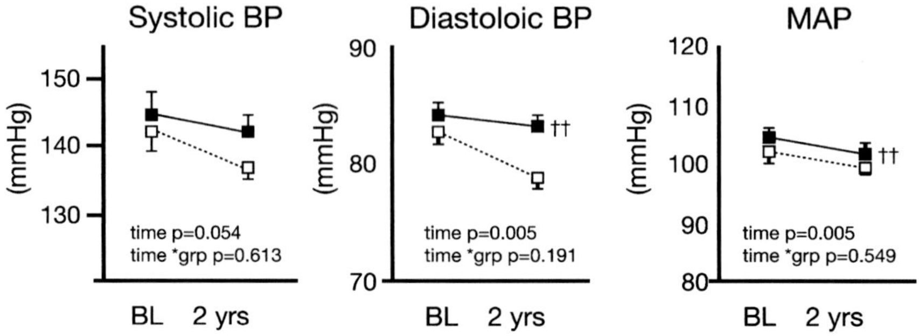

Fig. 9.1 Blood pressure (systolic, diastolic, and mean arterial pressure [MAP]) at baseline and 2 year follow-up with and without intervention in a randomized controlled trial of surgery in mild primary hyperparathyroidism. The *solid line* represents the group that underwent surgery and the *dotted line* represents the group that was observed. Adapted from Bollerslev et al. [62]

patients included in each group at the 15 year follow-up time-point was very small [61]. Another observational study of 62 patients who underwent parathyroidectomy and were followed for up to a mean of 9 years postoperatively, found no improvement in the patients with known hypertension ($N=18$), and 45% of those without a history of hypertension developed hypertension post-parathyroidectomy [60].

Data from more recent studies involving patients with less severe hyperparathyroidism are also inconsistent in their findings on resolution of hypertension with surgery. A retrospective review of patients with mild primary hyperparathyroidism (calcium 11.1 ± 0.6 mg/dL; PTH 136 ± 186 pg/mL) found a significant decrease in both systolic and diastolic blood pressure at 6 months post-parathyroidectomy among the subgroup of patients with known hypertension ($N=147$; blood pressure changes: 152 ± 10.5 to 140.3 ± 16.2 mmHg/94.5 ± 6.8 to 81.7 ± 10.3 mmHg). No significant change in blood pressure was seen postoperatively in the subgroup of patients without a history of hypertension ($N=145$) [62]. Once again, the finding that hypertensive patients respond to surgical cure differently than nonhypertensive patients with primary hyperparathyroidism is not consistent. Another study (preoperative calcium 10.8 mg/dL; PTH 90 pg/mL) found that ambulatory blood pressure actually increased post-parathyroidectomy in the subgroup of patients with a history of hypertension ($N=20$) [63]. A final observational study in 44 patients with very mild PHPT (mean serum calcium 10.5 mg/dl) found normal baseline blood pressure (123±1) that was unchanged at 12 months (122±2/76±1) and 24 months (125±3/78±1) after parathyroidectomy (28).

The best available data on the reversibility of hypertension in primary hyperparathyroidism is the only data that derives from a randomized controlled trial. These level I evidence-based data do not support the attribution of any decline in blood pressure to resolution of the primary hyperparathyroid state. The recent study of Bollerslev et al. reported on 116 Scandinavian patients with mild primary hyperparathyroidism (mean serum calcium 10.8 mg/dL) randomized to observation or surgery. At the 2 year time-point there was no difference in mean arterial pressure (MAP), or systolic or diastolic blood pressure, between the two groups (post-parathyroidectomy or follow-up with no intervention) [64]. It was, however, notable that both MAP and diastolic blood pressure declined significantly over time, with or without parathyroid surgery (see Fig. 9.1). Unfortunately, the results of Bollerslev et al. did not report separately on patients with primary hyperparathyroidism and a known history of hypertension. However, these data demonstrating similar declines in blood pressure with or without parathyroidectomy raise the possibility that the improvements in blood pressure reported in prior uncontrolled studies may not have been due to cure of the disease state.

Conclusions

A review of the available literature reveals that hypertension is common in patients with primary hyperparathyroidism, and that while several possible mechanisms have been proposed, no convincing theory has yet explained a possible link. In addition, the data on reversibility of hypertension with parathyroidectomy is conflicting, even in cases of more severe primary hyperparathyroidism. While many of the studies are small, short-term, or retrospective, recent data from a randomized trial in mild primary hyperparathyroidism (level I evidence) and a study with longer term follow-up of 15 years (level II-1 evidence) both showed no evidence that hypertension is reversible following surgical cure [61, 64]. At this time, the link between hypertension and primary hyperparathyroidism remains unclear and the data regarding reversibility with surgical cure is unconvincing. Review of available data provides no reason to reconsider the conclusions of the recent International Guidelines for Surgery in Asymptomatic Primary Hyperparathyroidism, which do not include hypertension as an indication for surgery [15].

References

1. Hellstrom J, Birke G, Edvall CA. Hypertension in hyperparathyroidism. Br J Urol. 1958; 30(1):13–24.
2. Silverberg SJ, Bilezikian JP. Primary hyperparathyroidism. In: Rosen CJ, editor. Primer on the metabolic bone diseases and disorders of mineral metabolism. 7th ed. Washington, DC: American Society for Bone and Mineral Research; 2008. p. 302–6.
3. Silverberg SJ, Bilezikian JP. Primary hyperparathyroidism. In: DeGroot LJ, Jameson JL, editors, JT Potts, section editor. Endocrinology. 6th ed. Philadelphia, PA: Elsevier Saunders; 2009.
4. Eastell R, Arnold A, Brandi ML, Brown EM, D'Amour P, Hanley DA, et al. Diagnosis of asymptomatic primary hyperparathyroidism: proceedings of the third international workshop. J Clin Endocrinol Metab. 2009;94(2):340–50.
5. Bilezikian JP, Khan AA, Potts JT, Jr and on behalf of the Third International Workshop on the Management of Asymptomatic Primary Hyperparathyroidism. Guidelines for the management of asymptomatic primary hyperparathyroidism: summary statement from the third international workshop. J Clin Endocrinol Metab. 2009;94(2):335–9.
6. Udelsman R, Pasieka JL, Sturgeon C, Young JE, Clark OH. Surgery for asymptomatic primary hyperparathyroidism: proceedings of the third international workshop. J Clin Endocrinol Metab. 2009;94(2):366–72.

7. Nilsson IL, Yin L, Lundgran E, Rastad J, Ekbom A. Clinical presentation of primary hyperparathyroidism in Europe—nationwide cohort analysis on mortality from nonmalignant causes. J Bone Miner Res. 2002;17 Suppl 2:N68–74.
8. Letizia C, Ferrari P, Cotesta D, Caliumi C, Cianci R, Cerci S, et al. Ambulatory monitoring of blood pressure (AMBP) in patients with primary hyperparathyroidism. J Hum Hypertens. 2005;19:901–6.
9. Kepez A, Harmanci A, Hazirolan T, Isildak M, Kocabas U, Ates A, et al. Evaluation of subclinical coronary atherosclerosis in mild asymptomatic primary hyperparathyroidism patients. Int J Cardiovasc Imaging. 2009;25:187–93.
10. Walker MD, Fleischer JB, Di Tullio MR, Homma S, Rundek T, Stein EM, et al. Cardiac structure and diastolic function in mild primary hyperparathyroidism. J Clin Endocrinol Metab. 2010;95:2172–9.
11. Stefenelli T, Abela C, Frank H, Koller-Strametz J, Globits S, Bergler-Klein J, et al. Cardiac abnormalities in patients with primary hyperparathyroidism: implications for follow-up. J Clin Endocrinol Metab. 1997;82:106–12.
12. Piovesan A, Molineri N, Casasso F, Emmolo I, Ugliengo G, Cesario F, et al. Left ventricular hypertrophy in primary hyperparathyroidsim. Effects of successful parathyroidectomy. Clin Endocrinol. 1999;50:321–8.
13. Vázquez-Díaz O, Casillo-Martínez L, Orea-Tejeda A, Orozco-Gutiérrez JJ, Asensio-Lafuente E, Reza-Alberrán A, et al. Reversible changes of electrocardiographic abnormalities after parathyroidectomy in patients with primary hyperparathyroidism. Cardiol J. 2009;16:241–5.
14. Walker MD, Fleischer J, Rundek T, McMahon DJ, Homma S, Sacco R, et al. Carotid vascular abnormalities in primary hyperparathyroidism. J Clin Endocrinol Metab. 2009;94:3849–56.
15. Silverberg SJ, Lewiecki EM, Mosekilde L, Peacock M, Rubin MR. Presentation of asymptomatic primary hyperparathyroidism: proceedings of the third international workshop. J Clin Endocrinol Metab. 2009;94(2):351–65.
16. Iwata S, Walker MD, Di Tullio MR, Hyodo E, Jin Z, Rui R, Homma S, Silverberg SJ. Aortic Valve Calcification in Mild Primary Hyperparathyroidism. J Clin Endocrinol Metab 2012 97(1):132–7.
17. Ronnie-Sivula H. Causes of death in patients previously operated on for primary hyperparathyroidism. Ann Chir Gynaecol. 1985;74:13–8.
18. Hedbäck G, Tisell LE, Bengtsson BA, Hedman I, Oden A. Premature death in patients operated on for primary hyperparathyroidism. World J Surg. 1990;14(6):829–35.
19. Palmér M, Adami HO, Bergström R, Akerström G, Ljunghall S. Mortality after surgery for primary hyperparathyroidism: a follow-up of 441 patients operated on from 1956 to 1979. Surgery. 1987;102(1):1–7.
20. Hedbäck G, Odén A, Tisell L. The influence of surgery on the risk of death in patients with primary hyperparathyroidism. World J Surg. 1991;15:399–407.
21. Söreide JA, van Heerden JA, Grant CS, Yau Lo C, Schleck C, Ilstrup DM. Survival after surgical treatment for primary hyperparathyroidism. Surgery. 1997;122:1117–23.
22. Wermers RA, Khosla S, Atkinson EJ, Grant CS, Hodgson SF, O'Fallon M, et al. Survival after the diagnosis of hyperparathyroidism: a population-based study. Am J Med. 1998;104:115–22.
23. Yu N, Donnan PT, Flynn RW, Murphy MJ, Smith D, Rudman A, et al. Increased mortality and morbidity in mild primary hyperparathyroid patients. The Parathyroid Epidemiology and Audit Research Study (PEARS). Clin Endocrinol. 2010;73:30–4.
24. Nainby-Luxmoore JC, Langford HG, Nelson NC, Watson RL, Barnes TY. A case-comparison study of hypertension and hyperparathyroidism. J Clin Endocrinol Metab. 1982;55(2):303–6.
25. Lueg M. Hypertension and primary hyperparathyroidism: a five-year case review. South Med J. 1982;75:1371–4.
26. Madhavan T, Frame B, Block MA. Influence of surgical correction of primary hyperparathyroidism on associated hypertension. Arch Surg. 1970;100:212–4.
27. Broulik PD, Horký K, Pacovský V. Blood pressure in patients with primary hyperparathyroidism before and after parathyroidectomy. Exp Clin Endocrinol. 1985;86(3):346–52.
28. Walker MD, Rundek T, Homma S, DiTullio M, Iwata S, Lee JA, Choi J, Liu R, Zhang C, McMahon DJ, Sacco RL, Silverberg SJ. Effect of Parathyroidectomy on Subclinical

Cardiovascular Disease in Mild Primary Hyperparathyroidism. Eur J Endocrinol. 2012;167:277–85.

29. Nilsson IL, Rastad J, Johansson K, Lind L. Endothelial vasodilatory function and blood pressure response to local and systemic hypercalcemia. Surgery. 2001;130:986–90.
30. Fardella C, Rodriguez-Portales JA. Intracellular calcium and blood pressure: comparison between primary hyperparathyroidism and essential hypertension. J Endocrinol Invest. 1995;18(11):827–32.
31. Suzuki T, Aoki K. Hypertensive effects of calcium infusion in subjects with normotension and hypertension. J Hypertens. 1988;6(12):1003–8.
32. Kamycheva E, Jorde R, Haug E, Sager G, Sundsfjord J. Effects of acute hypercalcaemia on blood pressure in subjects with and without parathyroid hormone secretion. Acta Physiol Scand. 2005;184:113–9.
33. Rambausek M, Ritz E, Rascher W, Kreusser W, Mann JF, Kreye VA, et al. Vascular effects of parathyroid hormone (PTH). Adv Exp Med Biol. 1982;151:619–32.
34. Hulter HN, Melby JC, Peterson JC, Cooke CR. Chronic continuous PTH infusion results in hypertension in normal subjects. J Clin Hypertens. 1986;2(4):360–70.
35. Fitzpatrick LA, Bilezikian JP, Silverberg SJ. Parathyroid hormone and the cardiovascular system. Curr Osteoporos Rep. 2008;6:77–83.
36. Perkovic V, Hewitson TD, Kelynack KJ, Martic M, Tait MG, Becker GJ. Parathyroid hormone has a prosclerotic effect on vascular smooth muscle cells. Kidney Blood Press Res. 2003;26:27–33.
37. Snijder MB, Lips P, Seidell JC, Visser M, Deeg DJH, Dekker JM, et al. Vitamin D status and parathyroid hormone levels in relation to blood pressure: a population based study in older men and women. J Intern Med. 2007;261:558–65.
38. Lumachi F, Ermani M, Luisetto G, Nardi A, Basso SM, Camozzi V, et al. Relationship between serum parathyroid hormone, serum calcium and arterial blood pressure in patients with primary hyperparathyroidism: results of a multivariate analysis. Eur J Endocrinol. 2002;146(5):643–7.
39. Maheswaran R, Beevers DG. Clinical correlates in parathyroid hypertension. J Hypertens Suppl. 1989;7(6):S190–1.
40. Diamond TW, Botha JR, Wing J, Meyers AM, Kalk JW. Parathyroid hypertension: a reversible disorder. Arch Intern Med. 1986;146:1709–12.
41. Sangal AK, Kevwitch M, Rao DS, Rival J. Hypomagnesemia and hypertension in primary hyperparathyroidism. South Med J. 1989;82:1116–8.
42. Zawada ET, Brautbar N. The possible role of magnesium in hypercalcemic hypertension. Magnesium. 1984;3:132–7.
43. Altura BM, Altura BT. New perspectives on the role of magnesium in the pathophysiology of the cardiovascular system. I. Clinical aspects. Magnesium. 1985;4(5–6):226–44.
44. Chakraborti S, Chakraborti T, Mandal M, Mandal A, Das S, Ghosh S. Protective role of magnesium in cardiovascular disease: a review. Mol Cell Biochem. 2002;238(1–2):163–79.
45. Pearson PJ, Evora PR, Seccombe JF, Schaff HV. Hypomagnesemia inhibits nitric oxide release from coronary endothelium: protective role of magnesium infusion after cardiac operations. Ann Thorac Surg. 1998;65:967–72.
46. Haenni A, Johansson K, Lind L, Lithell H. Magnesium infusion improves endothelium-dependent vasodilation in the human forearm. Am J Hypertens. 2002;15:10–5.
47. Saussine C, Judes C, Massfelder T, Musso MJ, Simeoni U, Hannedouche T, et al. Stimulatory action of parathyroid hormone on renin secretion in vitro: a study using isolated rat kidney, isolated rabbit glomeruli and superfused dispersed rat juxtaglomerular cells. Clin Sci. 1993;84(1):11–9.
48. Helwig JJ, Musso MJ, Judes C, Nickols GA. Parathyroid hormone and calcium: interactions in the control of renin secretion in the isolated, nonfiltering rat kidney. Endocrinology. 1991;129(3):1233–42.
49. Brinton GS, Jubiz W, Lagerquist LD. Hypertension in primary hyperparathyroidism: the role of the renin-angiotensin system. J Clin Endocrinol Metab. 1975;41(6):1025–9.
50. Zawada ET, Brickman AS, Maxwell MH, Tuck M. Hypertension associated with hyperparathyroidism is not responsive to angiotensin blockade. J Clin Endocrinol Metab. 1980;50: 912–5.

51. Ganguly A, Weinberger MH, Passmore JM, Caras JA, Khairi RM, Grim CE, et al. The renin-angiotensin-aldosterone system and hypertension in primary hyperparathyroidsim. Metabolism. 1982;31(6):595–600.
52. Kovács L, Góth MI, Szabolcs I, Dohán O, Ferencz A, Szilágyi G. The effect of surgical treatment on secondary hyperaldosteronism and relative hyperinsulinemia in primary hyperparathyroidism. Eur J Endocrinol. 1998;138:543–7.
53. Bernini G, Moretti A, Lonzi S, Bendinelli C, Miccoli P, Salvetti A. Renin-angiotensin-aldosterone system in primary hyperparathyroidism before and after surgery. Metabolism. 1999;48(3):298–300.
54. Gennari C, Nami R, Gonnelli S. Hypertension and primary hyperparathyroidism: the role of adrenergic and renin-angiotensin-aldosterone systems. Miner Electrolyte Metab. 1995; 21(1–3):77–81.
55. Pacak K, Keiser H, Eisenhofer G. Chapter 130: Pheochromocytomas. In: DeGroot LJ, Jameson JL, editors. Endocrinology. 5th ed. Philadelphia, PA: Elsevier Saunders; 2006.
56. Brandi ML, Gagel RF, Angeli A, Bilezikian JP, Beck-Peccoz P, Bordi C, et al. Consensus: guidelines for diagnosis and therapy of MEN type 1 and type 2. J Clin Endocrinol Metab. 2001;86:5658–71.
57. Thakker RV. Chapter 191: Multiple endocrine neoplasia type 1. In: DeGroot LJ, Jameson JL, editors. Endocrinology. 5th ed. Philadelphia, PA: Elsevier Saunders; 2006.
58. Jensen RT. Management of the Zollinger-Ellison syndrome in patients with multiple endocrine neoplasia type 1. J Intern Med. 1998;243:477–88.
59. Hoff AO, Gagel RF. Chapter 192: Multiple endocrine neoplasia type 2. In: DeGroot LJ, Jameson JL, editors. Endocrinology. 5th ed. Philadelphia, PA: Elsevier Saunders; 2006.
60. Jones DB, Jones JH, Lloyd JH, Lucas PA, Wilkins WE, Walker DA. Changes in blood pressure and renal function after parathyroidectomy in primary hyperparathyroidism. Postgrad Med J. 1983;59:350–3.
61. Lind L, Jacobsson S, Palmér M, Lithell H, Wengle B, Ljunghall S. Cardiovascular risk factors in primary hyperparathyroidism: a 15 year follow up of operated and unoperated cases. J Intern Med. 1991;230:29–35.
62. Heyliger A, Tangpricha V, Weber C, Sharma J. Parathyroidectomy decreases systolic and diastolic blood pressure in hypertensive patients with primary hyperparathyroidism. Surgery. 2009;146(6):1042–7.
63. Rydberg E, Birgander M, Bondeson AG, Bondeson L, Willenheimer R. Effect of successful parathyroidectomy on 24-hour ambulatory blood pressure in patients with primary hyperparathyroidism. Int J Cardiol. 2010;142(1):15–21.
64. Bollerslev J, Rosen T, Mollerup CL, Nordenström J, Baranowski M, Franco C, Pernow Y, Isaksen GA, Godang K, Ueland T, Jansson S and on behalf of the SIPH Study Group. Effect of surgery on cardiovascular risk factors in mild primary hyperparathyroidsim. J Clin Endocrinol Metab. 2009;94:2255–61.

Chapter 10
Hypertension, Vitamin D Deficiency, and Calcium Metabolism

M. Iftekhar Ullah, Christian A. Koch, and Vin Tangpricha

Abstract Vitamin D deficiency like many other chronic diseases such as diabetes, obesity, and hypertension is increasing in prevalence. Traditionally, vitamin D was thought to be only important for its role in bone and calcium homeostasis. With the improvement of vitamin D assays including utilization of liquid chromatography tandem mass spectrometry (LC-MS/MS), measuring serum levels of 25-hydroxyvitamin D [25(OH)D] has become more reliable. The optimal serum 25(OH)D concentration for skeletal health remains to be debated and is even less certain for extra-skeletal health such as hypertension. The target serum 25(OH)D concentration may differ according to the genetic make-up/profile of each individual, which may consist of different gene polymorphisms in the vitamin D receptor and proteins involved in vitamin D metabolism. Potential mechanisms of vitamin D deficiency causing hypertension involve the renin–aldosterone–angiotensin system (RAAS) and endothelial function. As many patients with obesity also have insulin resistance, one could consider insulin resistance as a mediator in causing elevated blood pressure. Based on data from cross-sectional and cohort studies, vitamin D deficiency increases the risk of incident hypertension. Although more definitive trials have not yet been completed to examine the role of vitamin D in hypertension, it seems prudent to recommend that patients with vitamin D deficiency be encouraged to modify their lifestyles and take vitamin D supplementation to achieve serum 25(OH)D concentrations that are optimal for skeletal health (at least 30 ng/mL). The completion

M.I. Ullah (✉)
Division of Internal Medicine and Hypertension, University of Mississippi Medical Center, 2500 N State Street, Jackson, MS 39216, USA
e-mail: mullah@umc.edu

C.A. Koch
Division of Endocrinology, University of Mississippi Medical Center, Jackson, MS, USA

V. Tangpricha
Section of Endocrinology, Division of Endocrinology, Diabetes & Lipids, Emory University School of Medicine, Atlanta VA Medical Center, Atlanta, GA, USA

C.A. Koch and G.P. Chrousos (eds.), *Endocrine Hypertension: Underlying Mechanisms and Therapy*, Contemporary Endocrinology, DOI 10.1007/978-1-60761-548-4_10,

of randomized controlled trials will inform whether vitamin D can influence the onset of hypertension and/or reduce blood pressure in individuals with established hypertension.

Keywords Vitamin D deficiency • Hypertension • Calcium metabolism • Metabolic syndrome • Vitamin D synthesis • VDR • Renin-Angiotensin system

Introduction

Vitamin D deficiency is increasing in prevalence throughout the world due to a number of reasons (Table 10.1) and is estimated to affect 42% of the general population and in higher proportions in different ethnic groups (82% and 69% for black and Hispanic individuals, respectively) [1, 2]. The importance of vitamin D in calcium homeostasis for the skeleton is generally well accepted. The role for vitamin D in other chronic diseases is becoming more recognized by recent experimental, clinical, and epidemiological studies. Hypertension, metabolic syndrome, diabetes, cardiovascular disease (CVD), certain types of malignancies including breast and colon cancer and immunologic dysfunctions have been associated with vitamin D deficiency [3–6]. Recent clinical studies have evaluated the hypothesis that hypovitaminosis D may trigger or worsen systemic hypertension, and supplementation with vitamin D may reduce blood pressure. Despite some encouraging results of vitamin D supplementation on hypertension, there has not been sufficient evidence

Table 10.1 Causes and risk factors for vitamin D deficiency [22, 23]

Gastrointestinal factors:
Insufficient oral intake
Malabsorption resulting from chronic pancreatitis, inflammatory bowel disease, celiac disease, cystic fibrosis, Whipple's disease, radiation enteritis, bariatric surgery
Metabolic factors:
Chronic renal insufficiency (from decreased 1alpha-hydroxylase activity)
Hypoalbuminemia (nephrotic syndrome, protein loosing enteropathy) due to decreased vitamin D binding protein
Hepatic failure
Medication Interactions: Antiepileptic medications, glucocorticoids, HAART, rifampin, ketoconazole, cholestyramine, St John's wart
Granulomatous diseases and malignancies: sarcoidosis, tuberculosis, lymphomas, histoplasmosis
Obesity (vitamin D is sequestered in fat)
Environmental factors:
decreased sun exposure due to increased distance from the equator, prolonged winter, covering of whole body with clothing, living mostly indoors, occupation or lifestyle
sun avoidance due to concern of skin cancer or risk for skin cancer, e.g., prolonged hospitalization, nursing home, advanced age

to show significant reduction in mortality, vascular disease, and cardiovascular risk with vitamin D [7–10].

Physiology of Vitamin D Synthesis and Metabolism

Vitamin D is a secosteroid hormone which may be produced in the human body from direct exposure of the skin to sunlight (Solar UV-B). This causes photochemical conversion of 7-dehydrocholesterol present in the skin to form previtamin D_3, which, in turn, converts rapidly to vitamin D_3. The oily fishes such as salmon, sardines and mackerel, egg yolks, and fish oils such as cod liver oil contain vitamin D naturally. Fortified milk, cereal, juice, and yogurt are common dietary sources in North America. The cutaneous synthesis of vitamin D may vary widely in different populations depending on latitude, season, and time of day. Skin pigmentation by melanin is a limiting factor in the cutaneous synthesis of vitamin D. Melanin acts as an effective natural sunscreen and, therefore, increased skin pigment can greatly reduce the solar UV-B mediated cutaneous synthesis of vitamin D3 by as much as 99% [11].

Vitamin D from the skin and diet is metabolized in the liver to form 25(OH)D. The circulating 25(OH)D is metabolized in the kidneys by the enzyme 25 (OH) vitamin D-1α-hydroxylase (1α-hydroxylase) to its active or hormonal form, 1,25-dihydroxyvitamin D [1,25$(OH)_2$D]. The renal production of 1,25$(OH)_2$D is closely regulated by serum parathyroid hormone (PTH) as well as serum calcium and phosphorus [12]. The absorption of renal calcium [13] as well as intestinal calcium and phosphorus is increased in the presence of 1,25$(OH)_2$D [14]. It was previously believed that the 1α-hydroxylase was present only in kidney cells; however, this enzyme has been found in variety of tissues which has led to investigation of the role of vitamin D in all of these extra-renal tissues [15].

Several vitamin D-dependent proteins in the enterocyte are regulated by 1,25$(OH)_2$D to increase intestinal absorption of both calcium and phosphorus. Vitamin D is also involved in bone formation, resorption, and mineralization as well as in maintaining neuromuscular function [12, 14]. Circulating 1,25$(OH)_2$D reduces the serum PTH level *directly* by negative feedback of parathyroid gland activity and *indirectly* by increasing serum calcium. It also regulates bone metabolism in part by interacting with the vitamin D receptor (VDR) in osteoblasts to release biochemical signals, leading to formation of mature osteoclasts. The osteoclasts release collagenase and hydrochloric acid to dissolve the matrix and mineral, releasing calcium into the blood [16].

Deficient vitamin D status impairs calcium and phosphorus homeostasis. Although the bone, small intestine, and kidneys are the classic organs responsive to vitamin D, the effects of vitamin D appear to involve several other organ systems. The VDR has been identified in numerous tissues and organs, including those not typically associated with calcium homeostasis and bone metabolism. This suggests that vitamin D may have a role in important biological processes beyond calcium homeostasis [17]. Some of the organs containing the VDR include the heart, vascular smooth muscle, endothelium, stomach, pancreas, brain, skin, gonads, as well as activated T and B lymphocytes, monocytes, and macrophages [18].

Vitamin D Receptor

The VDR is a steroid hormone nuclear receptor that binds to $1,25(OH)_2D$ with high affinity and mediates transcriptional gene regulation. It acts as a ligand-regulated "gene-switch" which regulates the transcription of specific genes, leading to a cascade of events in the cell [19]. This may play a vital role in disease prevention and maintenance of extra-skeletal health. A number of recent studies involving cell culture and VDR knockout mice have suggested that vitamin D plays a critical role in regulating the renin–angiotensin system (RAS) and thus, influencing the regulation of blood pressure [20, 21].

Consequences of Vitamin D Deficiency [24]

Biochemical consequences:

- Low serum 25(OH)D
- Normal or low serum calcium and phosphorus
- High normal or elevated PTH (secondary hyperparathyroidism (HPT))
- Normal or elevated serum alkaline phosphatase
- Decrease in 24 h urinary calcium excretion
- Decrease in calcium and phosphorus absorption from the intestine

Clinical consequences: Exacerbation or increased susceptibility to the following diseases

- Infections: Upper respiratory tract infections, tuberculosis
- Respiratory: Asthma, reactive airway disease
- Metabolic syndrome, increased insulin resistance and type 2 diabetes
- Cardiovascular: Systemic hypertension, pregnancy-induced hypertension, pre-eclampsia and eclampsia, increased mortality related to cardiovascular events
- Autoimmune diseases: Type 1 diabetes, multiple sclerosis, psoriasis, Crohn's disease, rheumatoid arthritis
- Malignancy: Breast, colon, prostate, pancreas
- Musculoskeletal: Muscle pain and weakness (leading to increased risk of fall and fracture), osteoarthritis, osteoporosis, osteomalacia and bone pain, rickets

Racial and Geographical Factors Influencing Vitamin D Nutritional Status

There are various cultural, social, racial, and geographical factors that may influence the vitamin D status. The amount of sunlight exposure is one of the most important factors in determining one's vitamin D status. A change in season or latitude may have a dramatic effect on the cutaneous production of cholecalciferol. Both systolic and diastolic blood pressures have been shown to be significantly and positively associated with distance from the equator [25, 26]. Above the latitude of approximately 33 °N, vitamin D3 synthesis in the skin becomes very low or nearly absent during most of the Winter. In Edmonton, Canada (52 °N), the photosynthesis of pre-cholecalciferol essentially ceases by mid-October and does not resume until mid-April, thus influencing the serum vitamin D concentration in that population [27]. Covering the entire body with clothing (as customary in women in some religions), use of sunscreen and glass shielding may significantly reduce or completely eliminate the production of vitamin D3 in the skin [28]. Biological factors that inhibit cutaneous vitamin D synthesis and bioavailability include skin pigmentation, medication use, body fat content, fat malabsorption, and age [29]. Increased skin pigmentation can reduce cutaneous vitamin D3 production as much as 99.9%, which may explain, at least in part, the higher prevalence of vitamin D deficiency in the African American population [11]. In addition, ethnicity-specific polymorphisms of the VDR gene and its promoter may influence the end-organ response to vitamin D, including individual calcium absorption.

Epidemiological Evidence of the Relationship Between Vitamin D and Hypertension

Several clinical and epidemiological studies have shown that there may be an association between hypertension and vitamin D status as well as calcium metabolism.

The abnormal calcium metabolism including HPT has been related to the development of hypertension [30]. In the early 1990s, Cooper et al. observed that individuals of African origin residing in the northern regions had higher blood pressure than those residing closer to the equator [31]. Langford and Watson [32] noted that children from rural Mississippi had higher blood pressure and low calcium intake compared to urban children. It has been also found that the intake of calcium in salt-sensitive blacks can reduce blood pressure and cause partial regression of left ventricular hypertrophy [33, 34]. Other investigators have found similar results [35, 36].

Several recent studies conducted by different investigators examining the data from the third National Health and Nutrition Examination Survey (NHANES III) showed an association between the serum 25 (OH)D concentration and blood pressure. In this study population, the serum 25(OH)D concentration was found to be inversely associated with blood pressure, even after adjustment for variables including age, gender, ethnicity, and physical activity. The 25(OH)D levels were considerably lower in women, elderly, racial/ethnic minorities, and persons with obesity, hypertension, and diabetes mellitus [37]. The adjusted prevalence of hypertension in this population was 30% higher in the lowest quartile compared to the highest quartile of serum 25(OH)D.

A recent prospective study investigating the independent association between serum 25(OH)D levels and risk of incident hypertension revealed similar findings [38]. In this study, the multivariable relative risk (RR) of incident hypertension among those with low vitamin D level (serum 25(OH)D levels were <15 ng/mL) was 6.13 in men and 2.67 in women (compared with those whose levels were >30 ng/mL). These findings suggest an association between vitamin D deficiency and the increased risk of hypertension. However, recent meta-analyses of different studies demonstrated mixed results. One meta-analysis of ten studies showed minimal improvement in blood pressure with vitamin D supplementation, whereas another meta-analysis showed 80% increase in the risk of incident hypertension with vitamin D deficiency [39].

Clinical Studies Showing Effect of Vitamin D Supplementation on Blood Pressure

Increasing the serum 25(OH)D concentration in the blood, directly or indirectly, has been shown to reduce blood pressure. Krause et al. demonstrated that exposure of persons to vitamin D producing UV-A three times a week for 6 weeks increased the circulating levels of 25(OH)D by 162% and reduced both systolic and diastolic blood pressure by 6 mm Hg, whereas hypertensive patients exposed to UV-A did not experience any increase in the blood level of 25(OH)D and had no change in their blood pressure (UV-A does not produce vitamin D) [40]. Another randomized, placebo-controlled study showed that 800 IU of vitamin D_3 plus 1,200 mg of calcium significantly reduced blood pressure by 9.3% after 8 week, whereas treatment with 1,200 mg of calcium alone reduced blood pressure by only 4.0% ($P=0.02$) [41]. Adults with significant vitamin D deficiency have been found to have a 50% higher risk of developing myocardial infarction and they are also more likely to die from these cardiac events [42, 43]. A very recent randomized placebo control pilot study showed a 9% reduction in systolic blood pressure ($p<0.001$) after treatment with calcitriol 0.5 μg twice daily for only 2 weeks. The blood pressure returned to its pretreatment level after one week of concluding the calcitriol therapy [44].

Vitamin D Deficiency and Hypertension: Potential Biological Mechanisms

(a) Regulation of the RAS
    The RAS is a regulatory cascade that plays a critical role in the regulation of blood pressure, electrolyte, and plasma volume homeostasis. Inappropriate stimulation of the RAS has been associated with hypertension. Vitamin D is a potent endocrine suppressor of renin biosynthesis to regulate the RAS [21]. Vascular smooth muscle and cardiac myocytes contain VDR and it has been estimated that there may be up to 200 genes regulating cardiovascular physiology

influenced by vitamin D [45, 46]. Mice lacking the VDR have elevated the production of renin and angiotensin II, leading to hypertension, cardiac hypertrophy, and increased water intake [20]. These abnormalities can be prevented by treatment with an ACE inhibitor or AT_1 receptor antagonist. Vitamin D suppression of renin expression is independent of calcium metabolism, the volume and salt-sensing mechanisms, and the angiotensin II feedback regulation. In normal mice, vitamin D deficiency stimulates renin expression, whereas injection of 1,25-dihydroxyvitamin D_3 [$1,25(OH)_2D_3$] reduces renin synthesis. In cell cultures, $1,25(OH)_2D$ directly suppresses renin gene transcription by a VDR-dependent mechanism. In a transgenic mouse model with mice over-expressing the human VDR in renin-producing cells, suppression of renin expression by $1,25(OH)_2$ D in vivo was found to be independent of PTH and calcium [47]. Vitamin D also has anti-inflammatory activity, reducing the production of IL-10 and CRP, and suppression of foam cell formation [45, 46, 48]. In the Framingham Offspring Cohort Study, the risk of developing cardiovascular events was found to be doubled with a low vitamin D level of <15 ng/mL (compared to those with vitamin D level >15 ng/mL) [42]. Thus, vitamin D deficiency may increase the risk of hypertension and CVD by up-regulating the renin–angiotensin–aldosterone system and correcting the deficiency status may be beneficial to cardiovascular health (Fig. 10.1).

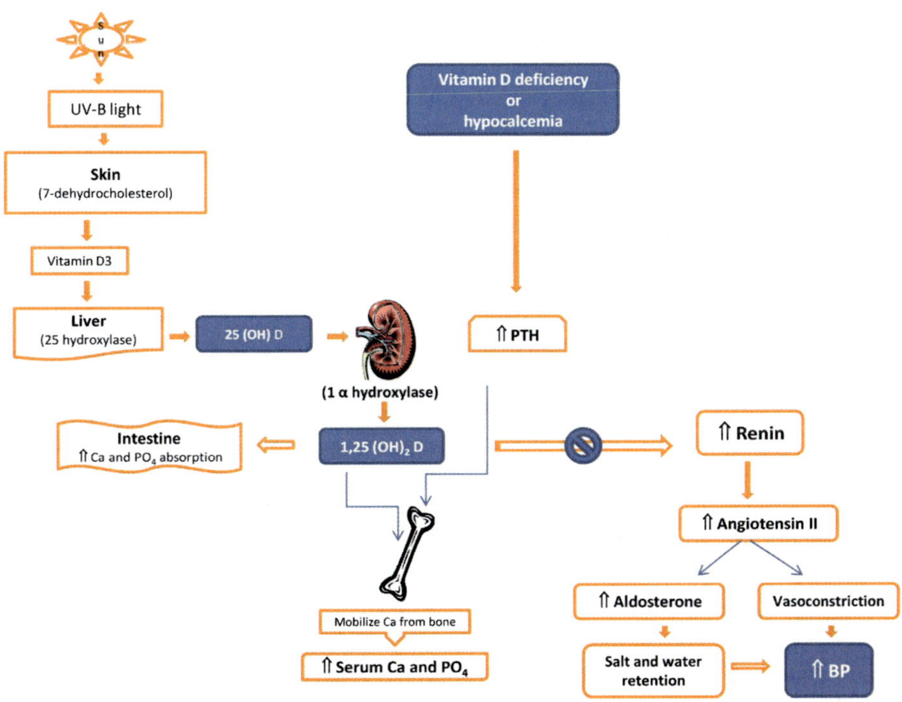

Fig. 10.1 Pathway of vitamin D metabolism and its relationship with PTH and renin–angiotensin–aldosterone system (modified from Ullah et al., Int J Endocrinol, 2010) [98]

(b) Hypertension, hyperparathyroidism, and vitamin D deficiency
Vitamin D deficiency is frequently seen in patients with primary HPT [49–51]. Hypovitaminosis D itself also causes decreased absorption of calcium from the intestine leading to hypocalcemia which triggers secondary elevation of PTH. Generally, the parathyroid level starts to rise when the serum 25(OH)D concentration drops below 30 ng/mL. Primary HPT with an inappropriately elevated PTH level has been shown to be associated with hypertension (in up to 40% of cases) but the mechanism of developing hypertension has remained controversial (see also chapter by Carrelli & Silverberg in this book). Low vitamin D status is associated with secondary elevation of PTH and increased arterial resistance leading to hypertension [52]. It has also been implicated directly and indirectly to affect cardiovascular risk by increasing susceptibility to arterial calcification [53]. The patients with mild primary HPT have been found to have increased stiffness measured in the radial artery [54]. Elevated PTH level may also contribute to vascular smooth muscle damage and cardiac hypertrophy and predisposition to valvular sclerosis as well as valvular and myocardial calcification [55, 56]. Hypertension generally persists in patients with primary HPT after parathyroidectomy [57]. Elevated PTH from vitamin D deficiency can increase the risk of inflammation with decreased levels of the anti-inflammatory cytokine interleukin-10 (IL-10) which increases after replacement of vitamin D [58, 59]. Increased vitamin D levels are associated with a TH2 shift and lack of vitamin D is proatherogenic because TH1 is stimulated [60–62]. A recent study found the combination of lower serum 25-OHD and higher serum PTH concentrations to be associated independently with sudden cardiac death risk among older adults without CVD disease [63].

Case studies showed improvement or complete resolution of systemic hypertension after parathyroidectomy [64]. In primary HPT with parathyroid adenoma, plasma renin activity and plasma aldosterone levels are higher among hypertensive patients and blood pressure, plasma renin activity, and plasma aldosterone levels normalize after parathyroidectomy [65]. These results are consistent with the hypothesis of a possible direct effect of PTH on renin secretion, which could contribute to the pathogenesis of hypertension.

(c) Vitamin D deficiency, calcium and endothelial function
Hypovitaminosis D has been shown to have direct effects on the vasculature causing increased vascular resistance [66]. It is also independently associated with increased carotid intima-media thickness [67], decreased arterial compliance, and endothelial dysfunction [68, 69]. Endothelial function (as assessed by flow-mediated dilation) and blood pressure were improved in diabetics after ingestion of only a single dose of vitamin D (100,000 IU) [70]. Elevated serum calcium and PTH levels can independently predict impaired endothelial function [71]. All of these above effects on vasculature may contribute to elevated blood pressure.

(d) Vitamin D deficiency and cardiovascular mortality
Numerous studies have suggested that vitamin D deficiency is associated with increased mortality from CVDs. Vitamin D deficiency is more prevalent in

patients with coronary artery disease. Lee et al. recently published a multicenter study which demonstrated that 96% of patients admitted in the hospital with acute coronary syndrome had inadequate vitamin D levels (<30 ng/mL) [72]. Low levels of serum 25(OH)D are independently associated with cardiovascular and all-cause mortality [73]. An analysis of Framingham study subpopulations showed an increased rate of cardiovascular adverse events (up to 80% higher) among those with vitamin D deficiency (defined in this study as a 25(OH) D < 15 ng/mL) [42]. Analysis of NHANES III study data yielded similar findings of an elevated mortality rate among people with the lowest quartile of vitamin D compared to those with the highest quartile [74]. A systematic review of studies assessing the effect of vitamin D supplementation on CVD events demonstrated a slight but statistically nonsignificant reduction in CVD risk [pooled relative risk, 0.90 (95% CI, 0.77–1.05)] with vitamin D supplementation (approximately 1,000 IU/day) [75]. In a meta-analysis of 18 randomized controlled trials, the intake of ordinary doses of vitamin D supplements (300–2,000 IU/day) was associated with decreases in total all-cause mortality rates (summary relative risk 0.93, 95% CI 0.87–0.99) [43].

Diagnosis of Vitamin D Deficiency

Even though vitamin D assays are now readily available in most laboratories in the USA, the clinicians are often confused about which test to order. Whereas individual immunoassays can easily deviate by 20% from those of LC-MS/MS, there is an outstanding precision between LC-MS/MS and the all method mean/mean of all the methods. LC-MS/MS can quantify vitamin D2 (ergocalciferol) and D3 (cholecalciferol) metabolites separately. This can help in assessing the patient's compliance with the intake of vitamin D supplements (consider LC-MS/MS if/when patient takes vitamin D2/ergocalciferol). Vitamin D produced cutaneously or ingested orally is quickly converted to 25(OH)D and this is the main storage form in the body. Only a fraction of this 25(OH)D is converted to its active metabolite $1,25(OH)_2D$ and is present in serum in a very low concentration compared to 25(OH)D. In mild to moderate vitamin D deficiency, the serum $1,25(OH)_2D$ may still be normal at the expense of 25(OH)D, which will be invariably low. Therefore, checking the serum 25(OH)D level is the most appropriate test in diagnosing vitamin D deficiency. However, the measurement of $1,25(OH)_2D$ may be useful where there is defect in metabolism of 25(OH)D and phosphate including pseudo vitamin D deficiency rickets, vitamin D resistant rickets, hereditary phosphate losing disorders, malignancy-related osteomalacia, sarcoidosis, and certain lymphomas.

There is no consensus yet as to what concentration of serum 25(OH)D constitutes optimal vitamin D status. Recent evidence suggests that the serum 25(OH)D concentration considered to be optimum for bone health may not be enough for cardiovascular and other extra-skeletal functions. The serum 25(OH)D concentration necessary to prevent rickets and osteomalacia (10–20 ng/mL) is lower than that which suppresses PTH levels (20–30 ng/mL) [76]. This level, in turn, is lower than the level needed to optimize intestinal calcium absorption (34 ng/mL) [77]. Lappe et al. recently reported that 25(OH)D levels of around 40 ng/mL were associated with a significant reduction in the incidence of internal cancers [78]. Finally, neuromuscular performance steadily improves as the serum 25(OH)D level increases and the maximum performance has been associated with a level around 50 ng/mL [79]. Levels for optimal brain development and function are still unclear. Although higher serum 25(OH)D concentrations have been associated with decreased risk of several diseases, these relationships have not been vigorously tested in clinical studies. There have not been many randomized controlled trials demonstrating treatment with vitamin D to achieve higher serum 25(OH)D concentrations improves outcomes. Therefore, these associations should be interpreted with caution. It would seem reasonable to target serum 25(OH)D concentrations above 30 ng/mL for optimal health benefits at least for skeletal health.

Treatment of Vitamin D Deficiency

Vitamin D deficiency can be easily treated with oral vitamin D supplements. However, the problem arises when someone asks: *when to treat, what is the optimum regimen, and how long to treat*. Based on the current level of evidence, vitamin D deficiency may be defined as a serum 25(OH)D level <20 ng/mL, insufficiency as a 25(OH)D level of 21–29 ng/mL and sufficiency as a 25(OH)D of 30–100 ng/mL [6]. A serum 25(OH)D level of 30–44 ng/mL is believed to be optimal for beneficial outcome for cardiovascular, musculoskeletal health, and malignancies [80]. Achieving a vitamin D level of at least 30 ng/mL has a significant efficacy in reducing the incidence of falls (up to 19%) and fractures in the elderly and the efficacy is highest when vitamin D levels reach 44 ng/mL [81, 82]. Patients with chronic kidney disease (stages 2–5) commonly have poorly controlled hypertension and they also suffer from vitamin D deficiency very frequently [83]. The vitamin D level is an independent predictor of disease progression and mortality in these patients and vitamin D supplementation decreases serum PTH without increasing phosphatemia or calcemia in dialysis patients [84, 85].

As a rule of thumb, serum 25(OH)D can be expected to rise by about 1 ng/mL for every 100 IU of additional vitamin D each day and up to 10,000 IU of vitamin D per day may be taken without significant toxicity for up to 3 months [86, 87]. In a healthy adult, sunbathing for prolonged periods in the summer can produce vitamin D doses equivalent to an oral supplementation of 20,000 IU daily but the serum 25(OH)D level rarely exceeds 100 ng/mL [88]. The risk of hypercalcemia related to vitamin D toxicity in healthy individuals increases when the daily vitamin D intake is >10,000 IU for a prolonged period or the serum 25(OH)D concentration exceeds 100 ng/mL [80]. Therefore, contrary to common misconceptions, vitamin D supplementation is relatively safe and toxicity is unlikely to develop unless a very high dose is used for a very prolonged period of time.

Vitamin D supplementation at a dose of 1,000–2,000 IU/day may be given empirically without a baseline serum 25(OH)D measurement to those likely to be vitamin D deficient including dark skinned or veiled persons, elderly and institutional subjects living mostly indoors [87, 89–91]. On the other hand, individuals with or at risk of cardiovascular, autoimmune disease and cancer may have their serum 25(OH)D level measured and appropriate treatment regimen should be initiated if the 25(OH)D level is <30 ng/mL. In these individuals, a large loading dose of 50,000 IU once a week may be given for 8–12 weeks, followed by a maintenance dose of 800–2,000 IU/day to prevent dropping of vitamin D level again to the pretreatment level [89–91]. The interval between initiating vitamin D supplementation and rechecking the vitamin D level should be at least 3 months to assess the treatment response and patient compliance.

The Institute of Medicine (IOM) [91] updated its guideline in 2010 regarding recommended daily allowances and tolerable upper limit of intake levels of vitamin D which is believed to be mostly inadequate by most experts. In this recent update, the IOM has concluded that in infants up to 12 months of age, 400 IU/day of vitamin D intake is adequate. In all other age groups, the estimated average requirement has been recommended to be also 400 IU daily. The tolerable upper intake levels have been set at 4,000 IU/day for everyone above age nine and older including pregnant and lactating females. In contrast, the *Endocrine Society released Clinical Practice Guidelines on Vitamin D* [87] that state the daily requirements for infants and children (up to 8 years) should be between 400 and 1,000 IU and for most adults it should be 1,500–2,000 IU daily. However, to maintain the serum 25(OH)D concentration constantly above 30 ng/mL, most adults (>18 years) will require at least 1,500–2,000 IU of vitamin D supplementation daily. The tolerable upper daily intake amounts have been suggested to be 2,000 IU for infants (0–12 months), 4,000 IU for children and adults up to 18 years and 10,000 IU for most other adults. Pregnancy and lactation requires special attention as the fetus is in utero exclusively dependent on vitamin D sufficiency of the mother. Maternal breast milk contains very little amount of vitamin D and thus, the infants who are exclusively breast fed are at a high risk of developing vitamin D deficiency. Vitamin D fortified formula and the sun exposure are the only ways to maintain vitamin D sufficiency in infants.

Conclusions

Hypertension is one of the most prevalent chronic disease conditions in the modern society. Adequate blood pressure control is the key to prevent complications related to poorly controlled hypertension. In clinical practice, the most common cause of uncontrolled hypertension is the lack of patient compliance. However, there are many instances when blood pressure is still very difficult to bring to/at the desired level despite using a modest regimen of medications with good patient compliance. This is when a clinician should begin to suspect an underlying secondary cause

Table 10.2 Subjects recommended to have their serum 25(OH)D level measured (modified from *Souberbielle* et al. *Vitamin D and musculoskeletal health, cardiovascular disease, autoimmunity and cancer: Recommendations for clinical practice. Autoimmun Rev, 2010.*) [88]

Patients with classical clinical conditions	Patients with nonclassical clinical conditions
Patients with or at risk of osteoporosis	Hypertension
Elderly with history of falls	Patients with autoimmune disease
Pregnancy	Subjects with high risk of autoimmune disease
Chronic kidney disease	Patients on corticosteroids
Transplant patients	Cancer patients undergoing treatment
Obesity	
Diabetes mellitus	
Hospitalized patients	
Patients with muscle and bone pain	

or other contributing causes. Vitamin D deficiency is not commonly considered in this regard. As discussed above, there is plenty of evidence from preclinical, epidemiological studies and early clinical to support a relationship between low vitamin D status and hypertension. The unique and complex interactions between hypovitaminosis D, PTH and calcium make it especially difficult to figure out how much of these effects are truly unique and distinct to vitamin D.

Even though there is evidence for the association between vitamin D deficiency and hypertension, it is not clear what degree of vitamin D deficiency may activate the RAS and trigger an increase in blood pressure. Most recent studies investigating the association of health conditions related to vitamin D suggest that a desirable 25(OH)D concentration may be at least 30 ng/mL (but less than 100 ng/mL) for optimum health, yet no consensus has been reached about its cutoff level [92–94]. This already represents a limiting factor in future studies, as each individual likely has a different cutoff, depending on ethnic group and/or polymorphisms in the VDR and other genes that regulate vitamin D metabolism. Therefore, more comprehensive studies may be needed including genetic profiling of study subjects with various levels of serum vitamin D to identify the most likely cutoff level that triggers clinical hypertension. The challenge remains that hypertension is multifactorial and some individuals with other comorbidities (like smoking, obesity, physical inactivity, metabolic syndrome) may have a lower threshold for vitamin D deficiency-induced clinical hypertension compared to those who do not have these risk factors.

Because of the increasing evidence in favor of an association between vitamin D deficiency and CVDs, it may be prudent to screen and correct hypovitaminosis D in high risk patients (see Table 10.2) including those with resistant hypertension. If screening is not available (especially in developing countries), supplementation with vitamin D 1,000–2,000 IU daily among this subpopulation may be safe and appropriate [85, 95, 96]. This can easily be achieved since vitamin D is widely available and inexpensive and is unlikely to cause any toxicity at this dosage. Finally, studies are underway to find vitamin D analogs with greater activity on RAS modulation but minimal calcemic potential. This may open a new horizon for a group of therapeutic inhibitors of the RAS, and potentially offer a new class of antihypertensive drugs that may be used in hypertensive individuals with or without vitamin D deficiency. Ongoing studies examining vitamin D and its effect on several clinical outcomes related to CVD will help shape the future role of vitamin D as therapy in patients at risk for or with hypertension or CVD [97].

References

1. Forrest KY, Stuhldreher WL. Prevalence and correlates of vitamin D deficiency in US adults. Nutr Res. 2011;31:48–54.
2. Lavie CJ, Lee JH, Milani RV. Vitamin D and cardiovascular disease will it live up to its hype? J Am Coll Cardiol. 2011;58:1547–56.
3. Ganji V, Zhang X, Shaikh N, Tangpricha V. Serum 25-hydroxyvitamin D concentrations are associated with prevalence of metabolic syndrome and various cardiometabolic risk factors in US children and adolescents based on assay-adjusted serum 25-hydroxyvitamin D data from NHANES 2001–2006. Am J Clin Nutr. 2011;94:225–33.
4. Judd SE, Tangpricha V. Vitamin d therapy and cardiovascular health. Curr Hypertens Rep. 2011;13:187–91.
5. Judd SE, Tangpricha V. Vitamin D deficiency and risk for cardiovascular disease. Am J Med Sci. 2009;338:40–4.
6. Holick MF. Vitamin D deficiency. N Engl J Med. 2007;357:266–81.
7. Elamin MB, Abu Elnour NO, Elamin KB, et al. Vitamin D and cardiovascular outcomes: a systematic review and meta-analysis. J Clin Endocrinol Metab. 2011;96:1931–42.
8. Avenell A, Maclennan GS, Jenkinson DJ, et al. Long-term follow-up for mortality and cancer in a randomized placebo-controlled trial of vitamin D3 and/or calcium (RECORD trial). J Clin Endocrinol Metab. 2012;97(2):614–22.
9. McGreevy C, Williams D. New insights about vitamin D and cardiovascular disease: a narrative review. Ann Intern Med. 2011;155:820–6.
10. Shapses SA, Manson JE. Vitamin D and prevention of cardiovascular disease and diabetes: why the evidence falls short. JAMA. 2011;305:2565–6.
11. Clemens TL, Adams JS, Henderson SL, Holick MF. Increased skin pigment reduces the capacity of skin to synthesise vitamin D3. Lancet. 1982;1:74–6.
12. DeLuca HF. Overview of general physiologic features and functions of vitamin D. Am J Clin Nutr. 2004;80:1689S–96.
13. Johnson JA, Kumar R. Vitamin D and renal calcium transport. Curr Opin Nephrol Hypertens. 1994;3:424–9.
14. Holick MF, Garabedian M. Vitamin D: photobiology, metabolism, mechanism of action, and clinical applications. In: Favus MJ, editor. Primer on the metabolic bone diseases and disorders of mineral metabolism. 6th ed. Washington, DC: American Society for Bone and Mineral Research; 2006. p. 129–37.
15. Zehnder D, Bland R, Williams MC, et al. Extrarenal expression of 25-hydroxyvitamin D(3)-1 alpha-hydroxylase. J Clin Endocrinol Metab. 2001;86:888–94.
16. Holick MF. Sunlight and vitamin D for bone health and prevention of autoimmune diseases, cancers, and cardiovascular disease. Am J Clin Nutr. 2004;80:1678S–88.
17. Holick MF. Vitamin D: a millenium perspective. J Cell Biochem. 2003;88:296–307.
18. Dusso AS, Brown AJ, Slatopolsky E. Vitamin D. Am J Physiol Renal Physiol. 2005;289: F8–28.
19. White JH. Vitamin D signaling, infectious diseases, and regulation of innate immunity. Infect Immun. 2008;76:3837–43.

20. Li YC, Qiao G, Uskokovic M, Xiang W, Zheng W, Kong J. Vitamin D: a negative endocrine regulator of the renin-angiotensin system and blood pressure. J Steroid Biochem Mol Biol. 2004;89–90:387–92.
21. Li YC, Kong J, Wei M, Chen ZF, Liu SQ, Cao LP. 1,25-Dihydroxyvitamin D(3) is a negative endocrine regulator of the renin-angiotensin system. J Clin Invest. 2002;110:229–38.
22. Kennel KA, Drake MT, Hurley DL. Vitamin D deficiency in adults: when to test and how to treat. Mayo Clin Proc. 2010;85:752–7.
23. Falk S, Kratzsch J, Paschke R, Koch CA. Hypercalcemia as a result of sarcoidosis with normal serum concentrations of vitamin D. Med Sci Monit. 2007;13(11):CS133–6.
24. Holick MF. Vitamin D: extraskeletal health. Endocrinol Metab Clin North Am. 2010;39:381–400.
25. Intersalt Cooperative Research Group. Intersalt: an international study of electrolyte excretion and blood pressure. Results for 24 hour urinary sodium and potassium excretion. BMJ. 1988;297:319–28.
26. Rostand SG. Ultraviolet light may contribute to geographic and racial blood pressure differences. Hypertension. 1997;30:150–6.
27. Lu Z, Chen TC, Kline L. Photosynthesis of previtamin D1 in cities around the world. In: Holick MF, Kligman A, editors. Proceedings of the Biologic Effects of Light Symposium. Berlin, Germany: Walter de Gruyter; 1992. p. 48–52.
28. Holick MF. McCollum Award Lecture, 1994: vitamin D–new horizons for the 21st century. Am J Clin Nutr. 1994;60:619–30.
29. Holick MF. High prevalence of vitamin D inadequacy and implications for health. Mayo Clin Proc. 2006;81:353–73.
30. McCarron DA, Pingree PA, Rubin RJ, Gaucher SM, Molitch M, Krutzik S. Enhanced parathyroid function in essential hypertension: a homeostatic response to a urinary calcium leak. Hypertension. 1980;2:162–8.
31. Cooper R, Rotimi C. Hypertension in populations of West African origin: is there a genetic predisposition? J Hypertens. 1994;12:215–27.
32. Langford HG, Watson RL. Potassium and calcium intake, excretion, and homeostasis in blacks, and their relation to blood pressure. Cardiovasc Drugs Ther. 1990;4 Suppl 2:403–6.
33. Zemel MB, Zemel PC, Bryg RJ, Sowers JR. Dietary calcium induces regression of left ventricular hypertrophy in hypertensive non-insulin-dependent diabetic blacks. Am J Hypertens. 1990;3:458–63.
34. Zemel MB, Gualdoni SM, Sowers JR. Reductions in total and extracellular water associated with calcium-induced natriuresis and the antihypertensive effect of calcium in blacks. Am J Hypertens. 1988;1:70–2.
35. Griffith LE, Guyatt GH, Cook RJ, Bucher HC, Cook DJ. The influence of dietary and nondietary calcium supplementation on blood pressure: an updated metaanalysis of randomized controlled trials. Am J Hypertens. 1999;12:84–92.
36. Allender PS, Cutler JA, Follmann D, Cappuccio FP, Pryer J, Elliott P. Dietary calcium and blood pressure: a meta-analysis of randomized clinical trials. Ann Intern Med. 1996;124: 825–31.
37. Martins D, Wolf M, Pan D, et al. Prevalence of cardiovascular risk factors and the serum levels of 25-hydroxyvitamin D in the United States: data from the Third National Health and Nutrition Examination Survey. Arch Intern Med. 2007;167:1159–65.
38. Forman JP, Giovannucci E, Holmes MD, et al. Plasma 25-hydroxyvitamin D levels and risk of incident hypertension. Hypertension. 2007;49:1063–9.
39. Pittas AG, Chung M, Trikalinos T, et al. Systematic review: vitamin D and cardiometabolic outcomes. Ann Intern Med. 2010;152:307–14.
40. Krause R, Buhring M, Hopfenmuller W, Holick MF, Sharma AM. Ultraviolet B and blood pressure. Lancet. 1998;352:709–10.
41. Pfeifer M, Begerow B, Minne HW, Nachtigall D, Hansen C. Effects of a short-term vitamin D(3) and calcium supplementation on blood pressure and parathyroid hormone levels in elderly women. J Clin Endocrinol Metab. 2001;86:1633–7.

42. Wang TJ, Pencina MJ, Booth SL, et al. Vitamin D deficiency and risk of cardiovascular disease. Circulation. 2008;117:503–11.
43. Autier P, Gandini S. Vitamin D supplementation and total mortality: a meta-analysis of randomized controlled trials. Arch Intern Med. 2007;167:1730–7.
44. Judd SE, Raiser SN, Kumari M, Tangpricha V. 1,25-dihydroxyvitamin D3 reduces systolic blood pressure in hypertensive adults: a pilot feasibility study. J Steroid Biochem Mol Biol. 2010;121:445–7.
45. Lee JH, O'Keefe JH, Bell D, Hensrud DD, Holick MF. Vitamin D deficiency an important, common, and easily treatable cardiovascular risk factor? J Am Coll Cardiol. 2008;52: 1949–56.
46. Zittermann A, Schleithoff SS, Tenderich G, Berthold HK, Korfer R, Stehle P. Low vitamin D status: a contributing factor in the pathogenesis of congestive heart failure? J Am Coll Cardiol. 2003;41:105–12.
47. Kong J, Qiao G, Zhang Z, Liu SQ, Li YC. Targeted vitamin D receptor expression in juxtaglomerular cells suppresses renin expression independent of parathyroid hormone and calcium. Kidney Int. 2008;74:1577–81.
48. Oh J, Weng S, Felton SK, et al. 1,25(OH)2 vitamin d inhibits foam cell formation and suppresses macrophage cholesterol uptake in patients with type 2 diabetes mellitus. Circulation. 2009;120:687–98.
49. Grey A, Lucas J, Horne A, Gamble G, Davidson JS, Reid IR. Vitamin D repletion in patients with primary hyperparathyroidism and coexistent vitamin D insufficiency. J Clin Endocrinol Metab. 2005;90:2122–6.
50. Silverberg SJ. Vitamin D deficiency and primary hyperparathyroidism. J Bone Miner Res. 2007;22 Suppl 2:V100–4.
51. Grubbs EG, Rafeeq S, Jimenez C, et al. Preoperative vitamin D replacement therapy in primary hyperparathyroidism: safe and beneficial? Surgery 2008;144:852–8; discussion 8–9.
52. Sambrook PN, Chen CJ, March L, et al. High bone turnover is an independent predictor of mortality in the frail elderly. J Bone Miner Res. 2006;21:549–55.
53. Watson KE, Abrolat ML, Malone LL, et al. Active serum vitamin D levels are inversely correlated with coronary calcification. Circulation. 1997;96:1755–60.
54. Rubin MR, Maurer MS, McMahon DJ, Bilezikian JP, Silverberg SJ. Arterial stiffness in mild primary hyperparathyroidism. J Clin Endocrinol Metab. 2005;90:3326–30.
55. Ogard CG, Engelmann MD, Kistorp C, Nielsen SL, Vestergaard H. Increased plasma N-terminal pro-B-type natriuretic peptide and markers of inflammation related to atherosclerosis in patients with primary hyperparathyroidism. Clin Endocrinol (Oxf). 2005;63:493–8.
56. Andersson P, Rydberg E, Willenheimer R. Primary hyperparathyroidism and heart disease–a review. Eur Heart J. 2004;25:1776–87.
57. Walker MD, Silverberg SJ. Cardiovascular aspects of primary hyperparathyroidism. J Endocrinol Invest. 2008;31:925–31.
58. Schleithoff SS, Zittermann A, Tenderich G, Berthold HK, Stehle P, Koerfer R. Vitamin D supplementation improves cytokine profiles in patients with congestive heart failure: a double-blind, randomized, placebo-controlled trial. Am J Clin Nutr. 2006;83:754–9.
59. Zittermann A. Vitamin D and disease prevention with special reference to cardiovascular disease. Prog Biophys Mol Biol. 2006;92:39–48.
60. Elenkov IJ, Wilder RL, Bakalov VK, Link AA, Dimitrov MA, Fisher S, Crane M, Kanik KS, Chrousos GP. IL-12, TNF-alpha, and hormonal changes during late pregnancy and early postpartum: implications for autoimmune disease activity during these times. J Clin Endocrinol Metab. 2001;86(10):433–8.
61. Al-Daghri NM, Alkharfy KM, Al-Saleh Y, Al-Attas OS, Alokail MS, Al-Othman A, Moharram O, El-Kholie E, Sabico S, Kumar S, Chrousso GP. Modest reversal of metabolic syndrome manifestations with vitamin D status correction: a 12-month prospective study. Metabolism. 2012;61(5):661–6.
62. Al-Daghri NM, Al-Attas OS, Alokail MS, Alkharfy KM, Al-Othman A, Draz HM, et al. Hypovitaminosis D associations with adverse metabolic parameters are accentuated in patients

with diabetes mellitus type 2: a BMI-independent role of adiponectin ? J Endocrinol Invest. 2011 Dec 15. [Epub ahead of print].

63. Deo R, Katz R, Shlipak MG, et al. Vitamin D, parathyroid hormone, and sudden cardiac death: results from the Cardiovascular Health Study. Hypertension. 2011;58:1021–8.
64. Puepet FH, Agaba EI, Chuhwak EK, Ugoya SO. Primary hyperparathyroidism presenting with severe hypertension in a middle aged Nigerian–a case report. Niger Postgrad Med J. 2008;15:58–60.
65. Gennari C, Nami R, Gonnelli S. Hypertension and primary hyperparathyroidism: the role of adrenergic and renin-angiotensin-aldosterone systems. Miner Electrolyte Metab. 1995;21:77–81.
66. Duprez D, De Buyzere M, De Backer T, Clement D. Relationship between vitamin D and the regional blood flow and vascular resistance in moderate arterial hypertension. J Hypertens Suppl. 1993;11:S304–5.
67. Targher G, Bertolini L, Padovani R, et al. Serum 25-hydroxyvitamin D3 concentrations and carotid artery intima-media thickness among type 2 diabetic patients. Clin Endocrinol (Oxf). 2006;65:593–7.
68. Al Mheid I, Patel R, Murrow J, et al. Vitamin D status is associated with arterial stiffness and vascular dysfunction in healthy humans. J Am Coll Cardiol. 2011;58:186–92.
69. London GM, Guerin AP, Verbeke FH, et al. Mineral metabolism and arterial functions in end-stage renal disease: potential role of 25-hydroxyvitamin D deficiency. J Am Soc Nephrol. 2007;18:613–20.
70. Sugden JA, Davies JI, Witham MD, Morris AD, Struthers AD. Vitamin D improves endothelial function in patients with Type 2 diabetes mellitus and low vitamin D levels. Diabet Med. 2008;25:320–5.
71. Ekmekci A, Abaci N, Colak Ozbey N, et al. Endothelial function and endothelial nitric oxide synthase intron 4a/b polymorphism in primary hyperparathyroidism. J Endocrinol Invest. 2009;32:611–6.
72. Lee JH, Gadi R, Spertus JA, Tang F, O'Keefe JH. Prevalence of vitamin D deficiency in patients with acute myocardial infarction. Am J Cardiol. 2011;107:1636–8.
73. Dobnig H, Pilz S, Scharnagl H, et al. Independent association of low serum 25-hydroxyvitamin d and 1,25-dihydroxyvitamin d levels with all-cause and cardiovascular mortality. Arch Intern Med. 2008;168:1340–9.
74. Melamed ML, Michos ED, Post W, Astor B. 25-hydroxyvitamin D levels and the risk of mortality in the general population. Arch Intern Med. 2008;168:1629–37.
75. Wang L, Manson JE, Song Y, Sesso HD. Systematic review: vitamin D and calcium supplementation in prevention of cardiovascular events. Ann Intern Med. 2010;152:315–23.
76. Lips P. Vitamin D deficiency and secondary hyperparathyroidism in the elderly: consequences for bone loss and fractures and therapeutic implications. Endocr Rev. 2001;22:477–501.
77. Heaney RP. Vitamin D depletion and effective calcium absorption. J Bone Miner Res 2003;18:1342; author reply 3.
78. Lappe JM, Travers-Gustafson D, Davies KM, Recker RR, Heaney RP. Vitamin D and calcium supplementation reduces cancer risk: results of a randomized trial. Am J Clin Nutr. 2007;85:1586–91.
79. Bischoff-Ferrari HA, Dietrich T, Orav EJ, et al. Higher 25-hydroxyvitamin D concentrations are associated with better lower-extremity function in both active and inactive persons aged>or = 60y. Am J Clin Nutr. 2004;80:752–8.
80. Bischoff-Ferrari HA, Shao A, Dawson-Hughes B, Hathcock J, Giovannucci E, Willett WC. Benefit-risk assessment of vitamin D supplementation. Osteoporos Int. 2009;21:1121–32.
81. Bischoff-Ferrari H. Vitamin D: what is an adequate vitamin D level and how much supplementation is necessary? Best Pract Res Clin Rheumatol. 2009;23:789–95.
82. Jean G, Souberbielle JC, Chazot C. Monthly cholecalciferol administration in haemodialysis patients: a simple and efficient strategy for vitamin D supplementation. Nephrol Dial Transplant. 2009;24:3799–805.
83. Barreto DV, Barreto FC, Liabeuf S, et al. Vitamin D affects survival independently of vascular calcification in chronic kidney disease. Clin J Am Soc Nephrol. 2009;4:1128–35.

84. Heaney RP. Vitamin D in health and disease. Clin J Am Soc Nephrol. 2008;3:1535–41.
85. Hathcock JN, Shao A, Vieth R, Heaney R. Risk assessment for vitamin D. Am J Clin Nutr. 2007;85:6–18.
86. Barger-Lux MJ, Heaney RP. Effects of above average summer sun exposure on serum 25-hydroxyvitamin D and calcium absorption. J Clin Endocrinol Metab. 2002;87:4952–6.
87. Holick MF, Binkley NC, Bischoff-Ferrari HA, et al. Evaluation, treatment, and prevention of vitamin D deficiency: an Endocrine Society clinical practice guideline. J Clin Endocrinol Metab. 2011;96:1911–30.
88. Souberbielle JC, Body JJ, Lappe JM, et al. Vitamin D and musculoskeletal health, cardiovascular disease, autoimmunity and cancer: recommendations for clinical practice. Autoimmun Rev. 2010;9:709–15.
89. Pepper KJ, Judd SE, Nanes MS, Tangpricha V. Evaluation of vitamin D repletion regimens to correct vitamin D status in adults. Endocr Pract. 2009;15:95–103.
90. Heaney RP. The Vitamin D requirement in health and disease. J Steroid Biochem Mol Biol. 2005;97:13–9.
91. IoM. Dietary Reference Intakes for Calcium and Vitamin D. Washington, DC: National Academies Press; 2011.
92. Bischoff-Ferrari HA, Giovannucci E, Willett WC, Dietrich T, Dawson-Hughes B. Estimation of optimal serum concentrations of 25-hydroxyvitamin D for multiple health outcomes. Am J Clin Nutr. 2006;84:18–28.
93. Hypponen E, Power C. Vitamin D status and glucose homeostasis in the 1958 British birth cohort: the role of obesity. Diabetes Care. 2006;29:2244–6.
94. Visser M, Deeg DJ, Puts MT, Seidell JC, Lips P. Low serum concentrations of 25-hydroxyvitamin D in older persons and the risk of nursing home admission. Am J Clin Nutr. 2006;84:616–22.
95. Costello RB. Vitamin D and health in the 21st century: federal initiatives to advance research. Am J Med Sci. 2009;338:34–9.
96. Food and Nutrition Board IoM. Standing Committee on the Scientific Evaluation of Dietary Reference Intakes: Dietary Reference Intakes: Calcium, Phosphorus, Magnesium, Vitamin D, and Fluoride. Washington, DC, USA: National Academy Press; 1997.
97. Manson JE, Bassuk SS, Lee IM, et al. The VITamin D and OmegA-3 TriaL (VITAL): rationale and design of a large randomized controlled trial of vitamin D and marine omega-3 fatty acid supplements for the primary prevention of cancer and 1cardiovascular disease. Contemp Clin Trials. 2012;33(1):159–71.
98. Ullah MI, Uwaifo GI, Nicholas WC, Koch CA. Does vitamin D deficiency cause hypertension? current evidence from clinical studies and potential mechanisms. Int J Endocrinol. 2010;2010:579640.

Chapter 11
Testosterone Deficiency or Male Hypogonadism

Christian A. Koch and Michael Zitzmann

Abstract Testosterone deficiency (TD) may represent a cardiovascular risk factor, as it has become a frequently diagnosed condition in the current obesity epidemic. Men diagnosed with TD often have comorbidities including hypertension, metabolic syndrome, and sleep apnea. Apart from sexual aspects including lack of sex drive and erectile dysfunction, challenging aspects in diagnosing and treating patients with TD include interindividual variation of symptoms combined with lack of symptom correlation with serum testosterone levels. Replacement therapy with testosterone has beneficial metabolic effects with an improved glycemic profile and improved cardiac function in selected patients.

Keywords Hypogonadism • 5-Alpha dihydro-T • Aging and testosterone • Senescence • Testosterone

Introduction

In men, testosterone (T) is essential for the development and maintenance of various tissues with reproductive and nonreproductive tasks. In general, T exerts widespread effects on the psyche, metabolism, and body composition. This is most obviously seen in the difference between men and women. T-deficiency is associated with a spectrum of pathophysiological symptoms, clinically termed hypogonadism. Physicians define this condition by adverse traits in physical appearance, disturbed

C.A. Koch
Division of Endocrinology, University of Mississippi Medical Center, Jackson, MS, USA

M. Zitzmann (✉)
Center for Reproductive Medicine and Andrology, Westfaelische Wilhelms University, Domagkstrasse 11, Muenster 48149, Germany
e-mail: Michael.Zitzmann@ukmuenster.de

C.A. Koch and G.P. Chrousos (eds.), *Endocrine Hypertension: Underlying Mechanisms and Therapy*, Contemporary Endocrinology, DOI 10.1007/978-1-60761-548-4_11,

mental and cognitive traits, shifts in body composition, namely increased body fat content and reduced muscle mass. Physical abilities in androgen-deficient men are further attenuated by lower oxygen supply to tissues due to decreased hemoglobin concentrations and by poor peripheral glucose utilization. Also, bone tissue is subject to strong regulation by T and its aromatization product, estradiol.

Among the main risk factors listed for cardiovascular disease (CVD) is male gender, most likely related to observations showing that men are at least twice as likely to suffer from coronary heart disease than women [1]. No clear reason for this observation exists although premenopausal women presumably may experience cardioprotective effects from estrogen [2]. One should consider that testosterone can be converted to estradiol in obese and nonobese men and women via aromatase, an enzyme that is expressed in adipocytes. Testosterone inhibits the development of preadipocytes and may exert vasodilatory effects via non-genomic mechanisms, primarily through the vascular smooth muscle [3].

Given the global epidemic of obesity and type 2 diabetes mellitus, as well as of patients with the metabolic syndrome, including hypertension, understanding the reasons and implications of recent meta-analyses that showed testosterone levels to be generally lower among patients with metabolic syndrome and type 2 diabetes becomes increasingly important [4–9]. Body mass index (BMI) and waist circumference have an inverse linear correlation with serum testosterone and insulin-like growth factor-1 concentrations, meaning the leaner someone is, the higher are the serum testosterone and IGF-1 levels [10].

Physiogenomic Background

T and its metabolite 5-alpha dihydro-T exert their effects on multiple gene expression and, thus, ultimately on maleness, via the androgen receptor (AR). A wide range of clinical conditions starting with complete androgen insensitivity are related to mutations in the AR. Subtle modulations of the transcriptional activity induced by the AR have also been described and can be assigned to a polyglutamine stretch of variable length within the N-terminal domain of the receptor. This stretch is encoded by CAG-triplets in exon 1 of the AR gene, which is located on the X-chromosome. Longer triplet residues mitigate binding of androgen receptor co-activators and, hence, facilitate decreased androgenicity. A marked relation to androgenic traits can be seen in men with an elongation of more than 37 CAG repeats, but also in those with CAG repeats within the normal range [11–13].

Aging and Testosterone: General Remarks

Senescence in males as such does not imply the necessity for testosterone substitution, whereas male hypogonadism is a prerequisite for testosterone substitution. As the incidence of hypogonadism increases with age, the terms “andropause,” “PADAM” meaning "partial androgen deficiency in aging men" or "male climacteric" have emerged in several publications, alluding to the female menopause and indicating that in men there could be an end to gonadal steroid production and fertility which occurs as precipitously and as definite as in women. However, a drastic decrease in androgen production cannot be observed in healthy men; androgen depletion is a rather slow process and "andropause" turns out to be a misnomer.

Unlike the impressive somatic character of symptoms encountered with diseases associated with "classical hypogonadism" such as Kallmann syndrome, pituitary insufficiency, Klinefelter's syndrome or conditions after bilateral orchiectomy, complaints of older men may be attributed to be "normal aging processes" or illnesses accumulating with advancing age, such as diabetes mellitus or atherosclerosis. The effects of these nosologic entities on libido, reactive erectile function, and nocturnal erections are well known, but low testosterone levels represent an additive negative factor [14].

Furthermore, androgens have psychotropic effects so that a deficiency may result in depressed mood and general fatigue, a decrease in cognitive functions and intellectual activity [15]. Older men in a hypogonadal state may also present with anemia, since testosterone acts positively on erythropoesis. Hypogonadism represents a risk factor for the loss of bone mass, and, can thus cause osteoporotic fractures in men [16–19]. Androgen depletion can also cause loss of muscle mass and increasing body fat content. A major sign of hypogonadism in younger men, a small prostate, is, however, rather unlikely in older males.

Testosterone levels rather exhibit great interindividual variability with advancing age; nevertheless, the proportion of men presenting with testosterone levels in the subnormal range (below 12 nmol/L or 350 ng/dL) increases significantly. Longitudinal studies as those in populations of aging men from Baltimore or Massachusetts demonstrate that such low levels can be found in fewer than 1% of men aged below 40 years, but in more than 20% of men older than 60 years and over 40% in men above 80 years [20].

Hence, subnormal testosterone levels are not a general, but frequent feature of aging men [21, 22]. This age-related deterioration of androgen production can be seen as a combined dysfunctionality of both the central and peripheral parts of the sex steroid regulation system and is named "late-onset hypogonadism" (LOH).

The direction as well as the weighting of pathological processes within such an imbalance may vary, and LOH presents with low to low-normal testosterone concentrations and LH levels which may be slightly decreased, normal, or elevated. In fact, the clinical entity might as well be named "mixed hypogonadism" as there is no clear-cut definition of age in relation to LOH. Usually described as disease met in "aging" men, the nosology with its typical hormone constellations can also be found in men of "younger age." In principle, it is a diagnosis made after exclusion of other causes for hypogonadism.

A central clinical question is whether the decrease of androgen levels described as LOH translates physiologically. Such clinical evidence could be sought in similarities between the symptoms of men with LOH and symptoms of other hypogonadal men as well as general symptoms of aging men. In this regard, one has to be aware that aging is most often accompanied by a decline of many physiological,

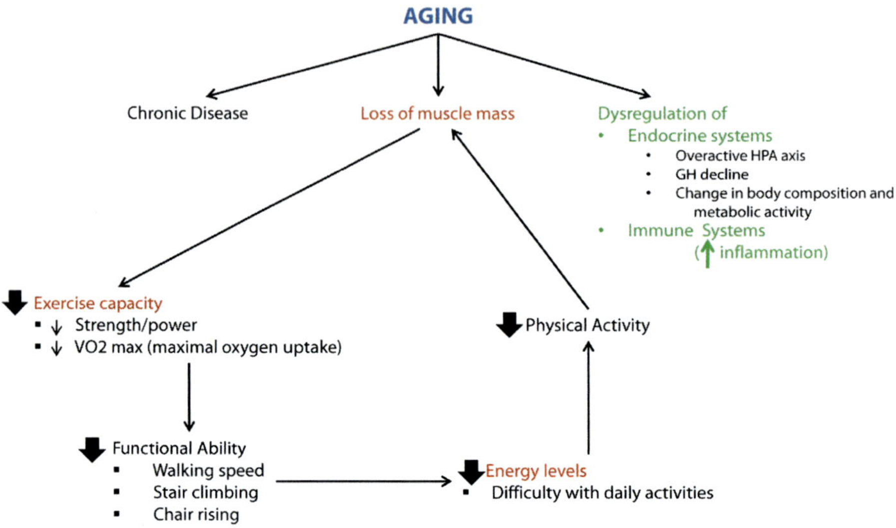

Fig. 11.1 The frailty cycle. Modified from ref. [21]

cognitive, and sexual functions since the incidence and prevalence of chronic diseases affecting these parameters increases with aging (Fig. 11.1).

Such chronic diseases are mainly atherosclerosis, diabetes mellitus, and obesity. Thus, in view of the multifactorial origin of aging symptoms, effects of LOH may not clearly be detectable. However, evidence from hypogonadism in younger men suggests a range of androgen-dependent functions, for which an adverse affection by LOH can be assumed. Especially the beneficial effects of testosterone substitution on these morbidities provide evidence for a significant role of androgens within the symptomatology of elderly men with LOH. These are discussed in the following.

Diagnostic Approaches to Male Hypogonadism

LOH is a diagnosis made by exclusion of other morbidities resulting in testosterone deficiency.

Hypogonadism manifests itself with a variety of symptoms, which can be of psychological, cognitive, sexual as well as somatic nature. The time of onset is significant in manifestation patterns of hypogonadism as well as the actual serum concentration of testosterone, leading to a stepwise increase of symptoms with decreasing testosterone levels. Older hypogonadal men usually exhibit characteristics similar to younger patients, but possibly to a lower degree. The pattern of complaints in older

Table 11.1 Symptoms and signs of testosterone deficiency (modified from ref. [23])

Classic symptoms and signs	Nonspecific symptoms and signs
Reduced libido and sexual activity	Decreased energy, self-confidence
Decreased spontaneous (morning) erections	Depressed mood or dysthymia
Gynecomastia	Poor concentration and memory
Loss of body (axillary and pubic) hair	Sleep disturbance, increased sleepiness
Small (especially <5 mL) or shrinking testes	Mild anemia
Infertility, low sperm count	Reduced muscle bulk and strength
Low trauma fracture, low bone mineral density	Increased body fat
Hot flushes, sweats	Diminished physical or work performance

men may be caused at least partly by various other chronic illnesses related to the aging process (Table 11.1).

Once a patient presents with symptoms causing clinical suspicion of testosterone deficiency, standardized patterns of diagnostics and therapy should be followed. Underlying causes of hypogonadism are disorders located at the testicular source of testosterone, the Leydig cells (primary hypogonadism) or at the central regulation unit, consisting of the hypothalamus and the pituitary gland (secondary hypogonadism), the latter secreting luteinizing hormone (LH), which stimulates Leydig cells.

Hypogonadal symptoms also occur in cases of target organ resistance, mostly due to inherited alterations of the androgen receptor; in this case, elevated concentrations of both testosterone and LH are found and the androgen-sensitivity index points to androgen resistance (see below, pharmacogenetic implications and ref. [24]).

For diagnostic purposes in men suspected of having male hypogonadism, assessment of total testosterone, luteinizing hormone, follicle stimulation hormone (FSH), prolactin, and estradiol is helpful, as well as calculation of free testosterone from total testosterone and sex hormone binding globulin (SHBG) (see Fig. 11.2); this complete overview of hormones classifies the clinical picture in regard to fertility and estrogen-related features of the phenotype (e.g., fat distribution, gynecomastia, bone density). Determination of androgen receptor genotype and concentrations of serum dihydrotestosterone should be performed in special cases of suspected androgen resistance.

Questionnaires related to possible androgen deficits have been utilized for screening purposes and may be useful for monitoring symptoms during testosterone substitution therapy. The androgen deficiency in aging male (ADAM) questionnaire, developed at St. Louis University and the aging male symptom scale (AMS) developed in Germany are two widely used clinical tools to assess clinical symptoms of androgen deficiency. Both of them have high sensitivities (88% and 83%, respectively) but they have very low specificities (60% and 39%, respectively) increasing the chance of false positive results [25–27].

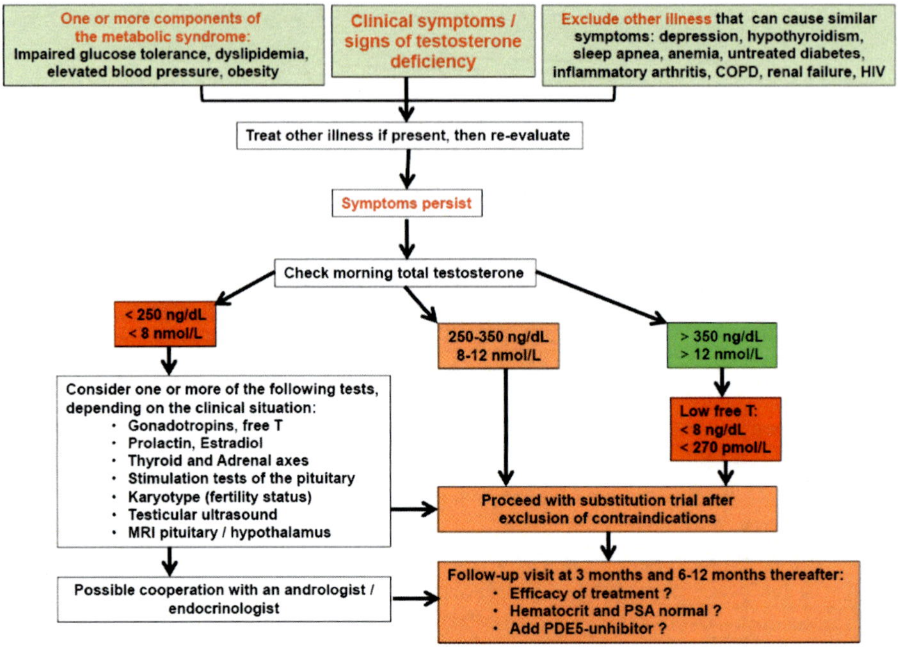

Fig. 11.2 Diagnostic algorithm for evaluating men with possible testosterone deficiency syndrome (TDS). Modified from ref. [8]

In addition, the effects of decreasing testosterone levels are enhanced by an age-dependent increase of levels of SHBG, further lowering the amount of bioavailable testosterone. Possibly reduced levels of growth hormone and insulin-like growth factor 1, which inhibit SHBG production in hepatocytes, are responsible for this phenomenon.

In cases of borderline total testosterone and existing symptoms (see below), low concentrations of bioavailable testosterone might be taken into consideration for an initiation of treatment. Notwithstanding, normal limits for bioavailable testosterone have not been defined.

Generally, there is no age-limit concerning the substitution of testosterone. Especially the short-acting, dose-titrable transdermal preparations provide the physician with the ability to treat men with LOH (as defined by low testosterone levels in combination with the major symptoms of hypogonadism such as depression, loss of vigor and libido, anemia). Testosterone levels in the low normal to mid-normal range should be aimed at. Reference ranges for healthy nonobese young men have recently been established [28]. In a study including 3,672 men from age 20 to age 98 years, mean age 59.7 years, it was shown that a total testosterone level should exceed 350 ng/dL to reliably predict normal free testosterone and that total testosterone levels have low specificity for the biochemical diagnosis of hypogonadism unless they are less than 150 ng/dL [29].

Body Composition as a Key Component in Understanding Testosterone Action on Metabolism And Blood Pressure

Muscle Tissue

In addition to the effects of T deficiency on body fat content, a loss of fat free mass and decrease in muscle protein synthesis is observed in hypogonadal men [30]. In agreement, when androgens are substituted such patients, fat-free mass increases significantly, which can be attributed to muscle growth [31, 32]. The growth of muscle tissue seems to follow a linear dose–response relationship over a wide range of T levels, as was demonstrated in healthy young men receiving androgen ablation by a GnRH agonist and subsequent T administration in various doses to achieve low to supraphysiological levels. As fat-free mass increased with the increasing T dose, so did volumes of thigh muscles [33]. Muscle biopsies in these men demonstrated a homogenous increase in cross-sectional areas of both type I and II muscle fibers, which maintained their proportion. As muscle fiber hypertrophy involves the addition of newly formed myonuclei via the fusion of myogenic cells, the myonuclear number increased in direct relation to the increase in muscle fiber diameter. Muscle cell hyperplasia did not play a significant role [34].

Body Fat

Cross-sectional investigations in healthy, eugonadal have demonstrated a negative relationship between body fat content and levels of total testosterone [35, 36], this applies in particular to abdominal fat tissue [37, 38]. In healthy obese men, the issue is complicated by simultaneously decreasing levels of SHBG, thus levels of free or bioavailable T are often maintained [39].

In hypogonadal men, an increased total BMI is regularly observed and as well a reduced lean BMI, measured with dual X-ray absorptiometry (DEXA) or bioimpedance, is found when compared to age-matched healthy controls, suggesting higher body weight due to increased fat mass in the presence of lower muscle mass [40, 41]. Testosterone treatment can significantly reduce body fat content in hypogonadal men and vice versa it can increase lean body mass, an observation which is not only due to shifts in proportions but also to growth of muscle tissue (*see below*) [32, 42–49].

This is exerted via a redistribution of body fat during which mainly visceral and intermuscular fat depots are affected, but subcutaneous tissue seems to be spared [50]; it is likely that fat cell size itself is modulated by androgens [51]. The process seems to follow a linear dose–response relationship to T [50], but the exact mechanism, by which fat cells are subject to androgen influence is not known. It can be speculated that this is mediated via increased insulin sensitivity and improved glucose utilization, resulting in lower insulin levels and, thus, a lower amount of lipid storage.

Visceral fat tissue plays a central role within the metabolic syndrome, which is mentioned in detail further below, acting as a source of inflammatory, anti-insulinergic and atherogenically relevant cytokines such as TNF-α and IL-6 [7, 52–55].

Fat tissue also functions as an endocrine organ: its product adiponectin plays an important role in metabolism and is related to cardiovascular risk factors. It is produced by fat cells in large quantities, yet its levels are inversely associated with total body fat mass, which is most likely caused by auto-/paracrine downregulation via inflammatory cytokines. Improvement of insulin sensitivity and inhibition of various atherogenic processes within the vessel wall are direct effects of adiponectin [55, 56].

Leptin is another hormone secreted by fat cells. Hypophagia to reduce fat mass is supported by leptin signals, but adipose tissue fosters further food intake by facilitating leptin resistance at the hypothalamic level via afferent nerve signals [57]. A vicious circle is thus induced as leptin resistance increases further adipocyte-related production of this hormone. There are indications that high levels of leptin can mitigate testosterone secretion, for instance via downregulating the action of kisspeptin through the Kiss1 gene [58, 59].

Testosterone seems to have various effects on fat cells and insulin resistance. A study in mouse pluripotent stem cells indicates that testosterone regulates body composition by promoting the commitment of these mesenchymal cells into the myogenic lineage and inhibiting their differentiation into the adipogenic lineage. This provides a unifying explanation for the reciprocal effects of androgens on muscle and fat mass in men [60]. A inhibiting effect of testosterone has also been described concerning the differentiation of preadipocytes: in 3T3-L1 cells that differentiate to form fat cells in adipogenic medium, testosterone inhibits adipocyte differentiation in vitro through an androgen receptor-mediated nuclear translocation of beta-catenin and activation of downstream Wnt signaling (such Wnt signals direct distinct fates of differentiation in precursor cell types) [60]. In addition, testosterone increases lipolysis and the number of adrenoreceptors in male rat adipocytes [61].

Testosterone may facilitate insulin sensitivity both in fat and muscle cells by upregulating the expression of insulin-induced downstream protein expression. Respective dose-dependent effects of testosterone on insulin receptor substrate-1 and glucose transporter 4 expression were seen in cells models [62]. Recent models of insulin resistance also suggest a pivotal role of mitochondrial function with the decreased transcription of oxidative phosphorylation genes in skeletal muscle of insulin-resistant subjects. This leads to decreased oxidative phosphorylation, decreased lipid oxidation, intracellular accumulation of triglycerides in skeletal muscle, and ultimately insulin resistance [63]. A study in 60 men demonstrated testosterone levels to correlate positively with mitochondrial capacity assessed by measuring maximal aerobic capacity and also expression of oxidative phosphorylation genes [64].

As discussed above, leptin resistance and consequently upregulated adipocyte leptin secretion play a pivotal role in obesity. Testosterone substitution in hypogonadal

Table 11.2 The International Diabetes Federation: updated criteria for the diagnosis of the metabolic syndrome (ref. [75])

New Criteria for the Definition of the Metabolic Syndrome
1. Waist circumference >94 cm (European Men)
2. Triglycerides >150 mg/dL or treatment
3. HDL-Cholesterol <40 mg/dL or treatment
4. Arterial blood pressure >130 mmHg systolic and/or >85 mmHg diastolic or treatment
5. Fasting glucose >100 mg/dL or known type 2 diabetes mellitus
3 of 5 criteria have to be met (Consensus IDF and NCEP ATP III)

men is able to reduce leptin secretion of fat cells, probably by an androgen receptor-mediated pathway (also see below ref. [65]), thus breaking the vicious cycle of leptin resistance and obesity [47, 66–68].

Metabolic Aspects and Glucose Metabolism

Within the last century, life circumstances have changed in developed countries as physical activity has decreased and, simultaneously, an oversupply of food is present. This results in an increasing prevalence of overweight and obesity, particularly over the past two decades. As a consequence, a complex disorder consisting of visceral obesity, dyslipidemia, insulin resistance, and hypertension emerges with increasing incidence: the so-called metabolic syndrome contributes to a symptomatology, which progressively may lead to the manifestation of type 2 diabetes in genetically predisposed subjects and CVD in all. While the pathogenesis of the metabolic syndrome and each of its components is complex and not well understood, central obesity and insulin resistance are acknowledged as important causative factors [69–72]. Persons affected are twice as likely to die from and three times as likely to suffer a heart attack or stroke compared to those free of the metabolic syndrome [73]. They also have a fivefold greater risk of developing type 2 diabetes mellitus, if not already present [74].

The International Diabetes Federation and the National Cholesterol Education Panel have recently updated and harmonized the criteria for diagnosis of the metabolic syndrome (Table 11.2).

In men, obesity as the central component of the metabolic syndrome is associated with low testosterone concentrations [37, 38, 65, 76].

On the other hand, in men, testosterone deficiency may contribute to the development of the metabolic syndrome. In turn, states of hyperinsulinemia and obesity lead to a reduction of testicular testosterone production. Testosterone has reciprocal effects on the generation of muscle and visceral adipose tissue by influencing the commitment of pluripotent stem cells and by inhibiting the development of preadipocytes. Insulin sensitivity of muscle cells is increased by augmenting mitochondrial capacity and fostering expression of oxidative phosphorylation genes. Testosterone has a protective effect on pancreatic β cells, which is possibly exerted by androgen receptor-mediated mechanisms and influence on inflammatory cytokines [77].

As some, but not all, epidemiological and interventional studies indicate, testosterone substitution might be helpful in preventing or attenuating the metabolic syndrome in aging men with LOH and in hypogonadal patients with type 2 diabetes mellitus, but larger controlled trials are needed to confirm such hypotheses [6, 7]. Meta-analyzing prospective (longitudinal, interventional) and cross-sectional studies of testosterone replacement therapy (TRT) in men with and without type 2 diabetes revealed that TRT significantly reduced fasting plasma glucose, hemoglobin A1C, fat mass, and triglyceride levels without significantly changing blood pressure [78]. Heterogeneous community-based studies showed low endogenous testosterone to be associated with an increased risk of all-cause and cardiovascular death [79, 80]. In men age 69–81 years, high serum testosterone levels predicted a reduced 5-year risk of cardiovascular events [81]. Men with normal testosterone concentrations appear to have lower rates of atherosclerosis and coronary artery disease. Men with congestive heart failure were more able to walk on testosterone therapy than such men on placebo [82–84].

Obesity is often associated with fatigue, excessive day time sleepiness and sleep apnea, although these manifestations may also occur in lean individuals. Proinflammatory cytokines, such as interleukin-6 and tumor necrosis factor alpha, are elevated in patients suffering from sleep apnea. Therapy with continuous positive airway pressure can improve sleepiness and blood pressure, as well as increase testosterone levels in men [5, 85–89].

General Metabolic Perspectives for Men

In an animal model using androgen receptor knock out (ARKO) mice, male ARKO mice were less dynamic and less oxygen consuming with increased secretion of adiponectin (exerting insulin sensitizing effects) and decreased lipolysis, partly explaining their adiposity [90]. Considering that burning calories mainly depends on the resting metabolism which is determined by muscle mass, physical activity to build/exercise muscle, and testosterone availability, this is not surprising. Additional apolipoprotein E-deficiency in ARKO mice accelerated atherosclerosis that could be reduced by testosterone treatment [91].

Looking at a human model of testosterone deficiency and its effects on metabolism, one could analyze individuals with androgen (complete) resistance syndrome. Women with complete androgen insensitivity syndrome are obese and have elevated total and LDL cholesterol levels as well as increased HOMA-IR indexes [92].

Hypogonadism in men with Klinefelter's syndrome (KFS) causes an unfavorable change in body composition leading to metabolic syndrome [93, 94]. Insulin resistance and metabolic syndrome in men with KFS are four times higher than in age-matched controls. In untreated KFS men, total fat mass and LDL cholesterol, triglyceride, CRP, and leptin levels are significantly increased, while HDL cholesterol levels are significantly decreased. KFS is associated with a significant increase in mortality risk of 40% (hazard ratio, 1.40; 95% confidence interval, 1.13–1.74), corresponding to a significantly reduced median survival of 2.1 years [95].

Special efforts to detect this underdiagnosed chromosome disorder and mitigate the increased mortality of these men due to complications of diabetes mellitus and cardiovascular events are necessary [93]. Although approaches examining the effects of testosterone on sub-parameters of the metabolic syndrome have been made (see above), prospective studies investigating its incidence in hypogonadal men receiving testosterone substitution therapy are needed. Such studies should take the modulatory effect of the androgen receptor into account to fully elucidate the putative potential of testosterone to attenuate or prevent the metabolic syndrome in men.

A Clinical Example to Elucidate the Andrologist's Approach to Metabolic Disorders in Hypogonadism

Key Question: Is There a Role for Testosterone Testing and Therapy in Obese Hypertensive Men?

Bob is a 52-year-old man complaining from mild erectile dysfunction (ED) and diminished libido. This may be an indicator of atherosclerosis or cardiovascular risk. Bob is 5 ft, 11 in. tall (180 cm) and gained 30 lb over the past 5 years. The physical examination showed that he is mildly hypertensive, with a blood pressure of 166/98 mm Hg, and weighs 217 lb (98.5 kg). You calculate his BMI to be 30.3 kg/m^2; and measure his waist circumference at 43 in. (109 cm), all signs indicating metabolic syndrome with late-onset obesity.

Laboratory values showed a serum total testosterone of 310 ng/dL (normal reference range, 350–1,030 ng/dL); bioavailable testosterone 90 ng/dL (normal reference range Males 50–69 years old, 95–285 ng/dL); Luteinizing hormone 4.3 mIU/mL (normal, 1.5–9.3); fasting blood sugar (FBS) 112 mg/dL (normal, 65–99 mg/dL); fasting insulin level: 19 μIU/mL (normal, <2); and a PSA of 1.1 ng/mL.

Based on the signs and symptoms exhibited by Bob, coupled with his blood laboratory values, is there any role for testosterone supplementation in his therapy, in addition to lifestyle changes including diet and exercise?

Rationale

A larger (2,314 men, aged 40–79 years), longer (average 7-year follow-up) nested case-control study found that every 173 ng/dL (6 nmol/L) increase in serum T was associated with a 21% lower risk of all-cause death (OR 0.79, 95% CI, 0.69–0.91, $P<0.01$) and CV death (OR 0.79, 95% CI, 0.64–0.97, $P=0.02$) after excluding deaths within the first 2 years and controlling for multiple variables (age, BMI, systolic blood pressure, cholesterol, cigarette smoking, diabetes, alcohol intake, physical activity, social class, education, and SHBG). These men had no CVD at baseline [96].

The Rancho Bernardo study (*N*=794 men, aged 50–91 years, average follow-up, 11.8 years, but up to 20 years) also found that total and bioavailable T were inversely related to risk of death. Men in the lowest quartile of total T (<241 ng/dL [8.4 nmol/L]) were 44% more likely to die during the follow-up period compared to those in highest quartile (>370 ng/dL [12.8 nmol/L]), independent of age, BMI, waist-to-hip ratio, alcohol use, current smoking, and exercise (HR 1.44, 95% CI, 1.12–1.84). Additional adjustment for prevalent diabetes, CVD, or the metabolic syndrome had minimal effect on the strength of this association. Low total T also predicted increased risk of death due to CV (HR 1.38, 95% CI 1.02–1.85) and respiratory disease (HR 2.29, 95% CI 1.25–4.20) [97–99].

Yet the association of T with death does not appear to operate through many risk factors and comorbidities, as the link between low T and shorter survival remains significant after adjustment for such covariates in multiple studies.

Possible explanations might include a separate association of the development of inflammatory cytokines and insulin resistance with the induction of hypogonadism (e.g., withdrawing testosterone therapy in men with known hypogonadism).

The Guidelines

The relations between testosterone deficiency syndrome (TDS; hypogonadism) and various health risk factors including metabolic syndrome, obesity, diabetes, vascular disease, frailty, and increased mortality in men has received renewed interest over the past decade.

In view of the growing interest from practitioners in TDS and improving men's health, several clinical guidelines on investigation, treatment, and monitoring of hypogonadism in men have been published by the Endocrine Society, American Association of Clinical Endocrinologists (AAEC), International Society of the Study of the Aging Male (ISSAM), International Society of Andrology (ISA), European Association of Urology (EAU), European Academy of Andrology (EAA), and the American Society of Andrology (ASA) [23, 100].

For maximum dissemination of this valuable information, the guidelines and recommendations were published in several journals to reach larger audiences.

The key recommendations of these guidelines were focused on:

1. Definition of TDS
2. Clinical diagnosis
3. Laboratory diagnosis
4. Assessment of treatment outcome and decision to continue therapy
5. Adverse effects and close monitoring

The guidelines recommended making a diagnosis of TDS in men consistent with signs and symptoms (e.g., low libido, erectile dysfunction, decreased muscle mass, decreased strength, increased body fat, decreased bone mineral density, decreased vitality, depressed mood) associated with low testosterone (less than 350 ng/dL; or 12 nmol/L according to the EAU Guidelines and less than 300 ng/dL or 10.3 nmol/L according to the Endocrine Society Guidelines) and some guidelines had provided an algorithm for diagnosis and treatment of men with TDS.

The recommendations also emphasized the need to discuss the benefit and risks of testosterone therapy with the patient and considering potential risks, including prostate cancer.

Further, the recommendations pointed strongly to close monitoring and assessment of the response to testosterone treatment. In the event lack of improvement in signs and symptoms are noted, the treatment is discontinued and other possible causes for the clinical presentation should be investigated.

One of the key areas of controversy in the recommendations and guidelines is the reliability and utility of the methods utilized in the measurements of total, bioavailable, free, and calculated free testosterone.

Also, there is disagreement on the lower limits of testosterone values that can be used in biochemically diagnosing TDS.

Thus, the uncertainty regarding which fraction of testosterone should be measured, and what the values mean clinically, remains the most urgent issue to be resolved.

Nevertheless, these recommendations and guidelines have provided many practitioners with imputes to diagnose and treat patients with TDS.

The guidelines also summarize the large amount of uncertainty that exists in male health care concerning symptoms of hypogonadism, and thresholds of testosterone concentrations that cause these symptoms.

From clinical experience in endocrinology, it is rather obvious that a universal, clear-cut threshold of testosterone concentrations cannot exist for all symptoms and in all men. Rather, there are strong indications that symptom-specificity exists concerning levels of testosterone. In general, mental problems seem to precede somatic/metabolic disorders, while erectile function seems to be maintained longest [101].

In addition, also the genetic background relating to the receptiveness of androgens, hence, androgen receptor polymorphisms are likely to play an interindividual role [12, 13].

Furthermore, a huge area of uncertainty exists regarding (a) the accuracy of testosterone assays, (b) the application of total or free testosterone, and (c) the subject of age stratification.

Such considerations have to be taken into account when taking care of patients like Bob, who definitely needs diagnosis and treatment: physicians have to use their clinical judgement and experience in such cases and handle each individual patient individually (instead of practicing "algorithm" or "cookbook" medicine). For a general practitioner, we suggest to approach men with symptoms of testosterone deficiency as outlined in Fig. 11.2, while considering factors mentioned in Fig. 11.3.

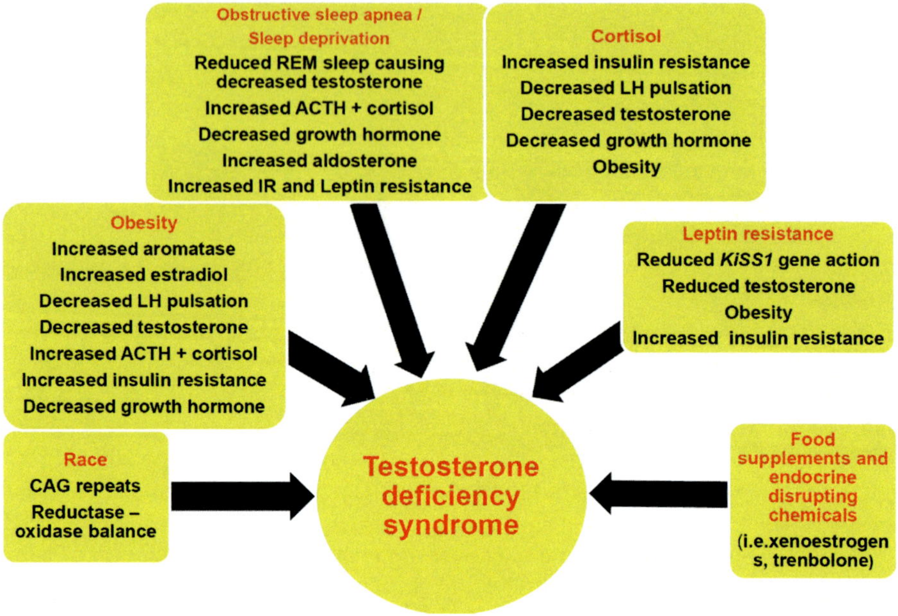

Fig. 11.3 Multiple determinants of the TDS. Modified from ref. [5]

Conclusion of the Case

According to generally accepted knowledge in medicine and cardiology, and quite apart from his testosterone levels, patient Bob has an increased risk for metabolic disorders/type 2 diabetes mellitus, arterial hypertension and is likely to die earlier from cardiovascular events than healthier men of his age. Indeed, he exhibits a sign of vascular compromise by the presence of erectile dysfunction, which may serve as a portal to his health: this is the reason why he came to consult the doctor!

In addition to that, we found low testosterone concentrations in his blood, as is quite typical for men of his age with his clinical profile. His complaints and the laboratory analysis allow the diagnosis: Bob has a TDS concomitant (and possibly causative) with/for his general clinical condition. There is enough evidence to start him on monitored testosterone substitution therapy, to improve both his mental problems, as well as to reduce the state of metabolic dyshomeostasis, including emerging glucose intolerance.

General Summary

1. Screening for testosterone levels in men of Bob's age with his matrix of mental and metabolic complaints is a state-of-the-art procedure and is strongly recommended.

2. TRT in hypogonadal men, following the guidelines, will most certainly improve mental and sexual problems and is likely to ameliorate metabolic dysfunction/ insulin resistance. A variety of testosterone therapies exist (see ref. [23].
3. Evidence is lacking that TRT prolongs the life span of hypogonadal men. Nevertheless, there is evidence that TRT is able to improve quality in men's life.

Contraindications to Testosterone Therapy According to ref. [23]

- Untreated severe obstructive sleep apnea (OSA)
- Hematocrit greater than 50%
- Uncontrolled or poorly controlled heart failure
- Patients with history of breast or prostate cancer
- Presence of palpable prostate nodule or induration
- Prostate-specific antigen greater than 4 ng/mL or greater than 3 ng/mL in men at high risk for prostate cancer such as African Americans, or men with first-degree relatives with prostate cancer, without further urological evaluation
- Severe lower urinary tract symptoms with International Prostate Symptom Score (IPSS) above 19

Benefits of Testosterone Replacement Therapy

As stated previously, symptoms that commonly improve with testosterone replacement include sex drive, erectile dysfunction, mood, energy, quality of life, muscle mass and strength, cognitive function, and bone mineral density [102].

There is a threshold level of testosterone above which there may be no further benefit in symptomatic improvement [46]. An adequate time period for changes in energy, mood, and sexual function on testosterone therapy seems to be 3 months [103]. Effects on body composition including waist circumference and serum lipid profiles likely require a longer period [103, 104]. Such effects depend on individual factors such as the degree of being above ideal body weight, individual body composition/adiposity, resting metabolism energy expenditure/calorie burning, and individual conditioning/oxygen consumption. In normal men, testosterone administration can increase IGF-1 levels [105].

Someone with a history of physical inactivity for a long period of time who has insidiously developed atherosclerotic plaques that are unstable may then experience harm as opposed to someone with rather stable or no atherosclerotic plaques. Therefore, it is advisable to have men (including diabetics) at increased risk for cardiovascular events consult a cardiologist, especially when having a history of being deconditioned, to design an individual stepwise physical activity program. This also accounts for sexual activity. A recent scientific statement from the American Heart Association outlines which steps should be taken and mentions that sexual activity with a person's usual partner is comparable to moderate physical activity in the range of four metabolic equivalents, i.e., the equivalent of climbing two flights of stairs or walking briskly [106]. Of note, this data and evidence level/recommendation derived from young married men and it is unknown how heart rate and blood pressure are responding in older individuals and men, especially when there is difficulty reaching an orgasm. Interestingly, this position paper from the AHA deals with sexual function and activity but does not mention testosterone in its therapeutic arsenal, although androgens can improve the response to slidenafil in men with erectile dysfunction [107].

When replacing sex steroids one has to consider that alteration of the clearance of thyroxine-binding globulin can occur in patients with thyroid disease, necessitating a dose change of patients on thyroid hormone replacement therapy. Therapy with sex steroids including testosterone might also unmask thyroid illness in previously undiagnosed individuals [108].

Risks and Barriers of Testosterone Replacement

Physicians (non-andrologists) are not generally comfortable starting TRT even if their patient meets all the criteria for TDS. Contrary to one common misconception that testosterone therapy in men causes cardiovascular problems, a systematic review and meta-analysis of randomized placebo-controlled trials found this not to be the case [109].

Another common misconception regarding risk of TRT concerns the perception that it will cause BPH or prostate cancer [100]. This is untrue, although TRT is absolutely contraindicated in patients who have been diagnosed with prostate cancer (as it is a androgen-sensitive disease). The revised Endocrine Society guidelines in 2010 lowered the PSA exclusion criteria to >3 ng/mL in men with higher risk of prostate cancer such as African Americans or men with first-degree relatives who had prostate cancer. Men who have been treated successfully for prostate cancer and are diagnosed later with "hypogonadism"/testosterone deficiency, may still be candidates for TRT after a prudent interval if no clinical or laboratory evidence of residual cancer can be found after a thorough urological evaluation [110, 111].

Regarding application forms of testosterone therapy, the following should be considered: The injectable administration of testosterone has a higher propensity to cause polycythemia compared to topical preparations. Intramuscular injection of testosterone causes a sudden supraphysiological increase in serum testosterone levels. Higher depot formulations such as those approved in Europe, may also cause pain at the injection site. Transdermal testosterone therapy can achieve more physiological sex hormone levels and profiles and minimize excessive stimulation of erythropoiesis [112]. On the other hand, transdermal preparations may cause skin reactions which are more commonly seen with patches than with gel preparations [46, 113].

Testosterone Deficiency Syndrome vs. Androgen Resistance

The Boston Area Community Health study ($n = 1,845$) has clearly shown that the prevalence of biochemical testosterone deficiency or low serum testosterone levels does not correlate well with the prevalence of TDS [114]. 9.3% of study participants had a serum total testosterone <300 ng/dL and free testosterone <5 ng/dL, whereas only 5.6% of the total study population had both symptoms and biochemical evidence of testosterone deficiency. Symptoms were more present in older than younger men (4.2% among men < age 50 years and 8.4% among men 50+ years).

This challenges the concept of using serum testosterone levels alone to diagnose TDS. A normal measured serum testosterone level can still be associated with TDS, depending on the action of testosterone at its receptor, introducing the concept of androgen (tissue) resistance, analogous to insulin resistance in patients with type 2 diabetes. As with insulin in patients with type 2 diabetes, there can be both in men with TDS, insufficient hormone (testosterone) production and variable degrees of resistance to the action of androgens (testosterone) operating at several tissue levels in the body, which may become progressively worse with aging (production/secretion of hormone), adverse lifestyle (more adiposity), or other disease processes (inflammation etc.) [24, 115], see Fig. 11.1.

Racial and Ethnic Variation in Physiological Response to Sex Hormone

The physiological response of the human body to sex hormones may significantly differ, depending on a person's genetic profile. Genetic polymorphism may be responsible for the variable response to any given level of hormone. Regarding testosterone, the number of CAG repeats in the testosterone receptor gene control the degree of end organ response to hormonal action and also determine how the hypothalamic pituitary axis will provide its feedback. Analyzing the NHANES III data demonstrated that the serum concentration of testosterone itself did not differ between black and white men. However, black men appeared to have higher estradiol levels than white men, after adjustments for percent body fat, activity, smoking, and age [116]. Black men tend to have significantly higher levels of dihydrotestosterone, suggesting that the peripheral 5α reductase activity may be higher in blacks than other racial groups [117].

Increased 5α reductase activity, as demonstrated by the higher 5α reduced products, has been suggested as a cause of higher prevalence of prostate cancer in black men [118]. Because of higher concentrations of dihydrotestosterone metabolites as well as shorter CAG repeats in the androgen receptor genes, black men may have an increased response to any given level of testosterone.

Special Considerations

Androgen Deprivation Therapy and Cardiovascular Risk

Treatment of prostate cancer with androgen deprivation therapy (ADT) has recently raised concerns about its effect on mortality among patients. Data from the Cancer of the Prostate Strategic Urologic Research Endeavor (CaPSURE) database [119] showed an increased risk of cardiovascular mortality over a median follow-up of 3.8 years in men with localized prostate cancer who were treated with radical prostatectomy and who received GnRH agonist and/or an antiandrogen before surgery compared with those who did not (adjusted HR, 2.6, 95% CI, 1.4–4.7). Prospective clinical trials suggest that ADT increases CVD risk by increasing body weight, reducing insulin sensitivity, and/or resulting in dyslipidemia [120]. ADT significantly decreases lean body mass, increases fat mass, increases serum cholesterol and triglyceride levels, significantly increases fasting plasma insulin by 26%, and decreases insulin sensitivity by 13% [121–124].

A cross-sectional study reported an increased prevalence of the metabolic syndrome in men receiving ADT than in age-matched control groups of both untreated men with prostate cancer and men without prostate cancer. They were more likely to have elevated fasting plasma glucose, increased abdominal girth as well as elevated triglycerides. Given the metabolic effects of ADT, the American Heart Association advisory paper recommended that men in whom ADT is initiated be referred to their primary care physician for periodic follow-up to evaluate their blood pressure, lipid profile, and glucose levels [120].

Testosterone Deficiency and Sleep Apnea

In the United States, OSA affects about 4–9% male adults. Sleep apnea is more prevalent among elderly, obese individuals, men and postmenopausal women. Signs and symptoms include loud snoring, excessive daytime sleepiness, and observed apneas. Signs and symptoms common to both sleep apnea and TDS include lack of energy, depression, and erectile dysfunction. (Fig. 11.3). In healthy adult men, circulating levels of testosterone have a distinct pattern, with an increase during sleep, a maximum around the time of awakening, and a drop during the day. Testosterone secretion is under a strong influence of sleep, and to a lesser extent, under circadian influence, resembling the regulation of prolactin. Thus, a healthy young man can expect a rise in his testosterone level during sleep independent of the time of the day. The appearance of the first REM sleep is highly correlated with the peak of testosterone. After restoring sleep in previously sleep deprived young adults, testosterone levels frequently normalize [125, 126].

Sleep apnea causes reversible neuroendocrine dysfunction in men, which is manifested by increased levels of ACTH, cortisol, leptin, and decreased concentrations of plasma growth hormone, IGF-I, and testosterone [59, 127, 128].

Low Testosterone and All-Cause Mortality and Cardiovascular Events in Women

A prospective study including 2,914 women between age 18 and 75 years assessed outcome measures including cardiovascular risk, CVD, and all-cause mortality [129]. Mean BMI was 26.7 ± 5.2 kg/m^2. Women with total testosterone values in the lowest quintile were found to have a higher risk to die of any cause or to develop a cardiovascular event within the follow-up period of 4.5 years compared to those women with higher testosterone quintiles. Interestingly, the women with lower testosterone levels also had lower IGF-1 levels that progressively increased with the higher quintiles. In contrast, other cross-sectional, longitudinal, and case–control studies have found that women with higher testosterone levels (such as many of those with polycystic ovarian syndrome) are at higher risk for diseases such as metabolic syndrome, type 2 diabetes, and coronary artery disease [130, 131].

Conclusion

With the widely spread global obesity epidemic one might expect an increased prevalence of testosterone deficiency and cardiovascular risk of such individuals [132]. Classic symptoms and signs of testosterone deficiency include sex drive and erectile function both of which may be reduced in obese individuals, especially in the presence of the metabolic syndrome or type 2 diabetes. The diagnosis of testosterone deficiency is challenging given the overlap of symptoms with features seen in patients with metabolic syndrome, type 2 diabetes, sleep apnea, and others, and the wide reference range of reportedly normal serum testosterone levels measured by a variety of currently available testosterone assays. Following the current guidelines for hypogonadal men, short-term replacement with exogenous testosterone improves clinical symptoms associated with testosterone deficiency and may ameliorate the features of the metabolic syndrome and insulin resistance, perhaps in the form of a kick-start which does not replace the need for long-term lifestyle changes, including increased physical activity with shrinking fat and building muscle mass. However, there is no consensus yet as to how long a person may be safely treated with exogenous androgen and whether TRT will prolong the life span of hypogonadal men [133].

References

1. Lerner DJ, Kannel WB. Patterns of coronary heart disease morbidity and mortality in the sexes: a 26-year follow-up of the Framingham population. Am Heart J. 1986;111:383–90.
2. Barrett-Connor E, Stuenkel C. Hormones and heart disease in women: heart and estrogen/progestin replacement study in perspective. J Clin Endocrinol Metab. 1999;84:1848–53.
3. Yildiz O, Seyrek M. Vasodilating mechanisms of testosterone. Exp Clin Endocrinol Diabetes. 2007;115:1–6.

4. Corona G, Monami M, Rastrelli G, Aversa A, Tishova Y, Saad F, et al. Testosterone and metabolic syndrome: a meta-analysis study. J Sex Med. 2011;8(1):272–83.
5. Ullah MI, Washington T, Kazi M, Tamanna S, Koch CA. Testosterone deficiency as a risk factor for cardiovascular disease. Horm Metab Res. 2011;43(3):153–64.
6. Zitzmann M. Testosterone deficiency, insulin resistance and the metabolic syndrome. Nat Rev Endocrinol. 2009;5(12):673–81.
7. Wang C, Jackson G, Jones TH, Matsumoto AM, Nehra A, Perelman MA, et al. Low testosterone associated with obesity and the metabolic syndrome contributes to sexual dysfunction and cardiovascular disease risk in men with type 2 diabetes. Diabetes Care. 2011;34(7):1669–75.
8. Traish AM, Miner MM, Morgentaler A, Zitzmann M. Testosterone deficiency. Am J Med. 2011;124(7):578–87.
9. Grossmann M. Low testosterone in men with type 2 diabetes: significance and treatment. J Clin Endocrinol Metab. 2011;96(8):2341–53.
10. Friedrich N, Rosskopf D, Brabant G, Völzke H, Nauck M, Wallaschofski H. Associations of anthropometric parameters with serum TSH, prolactin, IGF-I, and testosterone levels: results of the study of health in Pomerania (SHIP). Exp Clin Endocrinol Diabetes. 2010;118:266–73.
11. Canale D, Caglieresi C, Moschini C, Liberati CD, Macchia E, Pinchera A, et al. Androgen receptor polymorphism (CAG repeats) and androgenicity. Clin Endocrinol (Oxf). 2005; 63:356–61.
12. Zitzmann M. Pharmacogenetics of testosterone replacement therapy. Pharmacogenomics. 2009;10:1341–9.
13. Zitzmann M. The role of the CAG repeat androgen receptor polymorphism in andrology. Front Horm Res. 2009;37:52–61.
14. Liu PP, Fukuoka M. Sex hormones as novel risk biomarkers for atherosclerosis in peripheral vascular disease. J Am Coll Cardiol. 2007;50:1077–9.
15. Cherrier MM, Asthana S, Plymate S, Baker L, Matsumoto AM, Peskind E, et al. Testosterone supplementation improves spatial and verbal memory in healthy older men. Neurology. 2001;57:80–8.
16. Bours SP, van Geel PA, Geusens PP, et al. Contributors to secondary osteoporosis and metabolic bone diseases in patients presenting with a clinical fracture. J Clin Endocrinol Metab. 2011;96(5):1360–7.
17. Amin S, Zhang Y, Felson DT, Sawin CT, Hannan MT, Wilson PW, et al. Estradiol, testosterone, and the risk for hip fractures in elderly men from the Framingham Study. Am J Med. 2006;119(5):426–33.
18. Bellido T, Jilka RL, Boyce BF, Girasole G, Broxmeyer H, Dalrymple SA, et al. Regulation of interleukin-6, osteoclastogenesis, and bone mass by androgens. The role of the androgen receptor. J Clin Invest. 1995;95:2886–95.
19. Romagnoli E, Del Fiacco R, Russo S, Piemonte S, Fidanza F, Colapietro F, et al. Secondary osteoporosis in men and women: clinical challenge of an unresolved issue. J Rheumatol. 2011;38(8):1671–9.
20. Stellato R-K, Feldman H-A, Hamdy O, Horton E-S, McKinlay J-B. Testosterone, sex hormone-binding globulin, and the development of type 2 diabetes in middle-aged men: prospective results from the Massachusetts male aging study. Diabetes Care. 2000;23:490–4.
21. O'Connell MD, Ravindrarajah R, Tajar A, Wu FC. Low testosterone in ageing men: a modifiable risk factor for frailty? Trends Endocrinol Metab. 2011;22(12):491–8.
22. Kaufman JM, Vermeulen A. The decline of androgen levels in elderly men and its clinical and therapeutic implications. Endocr Rev. 2005;26:833–76.
23. Bhasin S, Cunningham GR, Hayes FJ, et al. Testosterone therapy in men with androgen deficiency syndromes: an endocrine society clinical practice guideline. J Clin Endocrinol Metab. 2010;95:2536–59.
24. Ly LP, Jimenez M, Zhuang TN, Celermajer DS, Conway AJ, Handelsman DJ. A double-blind, placebo-controlled, randomized clinical trial of transdermal dihydrotestosterone gel on muscular strength, mobility, and quality of life in older men with partial androgen deficiency. J Clin Endocrinol Metab. 2001;86(9):4078–88.

25. Morley JE. Testosterone replacement and the physiologic aspects of aging in men. Mayo Clin Proc. 2000;75 Suppl:S83–7.
26. Moore C, Huebler D, Zimmermann T, Heinemann LA, Saad F, Thai DM. The Aging Males' Symptoms scale (AMS) as outcome measure for treatment of androgen deficiency. Eur Urol. 2004;46:80–7.
27. Kazi M, Geraci SA, Koch CA. Considerations for the diagnosis and treatment of testosterone deficiency in elderly men. Am J Med. 2007;120:835–40.
28. Bhasin S, Pencina M, Jasuja GK, Travison TG, Coviello A, Orwoll E, et al. Reference ranges for testosterone in men generated using liquid chromatography tandem mass spectrometry in a community-based sample of healthy nonobese young men in the Framingham Heart Study and applied to three geographically distinct cohorts. J Clin Endocrinol Metab. 2011;96(8):2430–9.
29. Anawalt BD, Hotaling JM, Walsh TJ, Matsumoto AM. Performance of total testosterone measurement to predict free testosterone for the biochemical evaluation of male hypogonadism. J Urol. 2012;187(4):1369–73.
30. Mauras N, Hayes V, Welch S, Veldhuis J, Urban R. Testosterone deficiency in young men: marked alterations in whole body protein kinetics, strength, and adiposity. J Clin Endocrinol Metab. 1998;83:1886–92.
31. Brodsky IG, Balagopal P, Nair KS. Effects of testosterone replacement on muscle mass and muscle protein synthesis in hypogonadal men—a clinical research center study. J Clin Endocrinol Metab. 1996;81:3469–75.
32. Bhasin S, Storer TW, Berman N, Yarasheski KE, Cleveneger B, Casaburi RA. A replacement dose of testosterone increases fat-free mass and muscle size in hypogonadal men. J Clin Endocrinol Metab. 1997;82:407–13.
33. Bhasin S, Woodhouse L, Casaburi R, Singh AB, Bhasin D, Berman N, et al. Testosterone dose–response relationships in healthy young men. Am J Physiol Endocrinol Metab. 2001;281(6):E1172–81.
34. Sinha-Hikim I, Artaza J, Woodhouse L, Gonzalez-Cadavid N, Singh AB, Lee MI, et al. Testosterone-induced increase in muscle size in healthy young men is associated with muscle fiber hypertrophy. Am J Physiol Endocrinol Metab. 2002;283(1):E154–64.
35. Simon D, Charles MA, Nahoul K, et al. Association between plasma total testosterone and cardiovascular risk factors in healthy adult men: the Telecom Study. J Clin Endocrinol Metab. 1997;82:682–5.
36. Vermeulen A, Goemaere S, Kaufman JM. Testosterone, body composition and aging. J Endocrinol Invest. 1999;22(5 Suppl):110–6.
37. Khaw KT, Barrett-Connor E. Lower endogenous androgens predict central adiposity in men. Ann Epidemiol. 1992;2:675–82.
38. Marin P, Arver S. Androgens and abdominal obesity. Baillieres Clin Endocrinol Metab. 1998;12:441–51.
39. Vermeulen A, Kaufman JM, Giagulli VA. Influence of some biological indexes on sex hormone-binding globulin and androgen levels in aging or obese males. J Clin Endocrinol Metab. 1996;81(5):1821–6.
40. Katznelson L, Finkelstein JS, Schoenfeld DA, Rosenthal DI, Anderson EJ, Klibanski A. Increase in bone density and lean body mass during testosterone administration in men with acquired hypogonadism. J Clin Endocrinol Metab. 1996;81:4358–65.
41. Marin P. Testosterone and regional fat distribution. Obes Res. 1995;3 Suppl 4:609–12.
42. Marin P, Holmang S, Jonsson L, Sjostrom L, Kvist H, Holm G. The effects of testosterone treatment on body composition and metabolism in middle-aged obese men. Int J Obes Relat Metab Disord. 1992;16:991–7.
43. Marin P, Krotkiewski M, Bjorntorp P. Androgen treatment of middle-aged, obese men: effects on metabolism, muscle and adipose tissues. Eur J Med. 1992;1:329–36.
44. Behre HM, von Eckardstein S, Kliesch S, Nieschlag E. Long-term substitution therapy of hypogonadal men with transscrotal testosterone over 7–10 years. Clin Endocrinol. 1999;50:629–35.

45. Sih R, Morley JE, Kaiser FE, Perry III HM, Patrick P, Ross C. Testosterone replacement in older hypogonadal men: a 12-month randomized controlled trial. J Clin Endocrinol Metab. 1997;82(6):1661–7.
46. Wang C, Swedloff RS, Iranmanesh A, Dobs A, Snyder PJ, Cunningham G, et al. Transdermal testosterone gel improves sexual function, mood, muscle strength, and body composition parameters in hypogonadal men Testosterone Gel Study Group. J Clin Endocrinol Metab. 2000;85(8):2839–53.
47. Rolf C, von Eckardstein S, Koken U, Nieschlag E. Testosterone substitution of hypogonadal men prevents the age-dependent increases in body mass index, body fat and leptin seen in healthy ageing men: results of a cross-sectional study. Eur J Endocrinol. 2002;146:505–11.
48. Snyder PJ, Peachey H, Berlin JA, Hannoush P, Haddad G, Dlewati A, et al. Effects of testosterone replacement in hypogonadal men. J Clin Endocrinol Metab. 2000;85(8):2670–7.
49. McLachlan RI, O'Donnell L, Meachem SJ, Stanton PG, de Kretser DM, Pratis K, et al. Identification of specific sites of hormonal regulation in spermatogenesis in rats, monkeys, and man. Recent Prog Horm Res. 2002;57:149–79.
50. Woodhouse LJ, Gupta N, Bhasin M, Singh AB, Ross R, Phillips J, Bhasin S. Dose-dependent effects of testosterone on regional adipose tissue distribution in healthy young men. J Clin Endocrinol Metab. 2004;89(2):718–26.
51. Garaulet M, Perex-Llamas F, Fuente T, Zamora S, Tebar FJ. Anthropometric, computed tomography and fat cell data in an obese population: relationship with insulin, leptin, tumor necrosis factor-alpha, sex hormone-binding globulin and sex hormones. Eur J Endocrinol. 2000;143(5):657–66.
52. Grimble RF. Inflammatory status and insulin resistance. Curr Opin Clin Nutr Metab Care. 2002;5:551–9.
53. Guerre-Millo M. Adipose tissue hormones. J Endocrinol Invest. 2002;25:855–61.
54. Kyrou I, Chrousos GP, Tsigos C. Stress, visceral obesity, and metabolic complications. Ann N Y Acad Sci. 2006;1083:77–110.
55. Malkin CJ, Pugh PJ, Jones RD, Kapoor D, Channer KS, Jones TH. The effect of testosterone replacement on endogenous inflammatory cytokines and lipid profiles in hypogonadal men. J Clin Endocrinol Metab. 2004;89:3313–8.
56. Diez JJ, Iglesias P. The role of the novel adipocyte-derived hormone adiponectin in human disease. Eur J Endocrinol. 2003;148:293–300.
57. Yamada T, Katagiri H, Ishigaki Y, Ogihara T, Imai J, Uno K, et al. Signals from intra-abdominal fat modulate insulin and leptin sensitivity through different mechanisms: neuronal involvement in food-intake regulation. Cell Metab. 2006;3:223–9.
58. Lanfranco F, Motta G, Minetto MA, et al. Neuroendocrine alterations in obese patients with sleep apnea syndrome. Int J Endocrinol. 2010;2010:474518.
59. Isidori AM, Caprio M, Strollo F, Moretti C, Frajese G, Isidori A, et al. Leptin and androgens in male obesity: evidence for leptin contribution to reduced androgen levels. J Clin Endocrinol Metab. 1999;84:3673–80.
60. Singh R, Artaza JN, Taylor WE, Braga M, Yuan X, Gonzalez-Cadavid NF, et al. Testosterone inhibits adipogenic differentiation in 3T3-L1 cells: nuclear translocation of androgen receptor complex with beta-catenin and T-cell factor 4 may bypass canonical Wnt signaling to down-regulate adipogenic transcription factors. Endocrinology. 2006;147:141–54.
61. Xu XF, De Pergola G, Björntorp P. Testosterone increases lipolysis and the number of beta-adrenoreceptors in male rat adipocytes. Endocrinology. 1991;128:379–82.
62. Chen X, Li X, Huang HY, Li X, Lin JF. Effects of testosterone on insulin receptor substrate-1 and glucose transporter 4 expression in cells sensitive to insulin. Zhonghua Yi Xue Za Zhi. 2006;86:1474–7.
63. Mootha VK, Lindgren CM, Eriksson KF, Subramanian A, Sihag S, Lehar J, et al. PGC-1alpha-responsive genes involved in oxidative phosphorylation are coordinately downregulated in human diabetes. Nat Genet. 2003;34:267–73.
64. Pitteloud N, Mootha VK, Dwyer AA, Hardin M, Lee H, Eriksson KF, et al. Relationship between testosterone levels, insulin sensitivity, and mitochondrial function in men. Diabetes Care. 2005;28:1636–42.

65. Zitzmann M, Gromoll J, von Eckardstein A, Nieschlag E. The CAG repeat polymorphism in the androgen receptor gene modulates body fat mass and serum concentrations of leptin and insulin in men. Diabetologia. 2003;46:31–9.
66. Behre HM, Simoni M, Nieschlag E. Strong association between serum levels of leptin and testosterone in men. Clin Endocrinol (Oxf). 1997;47:237–40.
68. Jockenhövel F, Blum WF, Vogel E, et al. Testosterone substitution normalizes elevated serum leptin levels in hypogonadal men. J Clin Endocrinol Metab. 1997;82:2510–3.
68. Mayes JS, Watson GH. Direct effects of sex steroid hormones on adipose tissues and obesity. Obes Rev. 2004;5:197–216.
69. Anderson PJ, Critchley JA, Chan JC, Cockram CS, Lee ZS, Thomas GN, et al. Factor analysis of the metabolic syndrome: obesity vs insulin resistance as the central abnormality. Int J Obes. 2001;25:1782–8.
70. Eisenmann JC. Secular trends in variables associated with the metabolic syndrome of North American children and adolescents: a review and synthesis. Am J Hum Biol. 2003; 15:786–94.
71. Carr DB, Utzschneider KM, Hull RL. Intra-abdominal fat is a major determinant of the National Cholesterol Education Program Adult Treatment Panel III criteria for the metabolic syndrome. Diabetes. 2004;53:2087–94.
72. Cassells HB, Haffner SM. The metabolic syndrome: risk factors and management. J Cardiovasc Nurs. 2006;21:306–13.
73. Isomaa B, Almgren P, Tuomi T. Cardiovascular morbidity and mortality associated with the metabolic syndrome. Diabetes Care. 2001;24:683–9.
74. Stern M, Williams K, Gonzalez-Villalpando C. Does the metabolic syndrome improve identification of individuals at risk of type 2 diabetes and/or cardiovascular disease? Diabetes Care. 2004;27:2676–81.
75. Alberti KG, Eckel RH, Grundy SM, Zimmet PZ, Cleeman JI, Donato KA, Fruchart JC, James WP, Loria CM, Smith SC Jr; International Diabetes Federation Task Force on Epidemiology and Prevention; Hational Heart, Lung, and Blood Institute; American Heart Association; World Heart Federation; International Atherosclerosis Society; International Association for the Study of Obesity. Harmonizing the metabolic syndrome: a joint interim statement of the International Diabetes Federation Task Force on Epidemiology and Prevention; National Heart, Lung, and Blood Institute; American Heart Association; World Heart Federation; International Atherosclerosis Society; and International Association for the Study of Obesity. Circulation. 2009;120:1640–5.
76. van den Beld AW, de Jong FH, Grobbee DE, Pols HA, Lamberts SW. Measures of bioavailable serum testosterone and estradiol and their relationships with muscle strength, bone density, and body composition in elderly men. J Clin Endocrinol Metab. 2000; 85:3276–82.
77. Kapoor D, Goodwin E, Channer KS, Jones TH. Testosterone replacement therapy improves insulin resistance, glycaemic control, visceral adiposity and hypercholesterolaemia in hypogonadal men with type 2 diabetes. Eur J Endocrinol. 2006;154:899–906.
78. Corona G, Monami M, Rastrelli G, Aversa A, Storza A, Lenzi A, et al. Type 2 diabetes mellitus and testosterone: a meta-analysis study. Int J Androl. 2010;34:528–40.
79. Araujo AB, Dixon JM, Suarez EA, Murad MH, Guey LT, Wittert GA. Clinical review: endogenous testosterone and mortality in men: a systematic review and meta-analysis. J Clin Endocrinol Metab. 2011;96(10):3007–19.
80. Hyde Z, Norman PE, Flicker L, Hankey GJ, Almeida OP, McCaul KA, et al. Low free testosterone predicts mortality from cardiovascular disease but not other causes: the Health in Men Study. J Clin Endocrinol Metab. 2012;97(1):179–89.
81. Ohlsson C, Barrett-Connor E, Bhasin S, Orwoll E, Labrie F, Karlsson MK, et al. High serum testosterone is associated with reduced risk of cardiovascular events in elderly men. The MrOS (Osteoporotic Fractures in Men) study in Sweden. J Am Coll Cardiol. 2011; 58(16):1674–81.
82. Srinivas-Shankar U, Roberts SA, Connolly MJ, O'Connell MD, Adams JE, Oldham JA, et al. Effects of testosterone on muscle strength, physical function, body composition, and quality

of life in intermediate-frail and frail elderly men: a randomized, double-blind, placebo-controlled study. J Clin Endocrinol Metab. 2010;95(2):639–50.
83. Basaria S, Coviello AD, Travison TG, Storer TW, Farwell WR, Jette AM, et al. Adverse events associated with testosterone administration. N Engl J Med. 2010;363(2):109–22.
84. Caminiti G, Volterrani M, Iellamo F, Marazzi G, Massaro R, Miceli M, et al. Effect of long-acting testosterone treatment on functional exercise capacity, skeletal muscle performance, insulin resistance, and baroreflex, sensitivity in elderly patients with chronic heart failure: a double-blind, placebo-controlled randomized study. J Am Coll Cardiol. 2009;54(10): 919–27.
85. Kaltsas G, Vgontzas A, Chrousos G. Fatigue, endocrinopathies, and metabolic disorders. PM R. 2010;2(5):393–8.
86. Vgontzas AN, Bixler EO, Chrousos GP. Sleep apnoea is a manifestation of the metabolic syndrome. Sleep Med Rev. 2005;9(3):211–24.
87. Vgontzas AN, Pejovic S, Zoumakis E, Lin HM, Bentley CM, Bixler EO, et al. Hypothalamic-pituitary adrenal axis activity in obese men with and without sleep apnea: effects of continuous positive airway pressure therapy. J Clin Endocrinol Metab. 2007;92:4199–207.
88. Vgontzas AN, Zoumakis E, Bixler EO, Lin HM, Collins B, Basta M, et al. Selective effects of CPAP on sleep apnoea-associated manifestations. Eur J Clin Invest. 2008;38(8):585–95.
89. Trakada G, Chrousos G, Pejovic S, Vgontzas A. Sleep apnea and its association with the stress system, inflammation, insulin resistance, and visceral obesity. Sleep Med Clin. 2007;2(2):251–61.
90. Yanase T, Fan W, Kyoya K, Min L, Takayanagi R, Kato S, et al. Androgens and metabolic syndrome: lessons from androgen receptor knock out (ARKO) mice. J Steroid Biochem Mol Biol. 2008;109:254–7.
91. Bourghardt J, Wilhelmson AS, Alexanderson C, De Gendt K, Verhoeven G, Krettek A, et al. Androgen receptor-dependent and independent atheroprotection by testosterone in male mice. Endocrinology. 2010;151:5428–37.
92. Dati E, Baroncelli GI, Mora S, Russo G, Baldinotti F, Parrini D, et al. Body composition and metabolic profile in women with complete androgen insensitivity syndrome. Sex Dev. 2009;3:188–93.
93. Bojesen A, Kristensen K, Birkebaek NH, Fedder J, Mosekilde L, Bennett P, et al. The metabolic syndrome is frequent in Klinefelter's syndrome and is associated with abdominal obesity and hypogonadism. Diabetes Care. 2006;29:1591–8.
94. Ishikawa T, Yamaguchi K, Kondo Y, Takenaka A, Fujisawa M. Metabolic syndrome in men with Klinefelter's syndrome. Urology. 2008;71:1109–13.
95. Bojesen A, Juul S, Birkebaek N, Gravholt CH. Increased mortality in Klinefelter syndrome. J Clin Endocrinol Metab. 2004;89:3830–4.
96. Akishita M, Hashimoto M, Ohike Y, Ogawa S, Iijima K, Eto M, et al. Low testosterone level as a predictor of cardiovascular events in Japanese men with coronary risk factors. Atherosclerosis. 2010;210(1):232–6.
97. Laughlin GA, Barrett-Connor E, Bergstrom J. Low serum testosterone and mortality in older men. J Clin Endocrinol Metab. 2008;93:68–75.
98. Oh JY, Barrett-Connor E, Wedick NM, Wingard DL. Endogenous sex hormones and the development of type 2 diabetes in older men and women: the Rancho Bernardo study. Diabetes Care. 2002;25:55–60.
99. Barrett-Connor E, Von Mühlen DG, Kritz-Silverstein D. Bioavailable testosterone and depressed mood in older men: the Rancho Bernardo Study. J Clin Endocrinol Metab. 1999;84(2):573–7.
100. Wang C, Nieschlag E, Swerdloff RS, Behre H, Hellstrom WJ, Gooren LJ, et al. ISA, ISSAM, EAU, EAA and ASA recommendations: investigation, treatment and monitoring of late-onset hypogonadism in males. Aging Male. 2009;12:5–12.
101. Zitzmann M, Nieschlag E. Testosterone substitution: current modalities and perspectives. J Reprod Med Endocrinol. 2006;3:109–16.

102. Bassil N, Alkaade S, Morley JE. The benefits and risks of testosterone replacement therapy: a review. Ther Clin Risk Manag. 2009;5:427–48.
103. Saad F, Aversa A, Isidori AM, Zafalon L, Zitzmann M, Gooren L. Onset of effects of testosterone treatment and time span until maximum effects are achieved. Eur J Endocrinol. 2011;165(5):675–85.
104. Kalinchenko SY, Tishova YA, Mskhalaya GJ, Gooren LJ, Giltay EJ, Saad F. Effects of testosterone supplementation on markers of the metabolic syndrome and inflammation in hypogonadal men with the metabolic syndrome: the double-blinded placebo-controlled Moscow study. Clin Endocrinol (Oxf). 2010;73:602–12.
105. Hobbs CJ, Plymate SR, Rosen CJ, Adler RA. Testosterone administration increases insulin-like growth factor-I levels in normal men. J Clin Endocrinol Metab. 1993;77:776–9.
106. Levine GN, Steinke EE, Bakaeen FG, et al. Sexual activity and cardiovascular disease. A scientific statement from the American Heart Association. Circulation. 2012;125(8):1058–72.
107. Aversa A, Isidori AM, Spera G, Lenzi A, Fabbri A. Androgens improve cavernous vasodilation and response to sildenafil in patients with erectile dysfunction. Clin Endocrinol (Oxf). 2003;58:632–8.
108. Tahboub R, Arafah BM. Sex steroids and the thyroid. Best Pract Res Clin Endocrinol Metab. 2008;23(6):769–80.
109. Haddad RM, Kennedy CC, Caples SM, Tracz MJ, Boloña ER, Sideras K, et al. Testosterone and cardiovascular risk in men: a systematic review and meta-analysis of randomized placebo-controlled trials. Mayo Clin Proc. 2007;82:29–39.
110. Khera M, Lipshultz LI. The role of testosterone replacement therapy following radical prostatectomy. Urol Clin North Am. 2007;34:549–53, vi.
111. Sarosdy MF. Testosterone replacement for hypogonadism after treatment of early prostate cancer with brachytherapy. Cancer. 2007;109:536–41.
112. Dobs AS, Meikle AW, Arver S, Sanders SW, Caramelli KE, Mazer NA. Pharmacokinetics, efficacy, and safety of a permeation-enhanced testosterone transdermal system in comparison with bi-weekly injections of testosterone enanthate for the treatment of hypogonadal men. J Clin Endocrinol Metab. 1999;84:3469–78.
113. McGriff NJ, Csako G, Kabbani M, Diep L, Chrousos GP, Pucino F. Treatment options for a patient experiencing pruritic rash associated with transdermal testosterone: a review of the literature. Pharmacotherapy. 2001;21(11):1425–35.
114. Carruthers M. Time for international action on treating testosterone deficiency syndrome. Aging Male. 2009;12:21–8.
115. Carruthers M. The paradox dividing testosterone deficiency symptoms and androgen assays: a closer look at the cellular and molecular mechanisms of androgen action. J Sex Med. 2008;5:998–1012.
116. Rohrmann S, Nelson WG, Rifai N, Brown TR, Dobs A, Kanarek N, et al. Serum estrogen, but not testosterone, levels differ between black and white men in a nationally representative sample of Americans. J Clin Endocrinol Metab. 2007;92:2519–25.
117. Ross RK, Bernstein L, Lobo RA, Shimizu H, Stanczyk FZ, Pike MC, et al. 5-Alpha-reductase activity and risk of prostate cancer among Japanese and US white and black males. Lancet. 1992;339:887–9.
118. Wang C, Christenson P, Swerdloff R. Editorial: clinical relevance of racial and ethnic differences in sex steroids. J Clin Endocrinol Metab. 2007;92:2433–5.
119. Tsai HK, D'Amico AV, Sadetsky N, Chen M-H, Carroll PR. Androgen deprivation therapy for localized prostate cancer and the risk of cardiovascular mortality. J Natl Cancer Inst. 2007;99:1516–24.
120. Levine GN, D'Amico AV, Berger P, Clark PE, Eckel RH, Keating NL, et al. American Heart Association Council on Clinical Cardiology and Council on Epidemiology and Prevention, the American Cancer Society, and the American Urological Association. Androgen-Deprivation Therapy in Prostate Cancer and Cardiovascular Risk: a Science

Advisory from the American Heart Association, American Cancer Society, and American Urological Association: Endorsed by the American Society for Radiation Oncology. CA Cancer J Clin. 2010;60:194–201.

121. Smith MR. Changes in fat and lean body mass during androgen-deprivation therapy for prostate cancer. Urology. 2004;63:742–5.
122. Smith MR, Finkelstein JS, McGovern FJ, Zietman AL, Fallon MA, Schoenfeld DA, et al. Changes in body composition during androgen deprivation therapy for prostate cancer. J Clin Endocrinol Metab. 2002;87:599–603.
123. Smith MR, Lee H, Nathan DM. Insulin sensitivity during combined androgen blockade for prostate cancer. J Clin Endocrinol Metab. 2006;91:1305–8.
124. Hamilton EJ, Gianatti E, Strauss BJ, Wentworth J, Lim-Joon D, Bolton D, et al. Increase in visceral and subcutaneous abdominal fat in men with prostate cancer treated with androgen deprivation therapy. Clin Endocrinol (Oxf). 2011;74(3):377–83.
125. Axelsson J, Ingre M, Akerstedt T, Holmback U. Effects of acutely displaced sleep on testosterone. J Clin Endocrinol Metab. 2005;90:4530–5.
126. Penev PD. Association between sleep and morning testosterone levels in older men. Sleep. 2007;30:427–32.
127. Grunstein RR, Handelsman DJ, Lawrence SJ, Blackwell C, Caterson ID, Sullivan CE. Neuroendocrine dysfunction in sleep apnea: reversal by continuous positive airways pressure therapy. J Clin Endocrinol Metab. 1989;68:352–8.
128. Gianotti L, Pivetti S, Lanfranco F, Tassone F, Navone F, Vittori E, et al. Concomitant impairment of growth hormone secretion and peripheral sensitivity in obese patients with obstructive sleep apnea syndrome. J Clin Endocrinol Metab. 2002;87:5052–7.
129. Sievers C, Klotsche J, Pieper L, Schneider HJ, März W, Wittchen HU, et al. Low testosterone levels predict all-cause mortality and cardiovascular events in women: a prospective cohort study in German primary care patients. Eur J Endocrinol. 2010;163:699–708.
130. Ding EL, Song Y, Manson JE, Rifai N, Buring JE, Liu S. Plasma sex steroid hormones and risk of developing type 2 diabetes in women: a prospective study. Diabetologia. 2007; 50:2076–84.
131. Torrens JI, Sutton-Tyrrell K, Zhao X, Matthews K, Brockwell S, Sowers M, et al. Relative androgen excess during the menopausal transition predicts incident metabolic syndrome in midlife women: study of Women's Health Across the Nation. Menopause. 2009;16:257–64.
132. Jones TH, Saad F. The effects of testosterone on risk factors for, and the mediators of, the atherosclerotic process. Atherosclerosis. 2009;207:318–27.
133. Giannoulis MG, Martin FC, Nair KS, Umpleby AM, Sonksen P. Hormone replacement therapy and physical function in healthy older men. Time to talk hormones ? Endocr Rev. 2012;33(3):314–77.

Chapter 12
Insulin Resistance and Hypertension

Sudha S. Shankar and Helmut O. Steinberg

Abstract IR has been reported to be associated with elevated blood pressure and hypertension. It is reasonable to postulate that IR is causally related to increased rates of hypertension in IR, especially considering abnormalities in SNS activity, renal salt handling, and endothelial function. Other, albeit indirect, evidence for the causal role of IR in blood pressure elevation comes from studies where improvement in IR resulted in lowering of blood pressure. A likely mechanistic explanation for the association between IR and blood pressure is that adipocyte dysfunction, elevated free fatty acid levels and elevated insulin levels, over time, may adversely affect systems involved in blood pressure regulation. Since the association between IR and elevated blood pressure is not found in all populations, these studies also suggest that, depending on genetic and environmental factors, these IR-induced changes lead eventually to increased blood pressure, or diabetes, or cardiovascular disease, or any combination of these. Of these, the time-dependent effects on blood pressure, even if not detectable in all individuals as a measurable change, may be particularly significant from a population perspective. Importantly, improvement in IR will likely have significant overall beneficial effects, to prevent or postpone the development of diabetes, hypertension, and cardiovascular disease.

Keywords Insulin resistance • Hypertension • Attenuation pathways • Insulin signaling • IR assessment

The long-term regulation of blood pressure occurs via a complex interplay of multiple organ systems and their functions, such as the kidney, the sympathetic nervous system

---

S.S. Shankar
Department of Experimental Medicine, Merck Research Laboratories, Rahway, NJ, USA

H.O. Steinberg (✉)
Department of Diabetes and Endocrinology, Merck Research Laboratories, Rahway, NJ, USA
e-mail: helmut_steinberg@merck.com

C.A. Koch and G.P. Chrousos (eds.), *Endocrine Hypertension: Underlying Mechanisms and Therapy*, Contemporary Endocrinology, DOI 10.1007/978-1-60761-548-4_12,

(SNS), neurohormonal factors that determine sodium balance, and vascular responsiveness, in particular, peripheral vascular resistance. Simply put, blood pressure is proportional to the product of cardiac output and peripheral vascular resistance, with each of these determinants in turn being modulated by a number of other inputs. In health, various feedback loops operate in synchrony to maintain blood pressure within the normal range and prevent the development of hypertension.

It is important to note that while blood pressure itself is a continuous variable, in contrast, hypertension is a categorical variable defined by a set of criteria based on repeated measurements of blood pressure obtained under specific conditions. This is particularly important, since the risk of cerebrovascular and cardiovascular events correlates with blood pressure levels in a positive linear fashion, even at levels that do not qualify for a clinical diagnosis of hypertension. Therefore, even small increments in blood pressure over extended durations, whilst insufficient for a clinical diagnosis of hypertension, may be sufficient to significantly enhance the risk of strokes and myocardial infarctions within a population. Insulin resistance (IR) may be one of the factors that lead to such minor increments in blood pressure, developing and progressing insidiously over protracted periods of time, and thereby enhancing the risk of cardio- and cerebrovascular events.

Originally, the term insulin resistance (IR) was used to describe a phenotype characterized by reduced glucose uptake in response to prevailing levels of insulin. IR was quantified by the euglycemic hyperinsulinemic clamp [1]. Over time, it became clear that this phenotype was not restricted to defective insulin-mediated glucose uptake, and other characteristics such as elevated blood pressure and dyslipidemia, mainly elevated triglycerides and decreased HDL-cholesterol, were added. Coexistence of a number of these abnormalities defines the insulin resistance syndrome as outlined by Reaven. Clearly, not all characteristics are found in all subjects and the term "metabolic syndrome" has replaced IR in many instances to allow for this variable phenotype to be more inclusive, which is important, since the metabolic syndrome, like IR, has also been shown to be a predictor of cardiovascular disease.

Today, most assessments of IR are not based on the euglycemic hyperinsulinemic clamp but on other measurements such as fasting insulin levels, HOMA-IR, or indices derived from oral glucose or meal tolerance tests [2, 3] or frequently sampled intravenous glucose tolerance tests [4]. It is important to recognize the commonalities as well as the differences between these methods and the inherent limitations of each method when considering the effect of IR on blood pressure.

IR correlates highly with body mass index (BMI) and waist circumference [5]. However, although obesity (excess body fat mass) is a good surrogate marker for IR, obesity is not the only determinant of IR. Other factors such as hormones and/or physical fitness affect IR. This is clearly demonstrated when comparing IR between males and females. For the same BMI, premenopausal females tend to have more body fat than males but exhibit less IR [6, 7]. Furthermore, observations of metabolically obese normal weight subjects, and patients with lipodystrophy who have little to no adipose tissue but exhibit IR, suggest that the functional status of the adipose tissue rather than absolute fat mass modulates IR.

IR has been found to be not only associated with increased blood pressure and hypertension but also a predictor for the development of hypertension. This association has been found in children, adolescents, middle-aged adults, and the elderly. In some but not all studies, the strength of the association between IR and blood pressure decreased when adjusted for BMI or waist circumference, which is not surprising since BMI and waist circumference correlate highly with IR. However, other studies were not able to confirm the association between IR and increased blood pressure [8, 9]. This is most likely explained by environmental and genetic differences between those populations and the way these interact with blood pressure regulation. On the other hand, it is possible that IR and blood pressure may not be causally related but that the observed association between the two is due to another factor that leads to the development of both IR and elevated blood pressure.

If IR is causally related to increasing blood pressure and the development of hypertension, it must affect one or more of the systems that regulate blood pressure. IR could affect blood pressure (1) via attenuation of pathways related to and/or shared by insulin signaling, (2) via the effects of increased in insulin levels, required to compensate for IR and maintain near normal glucose homeostasis, on insulin signaling pathways that are not affected by IR, or (3) a combination of the two.

Autonomic Nervous System

The SNS contributes to the regulation of blood pressure by modulating cardiac contractility, heart rate, and peripheral vascular resistance. Small increases in contractility and heart rate (cardiac output) or vascular resistance can result in large blood pressure elevations. Therefore, any stimulatory effect of insulin resistance on the SNS can contribute to the development of hypertension. SNS activity can be assessed in humans by determining plasma or urine levels of catecholamines that originate from the synaptic spillover or by measuring the electric activity (microneurography) of peripheral sympathetic nerve fibers.

Numerous studies have assessed the relationship between obesity, IR, and SNS activity. There appears to be significant stepwise increases in SNS activity, measured by microneurography, from lean controls to obese subjects with peripheral obesity, and from obese subjects with peripheral obesity to obese subjects with central obesity [10], that occurs even before hypertension is diagnosed. Furthermore, SNS activity is even higher in hypertensive IR subjects as compared to non-hypertensive IR subjects, who also exhibit higher SNS activity as compared to BMI-matched subjects without IR [11]. In contrast to microneurography, which has shown consistent elevation in insulin resistance, results of catecholamine levels in IR have been conflicting, with high, normal, and low levels reported. However, studies examining weight loss have found that the fall in blood pressure (BP) was highly correlated with reductions in plasma NE.

The mechanism by which IR increases SNS activity is not well understood. It has been suggested that elevated insulin levels as seen in IR could be responsible for the increase in SNS activity. This rationale is based on observations showing that increases in insulin levels either via direct infusion or indirectly via administration of exogenous glucose that stimulates endogenous insulin secretion increase SNS activity. Unfortunately, no good data are available that define the dose–response relationship for insulin's effect to increase SNS activity in normal or IR subjects. Nevertheless, if hyperinsulinemia were to increase SNS activity, this would require that IR has to occur before the increase in SNS activity. In addition, it would also require IR not to blunt insulin's effect to stimulate SNS activity. Elevated free fatty acid levels have also been implicated in the increase of blood pressure via increased SNS activity [12]. Although the peak free fatty acid levels were very high, the study demonstrated that infusion of fatty acids resulted in both elevation of insulin levels and SNS activity.

In addition to IR's effect on the SNS, IR is likely to affect the parasympathetic nervous system. It has been reported that the vagal input to the heart is reduced in IR [13, 14], which may contribute to the increased heart rate observed in IR.

Sodium Balance and IR

The kidney contributes to the long-term regulation of blood pressure [15] via modulation of sodium balance which is one determinant of intravascular volume and cardiac output [16, 17]. A positive sodium balance will increase intra- and extravascular volume and blood pressure, whereas a negative sodium balance will result in the opposite set of outcomes. Total sodium balance reflects sodium intake from the diet and sodium loss (excretion), which is mainly determined by the net balance of sodium filtration vs. sodium uptake in the proximal and distal renal tubule.

Thus, theoretically, increases in blood pressure should, via increased filtration, result in excretion of sodium (pressure natriuresis), thereby lowering intravascular volume and cardiac output, and these effects in turn should restore blood pressure levels to normal over time. Sodium balance is affected by intra-renal as well as central mechanisms. At the level of the kidney, the glomerulo-tubular feedback loop, including the renin-angiotensin-aldosterone system modulate sodium balance and blood pressure. Moreover, based mainly on results from animal studies, the SNS also modulates sodium balance [18]. Therefore, any effect of IR on sodium balance can contribute to increases in blood pressure and the development of hypertension [18].

Indeed, results of the Olivetti Heart Study point to an effect of IR to increase sodium absorption in the proximal tubule [19]. In this study, after adjusting for age, fractional proximal, but not distal, sodium reabsorption was found to be directly associated with BMI, waist circumference, and triglycerides. Furthermore, fractional proximal sodium reabsorption was significantly greater in subjects with the metabolic syndrome as compared to subjects without. The metabolic syndrome was also associated with higher creatinine clearance and slightly lower fractional excretion of sodium. Finally, the study demonstrated a significant interaction between BMI and HOMA-IR, and a significantly greater fractional proximal tubule sodium reabsorption in obese subjects with IR.

A different way to assess the effect of the metabolic syndrome on blood pressure and renal salt handling is to measure changes in blood pressure in response to either a low dose (e.g., 3 g per day for 7 days) or a high dose (e.g., 18 g per day for 7 days) sodium diet. A number of studies have demonstrated different blood pressure responses to changes in sodium intake in subjects with the metabolic syndrome/IR as compared to subjects without IR. One large study [20] in Chinese individuals demonstrated that subjects with the metabolic syndrome as compared to subjects without the syndrome exhibited a more marked fall in blood pressure when on the low dose sodium diet, and a more pronounced increase in blood pressure when on the high dose sodium diet. Importantly, there was a significant and graded association between the number of metabolic risk factors and the age- and gender-adjusted proportion of study subjects with high salt sensitivity. Similar differences in the blood pressure responses to low and high sodium loads between subjects with and without the metabolic syndrome were observed in a large study from Venezuela [21].

Taken together, available evidence strongly suggests that IR may negatively affect handling of sodium by the kidneys, which could, over time, lead to increased blood pressure. The mechanisms by which IR changes sodium handling are not clear, but sympathetic activation and/or hyperinsulinemia, increased circulating adipokines, increased free fatty acid levels, and endothelial dysfunction have been implicated.

Peripheral Vasculature and IR

Change in the diameter of resistance vessels (small arteries and arterioles) under conditions of steady cardiac output affects blood pressure. If cardiac output is constant, increases in the diameter of resistance vessels lead to a reduction in blood pressure, whereas decreases in the diameter of resistance vessels lead to an elevation of blood pressure. Since effective resistance in a tube is inversely proportional to the fourth power of the radius, this means that even small changes in diameter will result in large effects on blood pressure.

The diameter of resistance vessels is determined by the balance of local and systemic inputs. The systemic input is provided by the SNS that mainly affects vascular smooth muscle tone. Local input originates from the endothelial cell and the vascular smooth muscle cell. Therefore, any effect of IR on endothelial cell function, vascular smooth muscle function, or SNS activity (as discussed already above) can contribute to elevation of blood pressure and the development of hypertension.

The endothelial cell produces a number of vasoactive substances; vasodilators including nitric oxide and prostacyclin, and vasoconstrictors including endothelin and possibly thromboxane A. It is well established that endothelial nitric oxide production is impaired in IR [22–24] although the mechanisms by which this occurs are less clear. Potential mechanisms of impaired nitric oxide production include decreased insulin signaling via Akt [25], decreased nitric oxide synthase activity due to impaired phosphorylation [26], or inhibition of nitric oxide synthase by asymmetric dimethyl-arginines (ADMAs) [27, 28]. Evidence for a reduction of prostacyclin production or augmentation of thromboxane A production in IR is less robust and comes mainly from studies in cell cultures, assessment of contractility of vascular strips from IR animals, or studies using specific inhibitors in animal models of IR and hypertension [24, 29].

Levels of endothelin have been found to be elevated in IR and type 2 DM [30–32]. It is possible that increased insulin levels in IR are, at least in part, responsible for the increased endothelin levels [33, 34]. However, despite a significant improvement in IR, endothelin levels did not change in type 2 diabetic subjects treated with pioglitazone [35] suggesting that endothelin levels may not be directly linked to IR.

Acute Effects of Insulin on Blood Pressure and Blood Flow

Increased levels of insulin are a hallmark of insulin resistance and often associated with elevated blood pressure. Therefore, it is logical to assess the effect of insulin to modulate blood pressure. Insulin acutely increases SNS activity [36, 37] and cardiac output [38, 39] and could therefore, if not compensated for by a fall in peripheral vascular resistance, increase blood pressure [40]. However, studies by some but not all groups [5, 41] have demonstrated that acute elevations in insulin levels, in normal insulin-sensitive subjects, lasting several hours do not increase blood pressure [39, 42] or actually result in small reductions in blood pressure [37, 39, 43]. In addition, in insulin-sensitive subjects, hyperinsulinemia is associated with increased rates of blood flow which correlates highly with insulin's effect to stimulate skeletal muscle glucose uptake [44]. These effects of insulin to increase nitric oxide production and skeletal muscle blood flow are impaired in IR [22]. The mechanism by which IR impairs insulin-mediated increments in nitric oxide production is not well understood. Increased levels of free fatty acids, at high physiologic levels as observed in IR and type 2 DM, have been shown to impair endothelial function [45–47]. Other factors such as increased cytokines (e.g., tumor necrosis factor alpha), increased leptin [48], and decreased adiponectin [49] levels have been proposed to contribute to the impaired vasodilatory action of insulin in IR.

Insulin-mediated increase in skeletal muscle blood flow can be completely abolished by L-NMMA [50], a mono-methyl-arginine and inhibitor of endothelial nitric oxide synthase, indicating that insulin mediates its effect on blood flow via increased production of nitric oxide. Importantly, it has been reported that hyperinsulinemia reduces levels of ADMA, an endogenous inhibitor of endothelial nitric oxide synthase [51]. Preliminary studies from our laboratory were able to reproduce these findings. Additionally, the result of our studies suggests that insulin's effect to lower ADMA levels is impaired in type 2 DM.

Since elevation of ambient insulin levels under euglycemic conditions did not result in increased blood pressure, one other explanation for the association between hyperinsulinemia and elevated blood pressure was proposed, namely that insulin increases the vascular response to vasopressors such as norepinephrine or angiotensin II. However, several studies addressing this possibility also failed to link hyperinsulinemia to increased vascular reactivity; hyperinsulinemia did not increase the pressor response to norepinephrine [52] in a group of lean insulin-sensitive subjects, and hyperinsulinemia did also not increase the pressor response to angiotensin II in a group of healthy subjects with a wide range of BMI [42].

Interestingly, hyperinsulinemia appeared to (1) shift the dose–response curve to systemically administered norepinephrine to the right in lean insulin-sensitive subjects [52], (2) reduce reflex forearm sympathetic vasoconstriction [53], and (3) also attenuate the blood pressure response to angiotensin II [42]. This attenuation of the response to pressor agents could be due to the increased production of nitric oxide and/or a reduction of Ca^{2+}-influx [23] into vascular smooth muscle cells. However, no shift in the dose–response curve to norepinephrine was observed in the obese IR subjects [52] in this study or in the study by Fujishima et al. [54]. It also appeared that, in response to similar norepinephrine plasma levels, the obese IR subjects had a more pronounced increase in blood pressure. Others [55] have observed a similar enhanced response to norepinephrine in obese type 2 diabetic patients. In our own studies, elevation of FFA levels in normal subjects by infusion of intralipid and heparin shifted the dose–response to norepinephrine to the left thus mimicking the response to vasopressors in IR.

Effects of Improving IR on Blood Pressure

If IR is mechanistically related to increased blood pressure and the development of hypertension, improvement in IR should result in lowering of blood pressure. Indeed, improvement of IR by means of weight loss [56, 57], exercise [58], or PPAR-gamma agents [59, 60] has been reported to reduce blood pressure by small to moderate degrees. However, the amount of weight loss reported in most studies was substantial, and changes in diet, especially reduced consumption of carbohydrates and sodium, may also play a role in the observed blood pressure reduction.

Furthermore, not all studies assessing the effect of PPAR-gamma agents on IR and blood pressure have been able to demonstrate a reduction in blood pressure [61].

Insulin Resistance, Incretins, and Blood Pressure

Incretins are gut-derived hormones that are secreted into the circulation. Incretin secretion is stimulated by food intake and involved in a number of physiologic actions ranging from the regulation of appetite and gastric emptying to stimulation of insulin release and SNS activity. The focus of this part will be on glucagon-like peptide-1 (GLP-1) because it is thought to be the most important incretin involved glucose homeostasis in response to a meal, the physiology of this incretin is better defined and known than most others, and there are currently two GLP-1 analogues, exenatide and liraglutide, marketed for the treatment of type 2 diabetes. Of interest, GLP-1 secretion has been reported to be diminished in insulin resistant and glucose intolerant subjects [62, 63]. However, GLP-1 action is thought to be normal in insulin resistance and type 2 diabetes [64].

In addition to the actions of GLP-1 on glucose homeostasis in response of a meal, which are mediated mainly via an augmentation of insulin secretion and suppression of glucagon secretion, GLP-1 has been reported to potentially affect the blood pressure and the cardiovascular system. Before providing more details regarding the effects of GLP-1 on blood pressure regulation, it is important to point out that GLP-1 administration resulting in pharmacologically high GLP-1 concentrations almost always results in increased insulin levels, even under euglycemic conditions, that may confound the interpretation of the observed cardiovascular effects.

GLP-1 receptors have been localized, amongst others, to cardiomyocytes, microvascular endothelium [65], the brain [66, 67], and the kidney [68], which all have the potential to affect blood pressure regulation. The notion that GLP-1 may affect blood pressure is supported by studies demonstrating the following responses to the administration of GLP-1: vasodilation, mediated via an endothelium-independent mechanism [69], and nitric oxide (NO) release [65, 70], activation of the SNS [71], and natriuresis [68]. However, the effects of GLP-1 and GLP-1 analogues on blood pressure in animals are dependent on the model used. For example, exenatide (also known as exendin-4) has been reported to decrease blood pressure in a salt-sensitive mouse model [68], and the exenatide analogue AC3174 has been shown to decrease blood pressure in a salt-sensitive rat model [72]. However, GLP-1 has been shown to acutely increase blood pressure in normotensive rats [73].

Data in humans regarding the effect of GLP-1 on vascular function, natriuresis, and the autonomic nervous system parallel, in part, the results from animal studies. For example, GLP-1 infusions increased flow-mediated vasodilation in type 2 diabetic patients [74]. GLP-1 also increased natriuresis in obese men [75]. In addition, GLP-1 was found to increase SNS activity in humans [76]. Given that GLP-1 appears to simultaneously affect systems involved in the regulation of blood pressure, which have opposing effects, it is clear that the net effect of GLP-1 on blood pressure might be rather small. This notion is supported by findings of short-term infusions where either no effect [77] or a slight increase [76] on blood pressure was observed. On the other hand, longer-term studies of approximately 6-month duration with exenatide [78] or liraglutide [79] demonstrated small decreases in blood pressure. However, it is unclear to what degree the decreased caloric (and salt) intake and the weight loss contributed to the observed lowering in blood pressure.

Summary and Conclusion

IR has been reported to be associated with elevated blood pressure and hypertension [80–83]. It is reasonable to postulate that IR is causally related to increased rates of hypertension in IR, especially in light of reports that IR is associated with abnormalities in SNS activity, renal salt handling, and endothelial function. Other, albeit indirect, evidence for the causal role of IR in blood pressure elevation comes from studies where improvement in IR resulted in lowering of blood pressure. A likely mechanistic explanation for the association between IR and blood pressure is that adipocyte dysfunction, elevated free fatty acid levels, and elevated insulin levels, over time, may adversely affect systems involved in blood pressure regulation. Since the association between IR and elevated blood pressure is not found in all populations, these studies also suggest that, depending on genetic and environmental factors, these IR-induced changes lead eventually to increased blood pressure, or diabetes, or cardiovascular disease, or any combination of these. Of these, the time-dependent effects on blood pressure, even if not detectable in all individuals as a measurable change, may be particularly significant from a population perspective. Importantly, improvement in IR will likely have significant overall beneficial effects, to prevent or postpone the development of diabetes, hypertension, and cardiovascular disease.

References

1. DeFronzo RA, Tobin JD, Andres R. Glucose clamp technique: a method for quantifying insulin secretion and resistance. Am J Physiol. 1979;237(3):E214–23.
2. Caumo A, Bergman RN, Cobelli C. Insulin sensitivity from meal tolerance tests in normal subjects: a minimal model index. J Clin Endocrinol Metab. 2000;85(11):4396–402.
3. Pillonetto G, Caumo A, Cobelli C. Dynamic insulin sensitivity index: importance in diabetes. Am J Physiol Endocrinol Metab. 2010;298(3):E440–8.
4. Bergman RN. Minimal model: perspective from 2005. Horm Res. 2005;64 Suppl 3:8–15.
5. Muscelli E, et al. Autonomic and hemodynamic responses to insulin in lean and obese humans. J Clin Endocrinol Metab. 1998;83(6):2084–90.
6. Steinberg HO, et al. Type II diabetes abrogates sex differences in endothelial function in premenopausal women. Circulation. 2000;101(17):2040–6.
7. Nuutila P, et al. Gender and insulin sensitivity in the heart and in skeletal muscles. Studies using positron emission tomography. Diabetes. 1995;44(1):31–6.
8. Saad MF, et al. Insulin and hypertension. Relationship to obesity and glucose intolerance in Pima Indians. Diabetes. 1990;39(11):1430–5.
9. Ferrannini E, et al. Insulin resistance, insulin response, and obesity as indicators of metabolic risk. J Clin Endocrinol Metab. 2007;92(8):2885–92.
10. Grassi G, et al. Effect of central and peripheral body fat distribution on sympathetic and baroreflex function in obese normotensives. J Hypertens. 2004;22(12):2363–9.
11. Huggett RJ, et al. Sympathetic neural activation in nondiabetic metabolic syndrome and its further augmentation by hypertension. Hypertension. 2004;44(6):847–52.
12. Florian JP, Pawelczyk JA. Non-esterified fatty acids increase arterial pressure via central sympathetic activation in humans. Clin Sci (Lond). 2010;118(1):61–9.
13. Quilliot D, et al. Impaired autonomic control of heart rate and blood pressure in obesity: role of age and of insulin-resistance. Clin Auton Res. 2001;11(2):79–86.
14. Valensi P, et al. Influence of parasympathetic dysfunction and hyperinsulinemia on the hemodynamic response to an isometric exercise in non-insulin-dependent diabetic patients. Metabolism. 1998;47(8):934–9.
15. Guyton AC. Roles of the kidneys and fluid volumes in arterial pressure regulation and hypertension. Chin J Physiol. 1989;32(2):49–57.
16. Charra B, Chazot C. Volume control, blood pressure and cardiovascular function. Lessons from hemodialysis treatment. Nephron Physiol. 2003;93(4):94–101.
17. Hall JE. Renal function in one-kidney, one-clip hypertension and low renin essential hypertension. Am J Hypertens. 1991;4(10 Pt 2):523S–33.
18. Hall JE. Mechanisms of abnormal renal sodium handling in obesity hypertension. Am J Hypertens. 1997;10(5 Pt 2):49S–55.

19. Strazzullo P, et al. Abnormalities of renal sodium handling in the metabolic syndrome. Results of the Olivetti Heart Study. J Hypertens. 2006;24(8):1633–9.
20. Chen J, et al. Metabolic syndrome and salt sensitivity of blood pressure in non-diabetic people in China: a dietary intervention study. Lancet. 2009;373(9666):829–35.
21. Hoffmann IS, Cubeddu LX. Increased blood pressure reactivity to dietary salt in patients with the metabolic syndrome. J Hum Hypertens. 2007;21(6):438–44.
22. Steinberg HO, et al. Obesity/insulin resistance is associated with endothelial dysfunction. Implications for the syndrome of insulin resistance. J Clin Invest. 1996;97(11):2601–10.
23. Sowers JR. Effects of insulin and IGF-I on vascular smooth muscle glucose and cation metabolism. Diabetes. 1996;45 Suppl 3:S47–51.
24. Du X, et al. Insulin resistance reduces arterial prostacyclin synthase and eNOS activities by increasing endothelial fatty acid oxidation. J Clin Invest. 2006;116(4):1071–80.
25. Okon EB, et al. Compromised arterial function in human type 2 diabetic patients. Diabetes. 2005;54(8):2415–23.
26. Symons JD, et al. Contribution of insulin and Akt1 signaling to endothelial nitric oxide synthase in the regulation of endothelial function and blood pressure. Circ Res. 2009;104(9):1085–94.
27. Perticone F, et al. Endothelial dysfunction, ADMA and insulin resistance in essential hypertension. Int J Cardiol. 2010;142(3):236–41.
28. Sydow K, Mondon CE, Cooke JP. Insulin resistance: potential role of the endogenous nitric oxide synthase inhibitor ADMA. Vasc Med. 2005;10 Suppl 1:S35–43.
29. Galipeau D, et al. Chronic thromboxane synthase inhibition prevents fructose-induced hypertension. Hypertension. 2001;38(4):872–6.
30. Ferri C, et al. Plasma endothelin-1 levels in obese hypertensive and normotensive men. Diabetes. 1995;44(4):431–6.
31. Piatti PM, et al. Relationship between endothelin-1 concentration and metabolic alterations typical of the insulin resistance syndrome. Metabolism. 2000;49(6):748–52.
32. Irving RJ, et al. Activation of the endothelin system in insulin resistance. QJM. 2001;94(6): 321–6.
33. Ferri C, De Mattia G. The effect of insulin on endothelin-1 (ET-1) secretion in human cultured endothelial cell. Metabolism. 1995;44(5):689–90.
34. Cardillo C, et al. Insulin stimulates both endothelin and nitric oxide activity in the human forearm. Circulation. 1999;100(8):820–5.
35. Fernandez M, et al. Addition of pioglitazone and ramipril to intensive insulin therapy in type 2 diabetic patients improves vascular dysfunction by different mechanisms. Diabetes Care. 2008;31(1):121–7.
36. Anderson EA, et al. Insulin increases sympathetic activity but not blood pressure in borderline hypertensive humans. Hypertension. 1992;19(6 Pt 2):621–7.
37. Anderson EA, et al. Hyperinsulinemia produces both sympathetic neural activation and vasodilation in normal humans. J Clin Invest. 1991;87(6):2246–52.
38. Laitinen T, et al. Effects of euglycaemic and hypoglycaemic hyperinsulinaemia on sympathetic and parasympathetic regulation of haemodynamics in healthy subjects. Clin Sci (Lond). 2003;105(3):315–22.
39. Fugmann A, et al. Central and peripheral haemodynamic effects of hyperglycaemia, hyperinsulinaemia, hyperlipidaemia or a mixed meal. Clin Sci (Lond). 2003;105(6):715–21.
40. Baron AD, et al. Skeletal muscle blood flow. A possible link between insulin resistance and blood pressure. Hypertension. 1993;21(2):129–35.
41. ter Maaten JC, et al. Relationship between insulin's haemodynamic effects and insulin-mediated glucose uptake. Eur J Clin Invest. 1998;28(4):279–84.
42. Buchanan TA, et al. Angiotensin II increases glucose utilization during acute hyperinsulinemia via a hemodynamic mechanism. J Clin Invest. 1993;92(2):720–6.
43. Baron AD, Brechtel G. Insulin differentially regulates systemic and skeletal muscle vascular resistance. Am J Physiol. 1993;265(1 Pt 1):E61–7.
44. Laakso M, et al. Kinetics of in vivo muscle insulin-mediated glucose uptake in human obesity. Diabetes. 1990;39(8):965–74.

45. Steinberg HO, et al. Elevated circulating free fatty acid levels impair endothelium-dependent vasodilation. J Clin Invest. 1997;100(5):1230–9.
46. Liu J, et al. Free fatty acids induce insulin resistance in both cardiac and skeletal muscle microvasculature in humans. J Clin Endocrinol Metab. 2011;96:438–46.
47. Mittermayer F, et al. Rosiglitazone prevents free fatty acid-induced vascular endothelial dysfunction. J Clin Endocrinol Metab. 2007;92(7):2574–80.
48. Galletti F, et al. High-circulating leptin levels are associated with greater risk of hypertension in men independently of body mass and insulin resistance: results of an eight-year follow-up study. J Clin Endocrinol Metab. 2008;93(10):3922–6.
49. Li HY, et al. The negative correlation between plasma adiponectin and blood pressure depends on obesity: a family-based association study in SAPPHIRe. Am J Hypertens. 2008;21(4):471–6.
50. Steinberg HO, et al. Insulin-mediated skeletal muscle vasodilation is nitric oxide dependent. A novel action of insulin to increase nitric oxide release. J Clin Invest. 1994;94(3):1172–9.
51. Eid HM, et al. Decreased levels of asymmetric dimethylarginine during acute hyperinsulinemia. Metabolism. 2007;56(4):464–9.
52. Baron AD, et al. Interactions between insulin and norepinephrine on blood pressure and insulin sensitivity. Studies in lean and obese men. J Clin Invest. 1994;93(6):2453–62.
53. Lembo G, et al. Insulin reduces reflex forearm sympathetic vasoconstriction in healthy humans. Hypertension. 1993;21(6 Pt 2):1015–9.
54. Fujishima S, et al. Effects of intra-arterial infusion of insulin on forearm vasoreactivity in hypertensive humans. Hypertens Res. 1995;18(3):227–33.
55. Huvers FC, et al. The enhanced pressor response in type 2 diabetes is not based upon a generalized increase in vascular responsiveness. Cardiovasc Res. 1998;38(1):206–14.
56. Su HY, et al. Effect of weight loss on blood pressure and insulin resistance in normotensive and hypertensive obese individuals. Am J Hypertens. 1995;8(11):1067–71.
57. Tiikkainen M, et al. Effects of equal weight loss with orlistat and placebo on body fat and serum fatty acid composition and insulin resistance in obese women. Am J Clin Nutr. 2004;79(1):22–30.
58. Dengel DR, et al. The independent and combined effects of weight loss and aerobic exercise on blood pressure and oral glucose tolerance in older men. Am J Hypertens. 1998;11(12):1405–12.
59. Basu A, et al. Effects of pioglitazone versus glipizide on body fat distribution, body water content, and hemodynamics in type 2 diabetes. Diabetes Care. 2006;29(3):510–4.
60. Yosefy C, et al. Rosiglitazone improves, while Glibenclamide worsens blood pressure control in treated hypertensive diabetic and dyslipidemic subjects via modulation of insulin resistance and sympathetic activity. J Cardiovasc Pharmacol. 2004;44(2):215–22.
61. Paradisi G, et al. Troglitazone therapy improves endothelial function to near normal levels in women with polycystic ovary syndrome. J Clin Endocrinol Metab. 2003;88(2):576–80.
62. Rask E, et al. Impaired incretin response after a mixed meal is associated with insulin resistance in nondiabetic men. Diabetes Care. 2001;24(9):1640–5.
63. Muscelli E, et al. Separate impact of obesity and glucose tolerance on the incretin effect in normal subjects and type 2 diabetic patients. Diabetes. 2008;57(5):1340–8.
64. Nauck MA. Unraveling the science of incretin biology. Eur J Intern Med. 2009;20 Suppl 2:S303–8.
65. Ban K, et al. Cardioprotective and vasodilatory actions of glucagon-like peptide 1 receptor are mediated through both glucagon-like peptide 1 receptor-dependent and -independent pathways. Circulation. 2008;117(18):2340–50.
66. Yamamoto H, et al. Glucagon-like peptide-1 receptor stimulation increases blood pressure and heart rate and activates autonomic regulatory neurons. J Clin Investig. 2002; 110(1):43–52.
67. Trapp S, Hisadome K. Glucagon-like peptide 1 and the brain: central actions-central sources? Auton Neurosci. 2011;161(1–2):14–9.

68. Hirata K, et al. Exendin-4 has an anti-hypertensive effect in salt-sensitive mice model. Biochem Biophys Res Commun. 2009;380(1):44–9.
69. Nystrom T, et al. Glucagon-like peptide-1 relaxes rat conduit arteries via an endothelium-independent mechanism. Regul Pep. 2005;125(1–3):173–7.
70. Gaspari T, et al. A GLP-1 receptor agonist liraglutide inhibits endothelial cell dysfunction and vascular adhesion molecule expression in an ApoE–/– mouse model. Diab Vasc Dis Res. 2011;8(2):117–24.
71. Perez-Tilve D, et al. Exendin-4 increases blood glucose levels acutely in rats by activation of the sympathetic nervous system. Am J Physiol. 2010;298(5):E1088–96.
72. Liu Q, et al. The exenatide analogue AC3174 attenuates hypertension, insulin resistance, and renal dysfunction in Dahl salt-sensitive rats. Cardiovasc Diabetol. 2010;9:32.
73. Gardiner SM, et al. Possible involvement of GLP-1(9–36) in the regional haemodynamic effects of GLP-1(7–36) in conscious rats. Br J Pharmacol. 2010;161(1):92–102.
74. Nystrom T, et al. Effects of glucagon-like peptide-1 on endothelial function in type 2 diabetes patients with stable coronary artery disease. Am J Physiol. 2004;287(6):E1209–15.
75. Gutzwiller JP, et al. Glucagon-like peptide 1 induces natriuresis in healthy subjects and in insulin-resistant obese men. J Clin Endocrinol Metab. 2004;89(6):3055–61.
76. Bharucha AE, et al. Effects of glucagon-like peptide-1, yohimbine, and nitrergic modulation on sympathetic and parasympathetic activity in humans. American J Physiol Regul Integr Comp Physiol. 2008;295(3):R874–80.
77. Halbirk M, et al. Cardiovascular and metabolic effects of 48-h glucagon-like peptide-1 infusion in compensated chronic patients with heart failure. Am J Physiol. 2010;298(3):H1096–102.
78. Okerson T, et al. Effects of exenatide on systolic blood pressure in subjects with type 2 diabetes. Am J Hypertens. 2010;23(3):334–9.
79. Sjoholm A. Impact of glucagon-like peptide-1 on endothelial function. Diabetes Obes Metab. 2009;11 Suppl 3:19–25.
80. Ferrannini E, et al. Insulin resistance, hyperinsulinemia, and blood pressure: role of age and obesity. European Group for the Study of Insulin Resistance (EGIR). Hypertension. 1997;30(5):1144–9.
81. DeFronzo RA, Ferrannini E. Insulin resistance. A multifaceted syndrome responsible for NIDDM, obesity, hypertension, dyslipidemia, and atherosclerotic cardiovascular disease. Diabetes Care. 1991;14(3):173–94.
82. Pinkney JH, et al. Insulin resistance, insulin, proinsulin, and ambulatory blood pressure in type II diabetes. Hypertension. 1994;24(3):362–7.
83. Reaven GM. Banting lecture 1988. Role of insulin resistance in human disease. Diabetes. 1988;37(12):1595–607.

Chapter 13
Obesity-Associated Hypertension

Gabriel I. Uwaifo

Abstract Both hypertension and obesity are highly prevalent chronic medical conditions that afflict an increasing portion of both the adult and the pediatric populations in clinical practice worldwide.

Based on the sheer prevalence of both of these conditions, it is not unexpected to discover that they often coexist. There is, however, considerable retrospective, cross-sectional and prospective data from various research studies and diverse populations which suggest that the association between obesity and so-called "essential hypertension" is significantly more prevalent than the result of chance co-occurrence. A growing body of data suggests that obesity has a direct, independent, and causal link to the onset and worsening of hypertension. This association now known as obesity-hypertension (OH) has also been shown to be significantly ameliorated by significant (>5% of baseline body weight) weight loss.

While the exact underlying etiopathogenesis of OH is still unclear, it appears to be multifactorial including both mechanical and humoral factors in its development. Among the identified putative contributory factors are renal salt retention, blood volume expansion, and sympathetic activation all of which can be induced by hyperinsulinemia and hyperleptinemia. Hypoadiponectinemia, activation of the renin-angiotensin-aldosterone system (RAAS) as well as the elevated levels of circulating endothelin and free fatty acids also likely play contributing roles. The high prevalence of obstructive sleep apnea (OSA) in the setting of obesity is another pathophysiologic link to the onset of hypertension in obese subjects whose importance is only recently being fully appreciated.

In addition to the well-established complications and comorbidities known to be associated with hypertension and obesity, OH as an entity appears to be associated with some distinctive cardiomyopathic features. This, in addition to issues related to

G.I. Uwaifo (✉)
Department of Medicine, Section of Endocrinology, Diabetes and Metabolism,
Louisiana State University Health Care System, New Orleans, LA, USA
e-mail: guwaif@lsuhsc.edu

C.A. Koch and G.P. Chrousos (eds.), *Endocrine Hypertension: Underlying Mechanisms and Therapy*, Contemporary Endocrinology, DOI 10.1007/978-1-60761-548-4_13,

accurate blood pressure measurement and tracking in obese subjects, requires some expertise and extra care on the part of clinical providers who care for these patients.

The management of OH while based on the same general principles applied to management of essential hypertension as a whole has the added blood pressure modulating effects that follow sustained weight loss. More research into the dominant pathophysiologic mechanisms and treatment strategies for drug-resistant OH is needed.

Keywords Hypertension • Obesity • Obesity-hypertension • SNS overactivity • Leptin • Renin–angiotensin-aldosterone system • Cortisol • Hyperinsulinemia • Endothelin • Free fatty acids • Atrial natriuretic peptide system

Introduction

Hypertension is a particularly common cardiovascular risk surrogate that has marked public health importance because of its association with cardiovascular, cerebrovascular, and renal risk in both adult and pediatric populations [1–4]. The current estimated prevalence of hypertension exceeds 980 million with estimates suggesting that this could exceed 1.5 billion by 2025 unless there are substantive public initiatives to change the present trajectory [4, 5]. The increasing prevalence of hypertension has been temporally associated with the relatively recent ongoing pandemic of obesity which has been apparent both within the United States and worldwide [6]. Obesity prevalence rates worldwide now exceed 300 million. Data from the Center of Disease Control's National Health and Nutrition Examination Survey reveal that rates of obesity in children ages 2–5 have more than doubled since 1980, to now 12.4%. Similar to adults, once a child becomes overweight, it is difficult to change. While the United States leads the world in obesity prevalence rates, the incidence rates in parts of the developing world including South America and the Middle East are likely to surpass those in the Western world within the next decade or less [6, 7].

Obesity is known to be independently associated with increased risk for various deleterious cardiovascular, renal, and metabolic outcomes including but not restricted to atherosclerotic vascular disease, heart failure, and type 2 diabetes [6, 7]. It has been estimated that obesity accounts for ~60% of all the newly diagnosed cases of type 2 diabetes worldwide [6, 7] and also increases overall all cause mortality rates across virtually all age and sex strata [8]. These risks are further accentuated when hypertension is found to cohabit with obesity in the same patient [7–10]. Overall it also appears that visceral adiposity as indicated by higher waist to hip ratios and higher waist circumference measures portends even greater potential atherovascular and metabolic risk [11, 12]. The ongoing obesity epidemic has become more than an adult-based problem, however, with recent published data documenting a similarly disturbing trend of increasing prevalence among children worldwide with a consequent increase in the prevalence of cardio-metabolic complications including hypertension which had hitherto been uncommon in pediatric populations [7, 13–16].

Beyond the individual consequences of the twin pandemics of obesity and hypertension however, the public health importance and expense resulting from these conditions and their coexistence is enormous. Some recent estimates show that despite the improvements in overall control rates for hypertension and the increased number of treatment options and their availability, suboptimal hypertension management still contributes to nearly 40,000 atherosclerotic events and nearly 9,000 related deaths annually in the United States alone [17]. This amounts to direct medical expenditure costs of ~964 million dollars annually based on 2002 dated estimates [17]. Estimates from Europe are even more staggering and were recently estimated at ~1.26 billion Euros [18]. The trends are also similar in the developing countries of the world with percentage of the gross domestic product being expended in management of obesity, hypertension, and their complications being even greater than in the developed world [6, 19].

The association between hypertension and obesity is one that exceeds the mere concurrence of two common chronic diseases in the same population. Data from prospective, cross-sectional and retrospective cohorts suggest that obesity often predates and has a significant causative role in the onset, development, progression, and worsening of hypertension [10, 20–26]. Estimates from the Framingham offspring cohort study suggest that ~78% of the hypertension burden in Caucasian men within that cohort and ~65% of the hypertension burden in women are directly the result of coexisting/antecedent obesity [27]. This finding has been replicated in various other populations and is probably of greater impact among some minority groups including African Americans (AA) and other groups of the African diaspora [5, 12, 28, 29]. Weight and blood pressure have been demonstrated to have a linear relationship in population-based blood pressure and body mass index (BMI) screening and this trend was observed in hypertensive, normotensive, obese, and non-obese subjects [30–34]. The NHANES and other studies have replicated these findings and trends in both adult and pediatric populations [35, 36]. Beyond the established association between measures of adiposity and hypertension, however, it is also apparent that body fat distribution is also important in the association between hypertension and obesity. Abdominal obesity and specifically visceral abdominal obesity has shown the strongest association with hypertension and this has been demonstrated in various study groups and ethnic cohorts [37–40]. Furthermore, weight gain has been shown to be associated with increased blood pressure. Estimates from the Framingham Heart study suggest that ~5%weight increases the risk for hypertension by ~30% over a 4-year period [41]. Contra wise, weight loss has been demonstrated to be associated with reduction in blood pressure (both diastolic and systolic) [31, 32, 42]. Other studies have confirmed and demonstrated similar findings. The Trials of hypertension prevention program for example which was a randomized multicenter prospective trial also demonstrated over an ~7-year period of follow-up that an 18-month weight loss intervention resulted in ~77% reduction in the new onset incidence of hypertension and this was more effective than a corresponding salt restriction program [43].

The rest of this manuscript concentrates on exploring the suggested putative mechanisms that underlie the development of OH and management strategies for ameliorating it.

Pathophysiology of Obesity-Hypertension

Central to the association of hypertension and obesity is the increased adiposity associated with obesity. Adipose tissue is now well established to be a prodigious endocrine organ and a host of the endocrine and paracrine products of the adipose tissue appear to play a role in the development of OH. Among the products of note in this regard are free fatty acids (FFAs), angiotensinogen, renin, tumor necrosis factor alpha (TNF α), leptin, resistin, plasminogen activator inhibitor one (PAI-1), adiponectin, interleukin-6, mineralocorticoid releasing factors, and 11 beta hydroxysteroid dehydrogenase (11 βHSD) to name a few [7, 20, 44–46]. Figure 13.1 highlights

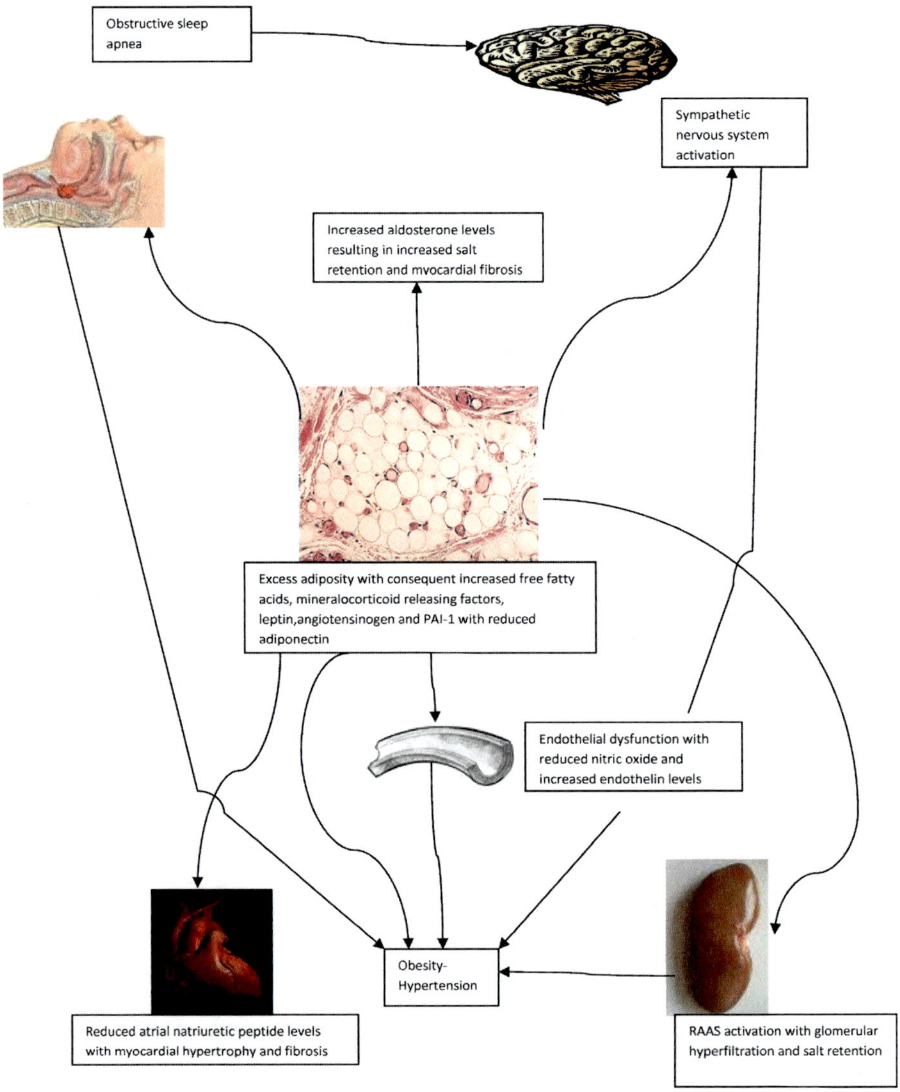

Fig. 13.1 Putative mechanisms for development of obesity-hypertension (OH)

Table 13.1 Mechanical and humoral factors implicated in OH

Hyperinsulinemia and insulin resistance
Chronic noninfective inflammation
Chronic adipocytokinemia (elevated local adipose and systemic interleukin 6 [IL-6], interleukin 1 [IL-1], tumor necrosis factor alpha [TNF-α], and plasminogen activator inhibitor 1 [PAI-1] levels)
RAAS activation (local adipose, renal, and systemic)
Sympathetic nervous system activation (local adipose, renal, and systemic)
Reduced atrial natriuretic peptide levels
Endothelial dysfunction and oxidative stress
Elevated endothelin levels
Elevated resistin levels
Hyperuricemia
Hypoadiponectinemia
Leptin resistance and hyperleptinemia
Elevated free fatty acids levels and hypertriglyceridemia
Overexpression of 11 beta hydroxysteroid dehydrogenase type 1 enzyme activity
Glomerular hyperfiltration and intraglomerular hypertension
Microalbuminuria
Increased renal capsular and intra-abdominal pressure
Renal sodium retention and impaired pressure natriuresis
Obesity-associated glomerulopathy (focal segmental glomerulosclerosis)
Obstructive sleep apnea

how these humoral agents are presumed to interrelate to result in OH while Table 13.1 details some of the humoral and mechanical factors that contribute to the development and evolution of OH. While these highlight the complexity involved in the development of OH, it also offers insight into the multiple therapeutic options available for its amelioration.

Increased renal sodium retention and expanded blood volume are central to OH. Among the means by which this is presumed to develop are increased sympathetic nervous system (SNS) activity as well as increased RAAS activity presumably augmented by the excessive production of angiotensinogen from the increased adipocyte cell mass [47, 48]. It also appears that increased intrarenal pressure associated with abdominal obesity contributes to this process [47–49]. The increased renal sodium retention impairs renal pressure natriuresis which in and of itself elevates systemic blood pressure but additionally obesity is associated with increased renal plasma flow, increased glomerular filtration rate, increased glomerular pressure, and increased renal tubular reabsorption which are the result at least in part of the hyperactivated RAAS and SNSs [48, 50–52]. These derangements all reduce overall glomerular reserve and encourage the early development of glomerular-based proteinuria even in the absence of the focal segmental glomerulosclerosis known to be associated with marked obesity [48, 50–52].

Sympathetic Nervous System Overactivity

SNS overactivity appears to play a central role in the development of OH. Cross-sectional data show that BMI and plasma norepinephrine levels are independent predictors of blood pressure levels especially among obese hypertensives [48, 50–52]. Obese subjects compared with age matched lean individuals have been shown to have elevated plasma norepinephrine levels and muscle sympathetic nerve activity [48, 50–52]. Beyond the systemic increased SNS activity, however, it has also been demonstrated that obesity is associated with local regional SNS overactivation in the kidneys and adipose tissue [53]. Furthermore, it has also been shown clinically that combined alpha and beta blockade results in better blood pressure control among obese than lean hypertensives [54]. It also appears that the SNS overactivation may play a role in the hyperleptinemia and hyperinsulinemia associated with obesity since the degrees of these improve with pharmacologic alpha and beta blockade [55]. Other potential mediators for the observed SNS overactivation include angiotensin 2, aldosterone, FFAs, and adiponectin.

Leptin

Leptin which is the product of the OB gene is predominantly expressed and produced by adipocytes in proportion to the total fat mass [45, 56–58]. While its established actions are mainly at the hypothalamus where it induces satiety and increased energy expenditure, it is known to have several other less well-characterized actions on various tissues including enablement of menarche, anabolic action on bone, and sympathetic activation of several tissues [45, 56–58]. This SNS hyperactivation is capable of inducing hypertension as has been demonstrated in rodent models where chronic leptin infusions cause sustained hypertension which can be prevented by combined beta and alpha blockade [59]. Several experimental models of obesity including the agouti obese and diet-induced obese mice both show selective leptin resistance involving its effects on metabolic rates and satiety in the hypothalamus but preservation of its SNS activatory effects and this appears to also often occur in typical human obesity [60–63].

Renin–Angiotensin-Aldosterone System

The renin–angiotensin-aldosterone system (RAAS) has been implicated in the etiopathogenesis of OH-based multiple clinical observations and the results of intervention trials using RAAS inhibitors and modulators in subjects with OH. Obese subjects are known to have elevated serum angiotensinogen, rennin, and angiotensin converting enzyme activity levels [64]. It has also been demonstrated that adipose tissue is capable of both paracrine and endocrine angiotensinogen production, thus providing one plausible mechanism for the increased angiotensinogen levels observed in obesity [65–68]. Angiotensin 2 which is the most vasoactive product of angiotensinogen exerts autocrine, paracrine, and endocrine effects that include increasing sodium retention, and inhibiting pressure natriuresis in addition to consequent volume expansion and blood pressure elevation [65–70]. It has also been shown that use of angiotensin concerting enzyme inhibitors (ACE-I) reduce not only sodium retention but also blood pressure in animal models of OH and in obese hypertensive human patients [71, 72]. Furthermore it has also been demonstrated that weight loss in obese subjects is associated with reduction in both the adipose tissue expression of angiotensinogen and circulating levels of angiotensinogen, renin, ACE-I, and aldosterone levels which is also accompanied with reduction in blood pressure levels [73, 74]. Aldosterone which is also known to be elevated in obesity and especially visceral obesity plays a critical role in the RAAS overactivity associated with obesity and in the development of OH [65, 73, 75, 76]. The basis of the hyperaldosteronism observed in OH is still the subject of ongoing investigation and speculation. The direct effect of adipocyte-derived angiotensinogen on systemic aldosterone production as well as the role of recently identified adipocyte-derived mineralocorticoid factors on adrenal aldosterone production appear to be among the underlying mechanisms involved [77]. There is also an emerging association now recognized between obstructive sleep apnea (OSA) which is quite prevalent in obesity and a clinical state of primary hyperaldosteronism [75, 76, 78]. The specific aldosterone receptor antagonist Eplerenone has been demonstrated to attenuate or prevent the onset of hypertension in obese dogs on a high fat diet [79] and adds to the available data that indicates the important role of aldosterone in OH. Similar findings in human cohorts confirm that this is also relevant to the pathophysiology of OH in humans [80–82].

Cortisol

The role of cortisol in the pathogenesis of OH is still unclear. Cushing's syndrome, a state of sustained systemic hypercortisolemia, is clearly associated with hypertension, visceral obesity, profound insulin resistance, and other features of the metabolic syndrome but sustained autonomous systemic hypercortisolemia has not been demonstrated in non-syndromic obesity [83]. There is, however, data that suggest overactivity of 11 beta hydroxysteroid dehydrogenase type 1 (11BHSD-1) in omental adipose tissue of obese subjects [84–86] which by increasing local tissue cortisol production may result in a "visceral Cushing's syndrome" like state sometimes referred to as "Omental Cushing's" [87]. The arena of tissue-specific inhibitors of 11BHSD-1 is still in phase 1 and 2 development but could ultimately prove to be another management option for management of resistant OH.

Hyperinsulinemia and Insulin Resistance

Hyperinsulinemia which is generally presumed to be compensatory for underlying tissue insulin resistance is highly prevalent though not universal to obesity. It has been suggested as another pathogenetic player in the development of OH [88, 89]. It is, however, difficult to tease apart the independent role of hyperinsulinemia in OH that is not interlinked to the often accompanying hyperleptinemia, RAAS activation, and SNS overactivation. In animal models, insulin is known to cause SNS activation in the absence of symptomatic hypoglycemia, RAAS activation, and increased renal sodium retention [25, 47]. The available human epidemiologic data, however, shows a less robust association between hyperinsulinemia and hypertension [90]. There is also human data that demonstrates that while hyperinsulinemia increases SNS activity, it is also associated with vasodilation and no accompanying blood pressure elevation [91]. One disease model that provides the opportunity to evaluate the potential role of hyperinsulinemia on its own without accompanying underlying insulin resistance and the metabolic syndrome is the clinic state of patients with insulinomas who have sustained fasting and postprandial hyperinsulinemia. Investigation of these patients has, however, not shown consistent SNS hyperactivation nor hypertension [92] suggesting that underlying insulin resistance rather than absolute hyperinsulinemia may be the critical basis for the observed association between hyperinsulinemia and OH. The elevated FFA levels that often accompany insulin resistance states are known to be associated with SNS hyperactivation and hyperglycemia often associated with insulin resistance can also deleteriously affect vascular compliance and increase the risk for development of hypertension [93, 94].

Adiponectin

Adiponectin is distinctive among adipokines in that in contrast to most others its adipose tissue expression is downregulated and its serum circulating levels reduced in the setting of excess adiposity associated with obesity [95]. Adiponectin has been suggested to be an independent risk factor for hypertension in both lean and obese subjects [95, 96]. It appears that hypoadiponectinemia induces activation of the adipose tissue RAAS and that SNS overactivity in turn reduces adiponectin gene expression providing links between hypoadiponectinemia and both RAAS and SNS overactivity [95, 96]. These may be the underlying basis for hypoadiponectinemia-associated hypertension.

Endothelin

Endothelial dysfunction is common in both obesity and hypertension [95–97]. It is also almost universally associated with systemic insulin resistance. The endothelial vascular tone is largely regulated by the balance between vasodilatory and vasoconstrictive endothelial vasoactive humoral agents of which nitric oxide (NO) and endothelin 1 (ET-1) are the major contributors [95–98]. ET-1 activity is known to be increased in subjects with OH and an association has been described between blood pressure levels and gene polymorphisms of ET-1 among obese Japanese subjects [99–102]. It appears that endothelin's role in the development of OH is the result of both the direct vasoconstrictive effects of the peptide and the reduced NO levels that occur in OH [98, 103]

Renal Capsular Pressure

The increased intra-abdominal and peritoneal fat has been demonstrated to mechanically induce increased intra-abdominal pressure [104]. Similarly, the increased perirenal fat has been implicated in inducing increased intra renal pressure [7]. This increased pressure has been demonstrated to be associated with impairment of renal-based pressure natriuresis and increased renal interstitial pressure as well as fluid retention all of which cause blood pressure elevation [105, 106]. The raised intrarenal pressure may also be part of the basis for the known better correlation between abdominal obesity and OH compared to lower body (so-called gynecoid) obesity (which is dominantly in the hips and thighs) and OH [49].

Other Renal Structural and Functional Changes

Beyond the known effects on the kidney from increased intrarenal pressure highlighted above, obesity induces a host of other structural changes which all conspire to result in blood pressure elevation. It has been shown amongst others that obesity causes marked afferent renal artery vasodilation and increased glomerular filtration as well as intraglomerular pressure [107]. It also appears however that the chronic renal vasodilation associated with obesity causes chronic elevated hydrostatic glomerular pressure which along with the hyperlipidemia and hyperglycemia often accompanying obesity induces glomerulosclerosis and progressive nephron loss which in time can lead to chronic renal disease and renal failure [49, 69, 107]. Focal segmental glomerulosclerosis is distinctively associated with obesity and is distinct from the idiopathic focal glomerulosclerosis seen in the general population [108, 109]. This distinct entity which is associated with a progression to end stage renal disease in the absence of intervention is also called the obesity-related glomerulopathy and is associated with coexisting glomerulomegaly and the development of hypertension [109]. Unlike the idiopathic form of focal segmental glomerulosclerosis it is far less commonly associated with the nephrotic syndrome and more indolent in clinical course. Clearly obesity is associated with development of renal damage, hypertension, and progressive nephron loss but this quickly initiates a positive reinforcing cycle whereby the progressive renal damage further worsens the blood pressure which accelerates the renal damage ultimately leading to end stage renal disease in the absence of clinical intervention.

Free Fatty Acids

Elevations in both fasting and postprandial FFA levels are well described in association with obesity and insulin resistance states [40, 110, 111]. It is believed that FFAs raise blood pressure by increasing SNS activity and also possibly by SNS vascular responses [44, 112]. It has been demonstrated that acute elevations in FFA following intravenous lipid infusions increase vascular reactivity to α agonists. Infusions of oleic acid for example either systemically or into the portal circulation in rat models increase both heart rate and blood pressure and these effects are ameliorated by adrenergic blockade [113, 114]. Portal vein infusions generally cause greater blood pressure elevations than systemic infusions suggesting an additional role for afferent pathways in the liver for mediating the hypertensive effect of FFAs. Similar findings though not as dramatic in effect size have been documented in humans following infusions of intralipid along with heparin [44, 115]. The long-term effects of chronic serum FFA elevation are still unclear and largely unstudied in humans [44, 115].

Resistin

Resistin is a relatively new identified adipocyte-derived peptide that has an insulin antagonistic effect in vivo and in vitro [116]. Serum levels of resistin are elevated in both dietary induced and genetic models of obesity. The exact role of resistin in OH is still controversial with reports on the level and degree of association yielding conflicting results [117, 118]. It does appear, however, that at least among the Chinese, certain resistin gene polymorphisms may be associated with a significantly increased blood pressure burden [117].

The Atrial Natriuretic Peptide System

The system of natriuretic peptides include the atrial natriuretic peptide (ANP) and the brain and C type natriuretic peptide. They are produced predominantly in the heart musculature, brain, blood vessels, and the kidney and are each encoded by separate genes and act on specific receptors [119–122]. The overall effects of these peptides include induction of natriuresis and diuresis with consequent reduction in plasma volume and renal sodium retention in clinical states associated with extracellular volume expansion. They also reduce sympathetic tone and blood pressure as part of their activity profile. Not unexpectedly based on this activity profile it is known that transgenic mice that overexpress the ANP gene have lower blood pressures while those with ANP gene knockout develop salt-sensitive hypertension [123–125]. It has been shown that compared to obese normotensive subjects, subjects with OH have lower ANP plasma levels. These patients also demonstrate a greater blood pressure reduction response to exogenously administered ANP [126]. These salutary effects are also even more pronounced in the setting of accompanying low calorie diet intake [127] In addition, it has been observed that the typical ANP surge associated with salt loading in lean subjects is markedly blunted. Plasma renin activity and aldosterone levels are typically suppressed in obese subjects following saline infusion, and these observations provide some mechanistic explanation for subjects with OH being particularly more salt sensitive than lean or non-hypertensive obese subjects [128]. The magnitude of the role ANP plays in the onset and development of OH is still the subject of ongoing study; however it is clear that impaired ANP action, overexpression of the natriuretic peptide C receptor (which increases ANP clearance), reduced ANP levels, and certain polymorphisms of the natriuretic peptide C receptor gene are all associated with hypertension [126, 127, 129].

The Role of Genetics

Genetics likely explains the clinical observation that while OH is common it is not universal to subjects with obesity. Ethnicity as a poor surrogate for genetic endowment shows some disparity in the degree and prevalence of OH even with comparable weight gain [44, 112, 130–132]. The Pima Indians are an example of a population with profound propensity for obesity and diabetes in whom the prevalence of hypertension is not correspondingly high unless they develop advanced diabetic nephropathy. African American women (probably consequent on their differences in adipose distribution) are also observed to show a lower prevalence and degree of hypertension than Caucasian women with similar degrees of weight gain [130–133].

Cardiovascular Consequences of Obesity-Hypertension

Sustained blood pressure elevation combined with coexisting obesity over a sustained period of time eventually results in deleterious hemodynamic and structural changes. Among the most prevalent structural change associated with OH is concentric or eccentric left ventricular hypertrophy (LVH) [23, 89, 111, 134, 135]. When pressure overload dominates the result is concentric LVH while eccentric LVH is the dominant pattern when volume overload is the major underlying hemodynamic feature. It appears that this LVH increases the risk for heart failure and dysrhythmias [23, 89, 111, 134, 135]. The dysrhythmias in particular may be the basis for the known increased risk for sudden cardiac death among persons with OH [136].

Because of the common coexistence of the distinctive dyslipidemia of the metabolic syndrome and insulin resistance in the setting of OH it is also not surprising that the risk for ASVD and in particular myocardial infarctions appears increased in

OH compared to subjects without hypertension as is eloquently demonstrated by data from the PROCAM study [112].

Beyond the effects of OH on the heart, its impact on the kidneys are also well documented. The association between obesity and progressive nephron loss as well as focal segmental glomerulosclerosis has already been previously highlighted. Data from the Framingham cohort suggest that for every unit increase in BMI after a mean follow-up of ~18.5 years, there is an accompanying 1.2× increase in the risk for accompanying renal disease [137–139].

OH is associated with a proinflammatory cytokine milieu which is largely driven by the host of inflammatory adipokines known to be overexpressed in the increased tissue fat mass associated with OH [112, 133]. Among the central players in this regard are TNF-α, C-reactive protein, IL-1 and 6, and the acute phase reactants fibrinogen and PAI-1 [112, 133, 140–142]. While the association between obesity and a chronic inflammatory state is well established, a direct cause and effect relationship has not been established and the relationship of these cytokines and adipokines to the development and onset of OH is unclear. It is also unclear if treatment with nonsteroidal anti-inflammatory or other anti-inflammatory agents would reduce the levels of these cytokines and adipokines and whether this would ultimately impact ASVD risk in obese subjects. What is apparent, however, is that this inflammatory milieu adds to the ASVD risk associated with obesity and OH. There is available data that demonstrates the ability of the anti-inflammatory agent salsalate in improving indices of insulin resistance and glycemic measures in diabetes [143–147].

Obesity and OH are also associated with hypercoagulability and increased risk for thromboembolism. This is multifactorial in origin including the association of obesity with polycythemia and the prothrombotic milieu resulting from the increased levels of fibrinogen, factor 7 antigen, protein C, and PAI-1 [148, 149]. Leptin appears to play an enabling role in the development of this prothrombotic mix. The complex interrelationships and consequences of OH on cardiovascular risk are further detailed in Fig. 13.2.

Differential Diagnostic Considerations

OH is quite prevalent, however, when a hypertensive subject under clinical evaluation is also found to be obese it is important for the clinician not to assume that this is simply OH with no other complicating issues involved. This is especially true if the patient's clinical presentation is with either resistant hypertension or a hypertensive urgency/emergency. Given the prevalence of obesity in the general population it is important to be aware that virtually all the identified causes of secondary hypertension including rarities like pheochromocytoma can and have been described in obese subjects and can thus be mistaken for regular OH if careful clinical inquiry by detailed history taking and comprehensive physical is not done. Among the important

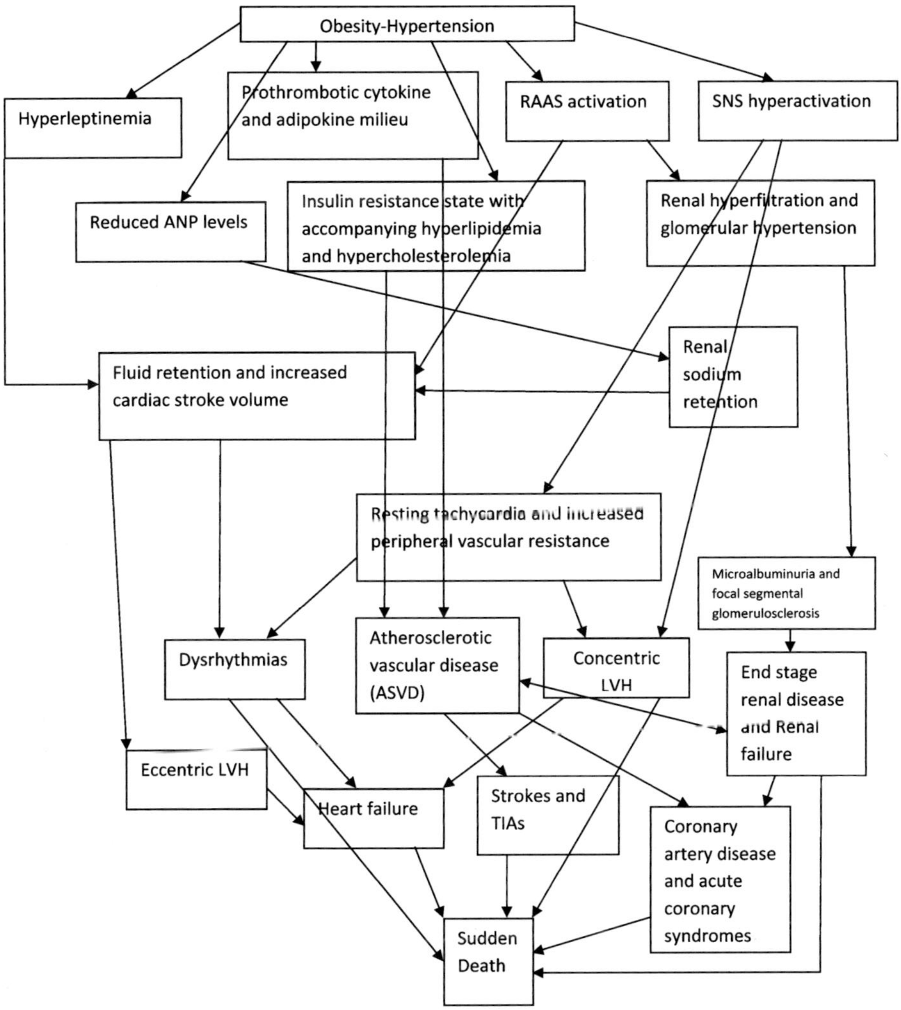

Fig. 13.2 Cardio-renal and cerebrovascular consequences of OH

endocrine considerations to be aware of that can present akin to typical OH are (a) clinical hypothyroidism which though not typically associated with marked obesity is often associated with a volume expanded hypertensive state, (b) Cushing's syndrome in which the degree of abdominal/visceral obesity and the relative atrophy of the extremities as well as the distinctive striae (violaceous, raised, and wide as opposed to the pale, thin striae albicante from mere abdominal distension), (c) acromegaly where the distinctive facial bony overgrowth, macroglossia, and spade like hands and feet may be the clinical findings which raise this possibility, (d) Hypopituitarism or hypothalamic obesity where the clinical history is critical in making the correct diagnosis as well as (e) insulinoma where the distinctive history of spells suggestive of recurrent hypoglycemia is central to the clinical suspicion.

While still poorly characterized, the entity of subclinical Cushing's syndrome is another diagnostic consideration that clinicians need to be aware of when evaluating the subject with obesity and hypertension [150–153]. These patients often clinically resemble subjects with typical obesity with features of the metabolic syndrome; however, careful testing of the hypothalamic–pituitary-adrenal axis demonstrates the presence of significant autonomous hypercortisolemia which has clinical consequences demonstrated the prevalence of dyslipidemia, insulin resistance, ASVD, osteopenia/osteoporosis, and hypertension in these subjects [154, 155]. These patients also have a prevalence of so-called "adrenal incidentalomas" exceeding that of the general population [152–155]. There is some controversy as to whether the adrenal nodules found in this setting are truly incidentalomas by strict definition as there are studies that show the resolution/improvement of the hypercortisolemia and many of its clinical sequelae including hypertension following adrenalectomy that removes the nodule(s) in question [152–155].

Obstructive Sleep Apnea and Obesity-Hypertension

Obesity and in particular upper body obesity is known to be a major risk factor for OSA [156]. Beyond this, however, OSA also often coexists with hypertension; while it has been estimated that ~5–10% of the general population have OSA it is estimated that ~50–60% of hypertensive subjects have OSA [156]. Furthermore, there is extensive evidence indicating that OSA is highly prevalent among subjects with obesity and the metabolic syndrome [157–160]. The association between hypertension and OSA is suggested to be possibly causative based on prospective observation of subjects in the Wisconsin Sleep cohort study which demonstrated that after adjustment for all major possible covariates, a prospective dose–response association exists between the degree of sleep disordered breathing at baseline and the degree of hypertension at follow-up ~4 years later [161–164]. There is also a considerable body of data that suggests that OSA is markedly under recognized and also often under- or untreated even when identified [161–164]. The clinical spectrum of presentation of OSA is quite broad and includes snoring, daytime somnolence, early morning headaches, fatigue, and frequent sleep time arousals with hypopnea and/or apneic spells [76, 78, 158]. On sleep laboratory testing findings may include demonstrable sleep time hypoxia, hypercapnia, restless leg syndrome, and frequent arousals. The frequent arousals are often associated with systolic blood pressure spikes and a loss of the normal physiologic blood pressure dip associated with sleep [76, 78, 158]. While polysomnography remains the gold standard method for confirmation of the diagnosis of OSA, there are several available and well-validated screening methods for assisting clinicians in identifying patients who should have more in-depth evaluation. Measurement of neck circumferences, inspection of the airways, and grading of the oropharynx using scales such as the

Mallampati scale as well as use of validated questionnaires such as the Epworth sleepiness scale are the most popular clinically accessible instruments [165, 166].

The exact means by which OSA induces hypertension is still the subject of ongoing clinical investigation. It does appear that the association between OSA and hypertension is beyond mere statistical association and seems to be such that OSA is associated not only with development of but also worsening of preexisting hypertension [76, 78, 158]. Among the suggested means by which OSA induces hypertension is its known association with SNS overactivity [167–170]. Animal models of OSA have also demonstrated that intermittent hypoxia is associated with sustained hypertension which can be ameliorated by surgical denervation of peripheral chemoreceptors, adrenal demedullation, and/or chemical denervation of the peripheral SNS [171–173]. It has also been shown that continuous positive airway pressure therapy (CPAP) using face masks which is the most reliably consistent treatment strategy for OSA is associated with reduction in SNS activity as well as improvement in resting tachycardia with consequent improvement in the degree of hypertension [156, 174].

Beyond the impact of SNS overactivity, however, it is also apparent that OSA is associated with endothelial dysfunction though it is still unclear whether this is an initiating factor or consequence of OSA [175]. Endothelium-dependent vasodilation is impaired in patients with OSA and improves with CPAP treatment [176, 177]. Endothelin-1 (ET-1) which is endothelium derived appears to play a causative role in the induction of hypertension in OSA [178]. It has been demonstrated that patients with OSA have higher plasma ET-1 levels than health controls and in addition the nocturnal ET-1 levels correlate significantly with the severity of the OSA [178]. Furthermore, CPAP treatment of OSA subjects has been demonstrated to reduce ET-1 levels and the degree of ET-1 level reduction also correlates significantly with the degree of salutary changes in mean arterial blood pressure and oxygen saturation [179].

Recent data also suggests that aldosterone and angiotensin 2 also play a prominent role in the development of hypertension in OSA. Plasma angiotensin 2 and aldosterone levels are elevated in OSA patients compared to controls. CPAP therapy has also been shown to be associated with correlated improvements in blood pressure, plasma renin activity, and plasma angiotensin levels [180]. The activation of the RAAS system in subjects with OSA has features consistent with primary hyperaldosteronism and the triad of hypertension, primary hyperaldosteronism, and OSA is now well recognized [181–184]. It has also been demonstrated that treatment with aldosterone antagonists ameliorates not only the hypertension associated with OSA but also indices of OSA severity as well [181–184]. Animal models of episodic hypoxia have also demonstrated that the hypertension associated with this is prevented when the renal arteries of such animals are denervated and angiotensin receptor blockade done chemically [185].

Hypoadiponectinemia also appears to have an independent role in the hypertension associated with OSA [186–188]. CPAP treatment has been shown to not only improve blood pressure (reduce degree of hypertension) but also proportionately increase serum adiponectin levels [189].

Management Strategies for Obesity-Hypertension

Lifestyle modification strategies are particularly important and central to the effective sustained management of OH. The trial of antihypertensive intervention and management (TAIM) demonstrated that weight loss of greater than 4.5 kg or ~5% of baseline weight in the studied cohort achieved blood pressure reductions comparable to that from a single optimally dosed antihypertensive agent [190]. There are other studies that have replicated these findings [43].

The Place of Weight Loss in OH Management

Sustained weight loss achieved has a salutary effect on blood pressure in OH irrespective of the means by which this is achieved. The central principle for dietary strategies for weight loss is the reduction of overall caloric content while increasing overall fiber content [191–195]. While there are many different strategies by which this may be achieved, reducing portion sizes, proper eating hygiene (regular meals and timing with minimized caloric snacking), and reduced fat and simple carbohydrate content in meals are the most robust strategies for achieving sustained weight loss [196, 197]. The Framingham study has demonstrated as also shown in the TAIM study that weight loss targets required to significantly impact blood pressure specifically and cardiovascular risk surrogates generally are relatively modest. Weight loss of 5 lbs or more can reduce ASVD risk estimates by ~40% [198]. The benefits of weight loss have also been documented in the Trial of Nonpharmacological Interventions in the elderly (TONE) study and the Trial of hypertension prevention (TOHP) study [199, 200]. These studies suggest that weight loss of ~2 kg is associated with 3.7/2.7 mmHg (systolic/diastolic blood pressure) reduction. The TOHP 2 study demonstrated that greater degree of weight loss, ~4.4 kg, was associated with greater degree of blood pressure improvement, 5/7 mmHg [42]. The blood pressure reduction has been shown to be robust as long as the weight loss is sustained. Neter and colleagues' meta-analysis of 25 studies that evaluated weight loss-dependent reduction in blood pressure suggested that on average each kg of weight loss resulted in ~1 mmHg reduction in both systolic and diastolic blood pressure [201]. Achieving and sustaining weight loss remains one of the central strategies for blood pressure control in OH. While in some patients sufficient weight loss can obviate the need for antihypertensives in others it can reduce the number and doses of required antihypertensives [202].

The Place of Dietary Modification in OH Management

While there are many aspects of dietary modification that can have a salutary effect on blood pressure, the DASH (dietary approaches to stop hypertension) strategy is one of the most robust for which substantive prospective data is available [195]. The DASH diet is rich in fruits and vegetables as well as low fat dairy products [195]. It appears that the major mode of action of DASH in blood pressure amelioration is by induction of pressure natriuresis and diuresis [7].

Salt restriction is another well-validated lifestyle management strategy that is particularly relevant to OH. The DASH study showed that when salt restriction to ~65 mmol/day in addition to the standard DASH program further improved blood pressure control [203–205]. It is now apparent though that the degree of responsivity to salt restriction is based on the salt sensitivity of the individual subject which appears to have strong genetic underpinnings [206]. The underlying basis for the salt-sensitive clinical phenotype is likely multifactorial and includes increased SNS activity, impaired response of the RAAS system and norepinephrine to sodium intake and volume depletion, suppression of the kallikrein–kinin system, and/or excess activity of the vasopressin pressor system [207]. It also appears that the salt-sensitive clinical phenotype most robustly identifies subjects with OH who respond best to weight-induced blood pressure improvement [207].

The Dietary intervention study in hypertension (DISH) was a prospective study that compared the weight loss achievement in three treatment groups: a weight reduction group, the sodium restriction group (daily intake of ~40 mEq), and a non-intervention usual care group [208, 209]. The weight reduction group who had a caloric reduction counseling strategy implemented lost on average 4.5 kg at the 1-year follow-up time point and ~60% of these subjects remained normotensive without requiring antihypertensive agents. This was in comparison to ~30% remaining normotensive in the control group [208, 209].

The Place of Exercise in OH Management

The place of increased daily exercise in weight loss and moreso in effective weight management is well established [191–193]. It is also important beyond establishing a culture of regular exercise to ensure consistency and to also encourage a culture of reducing sedentary activities and increasing over all physical activity levels [210, 211]. Sustained increased physical activity is essential to long-term weight loss and is the best predictor of sustained weight loss [22]. Estimates suggest that regular aerobic exercise can reduce blood pressure by up to 11/6 mmHg though other data suggest more conservative reductions [212, 213]. Based on the most robust available clinical trial data the general clinical consensus is to recommend regular physical activity for at least 30 min daily for most days of the week. This has been demonstrated to not only positively impact blood pressure in OH but also ameliorate overall ASVD risk and also assist with redistribution of adiposity away from the visceral adipose compartment [192, 214, 215]. The salutary effects of exercise of OH appear irrespective of age, speed of walking, and have been estimated to reduce overall ASVD outcomes by ~50% [192, 214–216]. It is also apparent from data and recommendations from the Institute of Medicine that for aerobic exercise "more is certainly better" as 60 min of moderately vigorous physical activity on a daily basis has been shown to impart even greater ASVD benefits including better blood pressure improvement and better impact on sustained weight management [217].

The Place of Alcohol Consumption Reduction in OH Management

Alcohol consumption is consistently associated with aggravation of hypertension and this is particularly relevant to OH as a lifestyle factor important for optimal blood pressure management. These findings have been replicated in multiple cross-sectional cohort studies [218]. Data suggests that constant daily consumption is associated with higher blood pressure than binge drinking [219–223]. Furthermore the degree of blood pressure elevation was not related to the type of alcoholic beverage taken [219–223]. Klatsky and colleagues suggest that the effect of alcohol on blood pressure has a "j" shaped curve so that alcohol abstainers tend to have higher blood pressures than those who imbibe between 1 and 3 drinks daily [222, 223]. It has been demonstrated prospectively that alcohol restriction does reduce blood pressure [224, 225]. The exact means by which alcohol elevates blood pressure is unclear but among the suggested mechanism are alterations in intracellular sodium flux, altered baroreflexes, altered intracellular calcium transport, magnesium deficiency (often nutritional related to poor caloric intake that often accompanies alcohol abuse), and altered insulin sensitivity [226]. Accepted clinical guidelines recommend alcohol restriction to no more than 20–30 g daily for men and 10–20 g daily for women in the general population. Whether even more stringent restrictions should apply to subjects with OH has not been directly studied.

Other Life Modification Strategies for OH Management

Behavior modification strategies and programs which have been used for decades in weight management of obese subjects if well deployed and sustained also have beneficial effects on blood pressure. Counseling that enables patients identify and address non-meal time eating cues is critical. In addition, encouraging subjects to keep a dietary intake inventory or food record helps with promoting self-monitoring and identification of deleterious eating patterns. Patients who can be convinced to keep detailed, consistent food records or diaries beyond providing valuable data to assist the dietician in prospective meal planning also often begin implementing appropriate behavioral change on their own volition [227]. Other behavioral modification strategies that may be useful in enabling weight loss as well as preventing weight regain include stimulus control, meal planning, stress and time management as well as deliberate reduction in sedentary time activities such as television watching and computer game playing.

Surgery and OH Management

Bariatric surgery is currently the most consistently effective weight loss strategy available for achieving sustained weight loss. Compared to other management modalities, its effectiveness is even more pronounced among subjects with severe obesity (BMIs $\geq$40 kg/m^2) [228–230]. The Swedish Obese Subjects study (SOS) has some of most robust data demonstrating that bariatric surgery is associated with significant improvements in most of the metabolic complications of severe obesity including improvements in blood pressure levels [31, 32, 228–230].

Pharmacotherapy of OH

Because of the difficulties associated with achieving sustained weight loss though this may be the ideal means of managing OH, pharmacotherapy is necessary in the vast majority of patients with OH. Considering the multifactorial etiology of OH it is not unexpected that monotherapy for OH is often unsuccessful. Though there are no studies that suggest one class of antihypertensives being superior or preferred in OH. Management strategies designed at addressing the multiple pathogenetic pathways involved in the etiology of OH are preferred and most effective. Blockade of the RAAS, of aldosterone action, and of SNS overactivity appear to be the dominant pathways to address in achieving effective management of OH [7]. There have been relatively few clinical trials that have deliberately explored the unique management of OH [71, 231]and so most of the management recommendations are based on data gleaned from subgroup analysis of data from large prospective antihypertensive trials that include significant obese subpopulations. The ideal therapeutic regimen for OH is one that addresses the multiple anomalies associated with OH onset while protecting the heart, brain, and kidneys while improving or at least not worsening the metabolic milieu associated with OH. While there are no absolutely contraindicated or indicated antihypertensives for OH, patient regimens need to be individualized based on individual comorbidities, degree of hypertension, and dominant pathophysiologic features [192, 193, 232, 233].

The RAAS Modulators

Included in this broad subgroup of antihypertensives are the ACE inhibitors (ACEI), angiotensin receptor blockers (ARBS), renin inhibitors (RI), and the Aldosterone Antagonists (AA). These agents are generally quite useful in OH as it is often associated with RAAS activation, systemic aldosterone excess, and salt retention [73, 79, 80, 156, 183, 184]. As a group, these agents have several pleiotropic effects that go beyond their blood pressure reducing properties and these include reduction in glomerular hypertension, improving insulin sensitivity, reducing LVH, and reducing microalbuminuria [73, 79, 80, 156, 183, 184]. These group of agents overall should be included in any therapeutic regimen for a patient with OH unless there are absolute contraindications to their use. There are several prospective clinical trials that support this assertion including the TROPHY trial which was a prospective multicenter double blind trial in patients with OH comparing the ACEI lisinopril and hydrochlorothiazide [71]. The TROPHY trial did show that the ACEI was more efficacious among Caucasian and younger subjects as compared to African American subjects. Data from a cohort of obese hypertensive Japanese subjects showed that the ACEI enalapril has a better metabolic profile compared to amlodipine which included reduction in circulating insulin, leptin, and norepinephrine levels [234]. Telmisartan and Irbesartan are unique among the ARBs in benign shown to increase adiponectin tissue expression from adipocytes by inducing peroxisome-proliferator activated receptor (PPAR) gamma [235]. The major recent ACEI and ARB trials did not specifically enroll obese subjects though there were subsets of patients from all these trials who were obese. None of these studies showed the response of obese subjects to be inferior to their non-obese counterparts and thus it is reasonable to presume that the cardioprotective and renoprotective effects of ACEIs and ARBs demonstrated in such trials as HOPE, LIFE, VALUE, Micro-HOPE, and IDNT are applicable to subjects with OH [236–243].

The Diuretics

While the initial dominant effect of diuretics is on reducing intravascular and extravascular volume, over time the main antihypertensive mechanism for diuretics becomes reduction in peripheral vascular resistance [244]. Diuretics as a whole are generally used for short periods as monotherapy in OH and rather high doses are typically required [71, 245]. Furthermore these higher doses of diuretics are associated with a greater chance of worsening the various metabolic derangements often associated with obesity. As a result, diuretics are not generally considered as preferred agents for the management of OH in the setting of monotherapy though they do have a place as adjunctive therapy whether as second or third steps in the therapeutic regimen.

The results of the Antihypertensive and Lipid lowering treatment to prevent Heart Attack Trial (ALLHAT) study do indicate a place for the use of diuretics in OH management. The nearly 34,000 patient strong ALLHAT study cohort included a substantial number of overweight and obese hypertensives but showed that low-dose diuretics, particularly 12.5–25 mg of chlorthalidone was non-inferior to calcium channel blockers (amlodipine) and ACEI (lisinopril), are initial therapy for uncomplicated hypertension [246]. Diuretics at this low dose also showed non-inferiority as far as capacity to amelioration of overall cardiovascular risk though a mildly elevated glucose level was apparent among diuretic users. This increase was not associated with any perceptible increase in ASVD morbidity or mortality among those subjects so treated [246].

The Beta Blockers

While beta blockade from a purely pathophysiologic stand point may be beneficial in OH because of their capacity to reduce SNS overactivity and improve overall ASVD morbidity and mortality risk, they are, however, associated with metabolic derangements often already apparent in obese subjects including insulin resistance, dyslipidemia, and dysglycemia while impeding weight loss efforts and increasing appetite [247, 248]. The Anglo-Scandinavian Cardiac output Trial (ASCOT) showed that atenolol was inferior to calcium channel blockers in blood pressure as far as mortality indices and was associated with a substantively greater risk for developing new onset diabetes [249]. Furthermore, the Atherosclerosis Risk in Communities (ARIC) Trial found essential similar findings regarding the risk for onset of diabetes among subjects treated with beta blockade [248] while meta-analyses of 13 large multicenter antihypertensive intervention trials showed that beta blockade with atenolol specifically was inferior compared to other therapeutic options as far as therapeutic efficacy [250, 251]. (While some studies suggest that beta blockers like metoprolol may be suboptimal for use in OH, others suggest that agents such as atenolol may be useful [252–254].) This inconsistency in data makes beta blockers not typically recommended as first line therapy in OH; however, it is critical to be aware of the different generations and types of beta blockers whose antihypertensive potencies and metabolic effects are not uniform. The newer generation beta blockers like carvedilol and nebivolol as well as the combined alpha/beta blocker labetalol may have a place in OH management though few cohort-specific trials in this regard have been completed and reported on so far [255–257]. One such trial investigating the glycemic effects in diabetes mellitus, Carvedilol-Metoprolol comparison in hypertensives trial, showed Carvedilol to be superior to Metoprolol as regards glycemic control and reduction of microalbuminuria among subjects with hypertension, diabetes, and overweight-obesity [258].

Despite this, however, it is important to be clear that beta blockade still has an important role in OH therapy as adjunctive therapy especially among subjects with known ASVD or recent acute coronary syndromes (ACS).

The Calcium Channel Blockers

Two major clinical trials, the Hypertension Optimal Treatment (HOT) trial and the Systolic hypertension in Europe (Syst-Eur) studies, have demonstrated that long acting dihydropyridine calcium channel blockers provide robust, sustained blood pressure control with no apparent deleterious effects [259, 260]. The ALLHALT study also corroborated these findings regarding amlodipine though there was an observation of higher heart failure rates compared to chlorthalidone-treated subjects was observed [246].

Another study using long acting nifedipine showed an efficacy in OH management among the studied cohort of 72–76% [261, 262]. The major presumed modes of action of calcium channel blockers in OH are systemic vasodilation and induction of mild natriuresis and diuresis while having a neutral metabolic profile.

Of note, dihydropyridine calcium channel blockers may increase glomerular hyperfiltration which may worsen microalbuminuria. This has not been demonstrated with non-dihydropyridine calcium channel blockers and long-term studies using the currently used long acting calcium channel blockers among subjects with OH who have incipient albuminuria are thus far unavailable to fully elucidate the potential clinical relevance of these observations [263].

The Alpha-1 Blockers

These agents assist with blocking the effects of SNS overactivity and generally have neutral to favorable metabolic effects [218]. One study showed a potential benefit of combined alpha and beta blockade in subjects with OH compared to lean hypertensive subjects [54]; however, alpha blockers as a whole are not first line antihypertensives in OH management but rather generally used as adjunctive therapy. The ALLHAT study results also suggest that alpha blockers are associated with higher risk for heart failure among treated subjects than patients on ACEI or diuretics [246, 264].

The Alpha-2 Blockers

These agents such as clonidine, reserpine, and alpha methyl dopa are generally much older antihypertensives which have generally fallen out of favor for antihypertensive therapeutics as a whole and thus have no place as first line therapy in OH. There are no large cohort trials of their use in OH and their use if desired by the individual clinician will need to be on a case by case basis with close clinical surveillance to avoid the well-documented significant side effect profile associated with these agents.

Other Antihypertensives

The plethora of other antihypertensives available for the management of clinical hypertension offer additional options to the clinician managing patients with OH. Other agents such as minoxidil, diazoxide, hydralazine, metyrosine, fenoldopam, sodium nitroprusside, and omapatrilat have unique clinical settings where they may be indicated as adjunctive therapy but are not mainstream agents for general blood pressure management and are certainly not first line agents for OH management. It is unlikely that there will ever be sufficiently powered clinical trials to investigate their specific utility in the setting of OH.

The Antiobesity Agents

Since sustained weight loss has been demonstrated to be associated with robust improvement in blood pressure, it is not surprising that certain antiobesity agents would have a role in the management of OH. It is, however, important to be knowledgeable about the specific properties of the individual antiobesity agent involved. Sibutramine was recently withdrawn from the market because of the reported excess ASVD risk associated with its use. This may not be unrelated to the well-established effect it had in increasing blood pressure [265–270].

Orlistat on the other hand which acts in the unique way of inhibiting gastrointestinal-based lipases and thus reducing fat absorption has been demonstrated to be associated with modest weight loss in addition to other salutary metabolic effects and a reduction in blood pressure (~2/1.64 mmHg) [271–273].

The potential utility of inhibition of the endogenous cannabinoid system on ameliorating obesity and its various comorbidities including OH was demonstrated by the results of the various RIO studies using the selective cannabinoid receptor antagonist Rimonabant. This agent has, however, been removed from the market due to psychiatric side effects including increased risk for depression and associated suicidal ideations. The clinical investigation of modulation of the endogenous cannabinoid system as a treatment strategy for the metabolic syndrome and obesity is ongoing [274–276].

Management of OSA

As detailed previously, OSA is commonly found in association with obesity and appears to confer an independent additional risk for the development of OH among obese subjects. The effective management of OH mainly by CPAP therapy but also less commonly by surgery such as uvulopalatopharyngoplasty (UVPPP) and certain medications [277–285] has been shown to be associated with improvement in various metabolic indices as well as OH [75, 76, 156]. The recognition, diagnosis, and effective management of OSA is a central piece to addressing resistant hypertension in obese subjects. There is also accumulating evidence that this impacts beyond blood pressure improvement also ASVD risk and overall quality of life [75, 76, 156, 191, 286–288].

Concluding Remarks

OH is increasingly recognized and represents a unique subset of the large body of essential hypertension that is seen in clinical medical practice. With the increasing worldwide prevalence of obesity and diabetes it is certain that the prevalence of OH is likely to increase. Effective prevention measures including predictive and biomarkers are needed [289, 290].

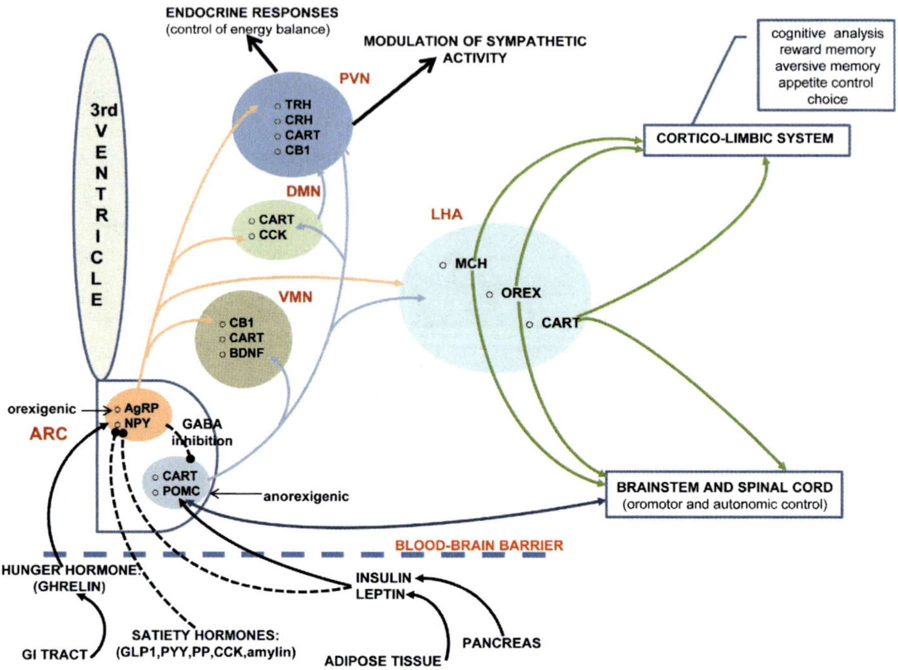

Fig. 13.3 Simplified overview of the relationship between hormonal and neural pathways that regulate energy homeostasis and body fat. Modified after Katherine AS, et al. Hypothalamic regulation of appetite: hypothalamic regions important in appetite regulation. Expert Rev Endocrinol Metab 2008;3(5):577–92; Natalie RA, et al. Central and peripheral regulation of food intake and physical activity: pathways and genes. Obesity (Silver Spring) 2008;16(Suppl 3): S11–22. *ARC* arcuate nucleus; *VMN* ventromedial nucleus; *DMN* dorsomedial nucleus; *PVN* paraventricular nucleus; *LHA* lateral/perifornical hypothalamic area; *α-MSH* α-melanocyte-stimulating hormone; *AgRP* Agouti-related protein; *CART* cocaine- and amphetamine-regulated transcript; *MCH* melanin concentrating hormone; *CCK* cholecystokinin; *DVC* dorsal vagal complex; *GLP-1* glucagon-like peptide-1; *NPY* neuropeptide Y; *OXM* oxyntomodulin; *POMC* proopiomelanocortin; *PP* pancreatic polypeptide; *PYY* peptide YY; OREX-orexin *light brown* circuits—orexigenic pathways; *light blue line* circuits—anorexigenic pathways; *black dashed lines*—inhibitory signaling for various neuropeptides; *green circuits*—interactions among LHA and other structures from CNS

Available data suggest that OH is a complex entity with multiple contributing mechanisms including activation of the SNS, RAAS, and cytokine-adipokine systems [289, 291, 292] (Fig. 13.3). OH has significant consequences both to the cardiovascular and cardiorenal systems as well as to the cerebrovascular system that can have significant morbidity and mortality burdens hence the need for its early recognition and effective treatment. The mixed metabolic milieu associated with OH adds a degree of redundancy to the sustenance of blood pressure which often requires a multifaceted management approach.

Strategies for OH management must include interventions aimed at appropriate weight management, improvement of the associated metabolic derangements, and protection of the major end organs impacted by the disease; especially the heart, kidneys, and the brain. The high prevalence of OSA in OH makes the recognition and effective management of OSA often with aldosterone antagonism an important facet of OH management as are careful consideration of pharmacotherapeutic choices. RAAS modulators and calcium channel blockers appear to be the best preferred agents with beta blockers, diuretics, alpha-1 blockers, and other antihypertensives as adjunctive options to be considered on an individual case by case basis.

Considering the prevalence of OH there is certainly lingering need for more focused clinical trials to investigate specific antihypertensive strategies exclusively in OH especially among minority populations, in children, and other unique cohorts such as pregnancy. Based on the known pathophysiology of the condition, better therapeutic approaches to the management of OH may result from future availability of adiponectin analogues or receptor agonists as well leptin receptor sensitizers.

The management of OH often requires careful consideration of factors that may underlie resistant hypertension including sodium retention, hyperaldosteronism, OSA, development of focal segmental glomerulosclerosis, etc. The possibility of underlying secondary entities which may camouflage as OH including Cushing's syndrome, hypothyroidism, acromegaly, etc. also need to be considered. The clinician involved in caring for these patients needs to be aware of these possibilities and investigate appropriately to be able to achieve optimal patient outcomes.

Acknowledgments We are grateful to Dr. Eugen Melcescu who has helped with illustrations.

References

1. Whelton PK, He J, Muntner P. Prevalence, awareness, treatment and control of hypertension in North America, North Africa and Asia. J Hum Hypertens. 2004;18:545–51.
2. Muntner P, He J, Chen J, Fonseca V, Whelton PK. Prevalence of non-traditional cardiovascular disease risk factors among persons with impaired fasting glucose, impaired glucose tolerance, diabetes, and the metabolic syndrome: analysis of the Third National Health and Nutrition Examination Survey (NHANES III). Ann Epidemiol. 2004;14:686–95.
3. Muntner P, He J, Cutler JA, Wildman RP, Whelton PK. Trends in blood pressure among children and adolescents. JAMA. 2004;291:2107–13.
4. Kearney PM, Whelton M, Reynolds K, Whelton PK, He J. Worldwide prevalence of hypertension: a systematic review. J Hypertens. 2004;22:11–9.
5. Kearney PM, Whelton M, Reynolds K, Muntner P, Whelton PK, He J. Global burden of hypertension: analysis of worldwide data. Lancet. 2005;365:217–23.
6. Obesity: preventing and managing the global epidemic. Report of a WHO consultation. World Health Organ Tech Rep Ser. 2000;894:i–xii; 1–253.
7. Francischetti EA, Genelhu VA. Obesity-hypertension: an ongoing pandemic. Int J Clin Pract. 2007;61:269–80.
8. Calle EE, Thun MJ, Petrelli JM, Rodriguez C, Heath Jr CW. Body-mass index and mortality in a prospective cohort of U.S. adults. N Engl J Med. 1999;341:1097–105.
9. Banegas JR, Lopez-Garcia E, Graciani A, et al. Relationship between obesity, hypertension and diabetes, and health-related quality of life among the elderly. Eur J Cardiovasc Prev Rehabil. 2007;14:456–62.

10. Aneja A, El-Atat F, McFarlane SI, Sowers JR. Hypertension and obesity. Recent Prog Horm Res. 2004;59:169–205.
11. Yusuf S, Hawken S, Ounpuu S, et al. Obesity and the risk of myocardial infarction in 27,000 participants from 52 countries: a case-control study. Lancet. 2005;366:1640–9.
12. Steyn K, Sliwa K, Hawken S, et al. Risk factors associated with myocardial infarction in Africa: the INTERHEART Africa study. Circulation. 2005;112:3554–61.
13. Larsson S, Alicja W. Epidemiology of obesity and diabetes. In: Mantzoros C, editor. Obesity and diabetics. Totowa: Humana; 2006. p. 15–30.
14. Sorof J, Daniels S. Obesity hypertension in children: a problem of epidemic proportions. Hypertension. 2002;40:441–7.
15. Virdis A, Ghiadoni L, Masi S, et al. Obesity in the childhood: a link to adult hypertension. Curr Pharm Des. 2009;15:1063–71.
16. Zhang L, Zhang WH, Zhang L, Wang PY. Prevalence of overweight/obesity and its associations with hypertension, diabetes, dyslipidemia, and metabolic syndrome: a survey in the suburban area of Beijing, 2007. Obes Facts. 2011;4(4):284–9.
17. Flack JM, Casciano R, Casciano J, et al. Cardiovascular disease costs associated with uncontrolled hypertension. Manag Care Interface. 2002;15:28–36.
18. Hansson L, Lloyd A, Anderson P, Kopp Z. Excess morbidity and cost of failure to achieve targets for blood pressure control in Europe. Blood Press. 2002;11:35–45.
19. Yach D, Stuckler D, Brownell KD. Epidemiologic and economic consequences of the global epidemics of obesity and diabetes. Nat Med. 2006;12:62–6.
20. Abstracts of the fourth international symposium on obesity and hypertension: genetics, molecular mechanisms, metabolic syndrome and cardiovascular risk. 27-29 October 2005, Berlin, Germany. Int J Obes (Lond). 2005;29 Suppl 3:S1–19.
21. Diaz ME. Hypertension and obesity. J Hum Hypertens. 2002;16 Suppl 1:S18–22.
22. El-Atat F, Aneja A, McFarlane S, Sowers J. Obesity and hypertension. Endocrinol Metab Clin North Am. 2003;32:823–54.
23. Faloia E, Giacchetti G, Mantero F. Obesity and hypertension. J Endocrinol Invest. 2000;23: 54–62.
24. Kotchen TA. Obesity-related hypertension: epidemiology, pathophysiology, and clinical management. Am J Hypertens. 2010;23:1170–8.
25. Kotchen TA. Obesity-related hypertension?: weighing the evidence. Hypertension. 2008;52:801–2.
26. Kurukulasuriya LR, Stas S, Lastra G, Manrique C, Sowers JR. Hypertension in obesity. Med Clin North Am. 2011;95(5):903–17.
27. Garrison RJ, Kannel WB, Stokes III J, Castelli WP. Incidence and precursors of hypertension in young adults: the Framingham Offspring Study. Prev Med. 1987;16:235–51.
28. Okosun IS, Rotimi CN, Forrester TE, et al. Predictive value of abdominal obesity cut-off points for hypertension in blacks from west African and Caribbean island nations. Int J Obes Relat Metab Disord. 2000;24:180–6.
29. Harris MM, Stevens J, Thomas N, Schreiner P, Folsom AR. Associations of fat distribution and obesity with hypertension in a bi-ethnic population: the ARIC study. Atherosclerosis Risk in Communities Study. Obes Res. 2000;8:516–24.
30. Stamler R, Stamler J, Riedlinger WF, Algera G, Roberts RH. Weight and blood pressure. Findings in hypertension screening of 1 million Americans. JAMA. 1978;240:1607–10.
31. Heneghan HM, Meron-Eldar S, Brethauer SA, Schauer PR, Young JB. Effect of bariatric surgery on cardiovascular risk profile. Am J Cardiol. 2011;108:1499–507.
32. Benraouane F, Litwin SE. Reductions in cardiovascular risk after bariatric surgery. Curr Opin Cardiol. 2011;26:555–61.
33. Johnson WD, Brashear MM, Gupta AK, Rood JC, Ryan DH. Incremental weight loss improves cardiometabolic risk in extremely obese adults. Am J Med. 2011;124(10):931–8.
34. Masuo K, Rakugi H, Ogihara T, Lambert GW. Different mechanisms in weight loss-induced blood pressure reduction between a calorie-restricted diet and exercise. Hypertens Res. 2012;35:41–7.

35. Weiss R, Dziura J, Burgert TS, et al. Obesity and the metabolic syndrome in children and adolescents. N Engl J Med. 2004;350:2362–74.
36. Must A, Spadano J, Coakley EH, Field AE, Colditz G, Dietz WH. The disease burden associated with overweight and obesity. JAMA. 1999;282:1523–9.
37. Cassano PA, Segal MR, Vokonas PS, Weiss ST. Body fat distribution, blood pressure, and hypertension. A prospective cohort study of men in the normative aging study. Ann Epidemiol. 1990;1:33–48.
38. Troisi RJ, Weiss ST, Segal MR, Cassano PA, Vokonas PS, Landsberg L. The relationship of body fat distribution to blood pressure in normotensive men: the normative aging study. Int J Obes. 1990;14:515–25.
39. Hayashi T, Boyko EJ, Leonetti DL, et al. Visceral adiposity is an independent predictor of incident hypertension in Japanese Americans. Ann Intern Med. 2004;140:992–1000.
40. Canoy D, Luben R, Welch A, et al. Fat distribution, body mass index and blood pressure in 22,090 men and women in the Norfolk cohort of the European Prospective Investigation into Cancer and Nutrition (EPIC-Norfolk) study. J Hypertens. 2004;22:2067–74.
41. Vasan RS, Larson MG, Leip EP, Kannel WB, Levy D. Assessment of frequency of progression to hypertension in non-hypertensive participants in the Framingham Heart Study: a cohort study. Lancet. 2001;358:1682–6.
42. Stevens VJ, Obarzanek E, Cook NR, et al. Long-term weight loss and changes in blood pressure: results of the Trials of Hypertension Prevention, phase II. Ann Intern Med. 2001;134:1–11.
43. He J, Whelton PK, Appel LJ, Charleston J, Klag MJ. Long-term effects of weight loss and dietary sodium reduction on incidence of hypertension. Hypertension. 2000;35:544–9.
44. Hall JE, Hildebrandt DA, Kuo J. Obesity hypertension: role of leptin and sympathetic nervous system. Am J Hypertens. 2001;14:103S–15.
45. Haynes WG. Role of leptin in obesity-related hypertension. Exp Physiol. 2005;90:683–8.
46. Hall JE, da Silva AA, do Carmo JM, et al. Obesity-induced hypertension: role of sympathetic nervous system, leptin, and melanocortins. J Biol Chem. 2010;285(23):17271–6.
47. Hall JE. Pathophysiology of obesity hypertension. Curr Hypertens Rep. 2000;2:139–47.
48. Hall JE, Kuo JJ, da Silva AA, de Paula RB, Liu J, Tallam L. Obesity-associated hypertension and kidney disease. Curr Opin Nephrol Hypertens. 2003;12:195–200.
49. Hall JE. The kidney, hypertension, and obesity. Hypertension. 2003;41:625–33.
50. Pecly IM, Genelhu V, Francischetti EA. Renal functional reserve in obesity hypertension. Int J Clin Pract. 2006;60:1198–203.
51. Hsu CY, McCulloch CE, Iribarren C, Darbinian J, Go AS. Body mass index and risk for end-stage renal disease. Ann Intern Med. 2006;144:21–8.
52. Parati G. Obesity, hypertension and the sympathetic nervous system. J Hypertens. 2002;20:835–7.
53. Rumantir MS, Vaz M, Jennings GL, et al. Neural mechanisms in human obesity-related hypertension. J Hypertens. 1999;17:1125–33.
54. Wofford MR, Anderson Jr DC, Brown CA, Jones DW, Miller ME, Hall JE. Antihypertensive effect of alpha- and beta-adrenergic blockade in obese and lean hypertensive subjects. Am J Hypertens. 2001;14:694–8.
55. Sanjuliani AF, de Abreu VG, Francischetti EA. Selective imidazoline agonist moxonidine in obese hypertensive patients. Int J Clin Pract. 2006;60:621–9.
56. Haynes WG, Sivitz WI, Morgan DA, Walsh SA, Mark AL. Sympathetic and cardiorenal actions of leptin. Hypertension. 1997;30:619–23.
57. Sivitz WI, Walsh SA, Morgan DA, Thomas MJ, Haynes WG. Effects of leptin on insulin sensitivity in normal rats. Endocrinology. 1997;138:3395–401.
58. Haynes WG, Morgan DA, Walsh SA, Mark AL, Sivitz WI. Receptor-mediated regional sympathetic nerve activation by leptin. J Clin Invest. 1997;100:270–8.
59. Carlyle M, Jones OB, Kuo JJ, Hall JE. Chronic cardiovascular and renal actions of leptin: role of adrenergic activity. Hypertension. 2002;39:496–501.
60. Rahmouni K, Haynes WG, Morgan DA, Mark AL. Selective resistance to central neural administration of leptin in agouti obese mice. Hypertension. 2002;39:486–90.

61. Eikelis N, Schlaich M, Aggarwal A, Kaye D, Esler M. Interactions between leptin and the human sympathetic nervous system. Hypertension. 2003;41:1072–9.
62. Rahmouni K. Obesity, sympathetic overdrive, and hypertension: the leptin connection. Hypertension. 2010;55:844–5.
63. Rahmouni K, Morgan DA, Morgan GM, Mark AL, Haynes WG. Role of selective leptin resistance in diet-induced obesity hypertension. Diabetes. 2005;54:2012–8.
64. Umemura S, Nyui N, Tamura K, et al. Plasma angiotensinogen concentrations in obese patients. Am J Hypertens. 1997;10:629–33.
65. Rahmouni K, Correia ML, Haynes WG, Mark AL. Obesity-associated hypertension: new insights into mechanisms. Hypertension. 2005;45:9–14.
66. Chan NN, Tong PC, Kong AP, Chan JC. Obesity hypertension: the rationale for renin-angiotensin system blockade. Hong Kong Med J. 2005;11:217–20.
67. Segura J, Ruilope LM. Obesity, essential hypertension and renin-angiotensin system. Public Health Nutr. 2007;10:1151–5.
68. Sibley S. Hypertension, obesity, and the renin-angiotensin system: a tale of tight associations. Minn Med. 2003;86:46–8.
69. Hall JE, Brands MW, Henegar JR. Mechanisms of hypertension and kidney disease in obesity. Ann N Y Acad Sci. 1999;892:91–107.
70. Hall JE, Brands MW, Henegar JR. Angiotensin II and long-term arterial pressure regulation: the overriding dominance of the kidney. J Am Soc Nephrol. 1999;10 Suppl 12:S258–65.
71. Reisin E, Weir MR, Falkner B, Hutchinson HG, Anzalone DA, Tuck ML. Lisinopril versus hydrochlorothiazide in obese hypertensive patients: a multicenter placebo-controlled trial. Treatment in Obese Patients With Hypertension (TROPHY) Study Group. Hypertension. 1997;30:140–5.
72. Robles RG, Villa E, Santirso R, et al. Effects of captopril on sympathetic activity, lipid and carbohydrate metabolism in a model of obesity-induced hypertension in dogs. Am J Hypertens. 1993;6:1009–15.
73. Engeli S, Bohnke J, Gorzelniak K, et al. Weight loss and the renin-angiotensin-aldosterone system. Hypertension. 2005;45:356–62.
74. Barbato KBG, Martins RCV, Rodrigues MLG, Braga JU, Francischetti EA, Genelhu V. [Effects of greater-than-5% weight reduction on hemodynamic, metabolic and neuroendocrine profiles of grade I obese subjects]. Arq Bras Cardiol. 2006;87:12–21.
75. Goodfriend TL, Calhoun DA. Resistant hypertension, obesity, sleep apnea, and aldosterone: theory and therapy. Hypertension. 2004;43:518–24.
76. Goodfriend TL. Obesity, sleep apnea, aldosterone, and hypertension. Curr Hypertens Rep. 2008;10:222–6.
77. Ehrhart-Bornstein M, Lamounier-Zepter V, Schraven A, et al. Human adipocytes secrete mineralocorticoid-releasing factors. Proc Natl Acad Sci U S A. 2003;100:14211–6.
78. Di Guardo A, Profeta G, Crisafulli C, et al. Obstructive sleep apnoea in patients with obesity and hypertension. Br J Gen Pract. 2010;60:325–8.
79. de Paula RB, da Silva AA, Hall JE. Aldosterone antagonism attenuates obesity-induced hypertension and glomerular hyperfiltration. Hypertension. 2004;43:41–7.
80. Bomback AS, Muskala P, Bald E, Chwatko G, Nowicki M. Low-dose spironolactone, added to long-term ACE inhibitor therapy, reduces blood pressure and urinary albumin excretion in obese patients with hypertensive target organ damage. Clin Nephrol. 2009;72:449–56.
81. Kotchen TA, Kotchen JM, Grim CE, Krishnaswami S, Kidambi S. Aldosterone and alterations of hypertension-related vascular function in African Americans. Am J Hypertens. 2009;22:319–24.
82. Kidambi S, Kotchen JM, Krishnaswami S, Grim CE, Kotchen TA. Aldosterone contributes to blood pressure variance and to likelihood of hypertension in normal-weight and overweight African Americans. Am J Hypertens. 2009;22:1303–8.
83. Peeke PM, Chrousos GP. Hypercortisolism and obesity. Ann N Y Acad Sci. 1995;771: 665–76.

84. Rask E, Walker BR, Soderberg S, et al. Tissue-specific changes in peripheral cortisol metabolism in obese women: increased adipose 11beta-hydroxysteroid dehydrogenase type 1 activity. J Clin Endocrinol Metab. 2002;87:3330–6.
85. Goedecke JH, Wake DJ, Levitt NS, et al. Glucocorticoid metabolism within superficial subcutaneous rather than visceral adipose tissue is associated with features of the metabolic syndrome in South African women. Clin Endocrinol (Oxf). 2006;65:81–7.
86. Wake DJ, Walker BR. Inhibition of 11beta-hydroxysteroid dehydrogenase type 1 in obesity. Endocrine. 2006;29:101–8.
87. Bujalska IJ, Kumar S, Stewart PM. Does central obesity reflect "Cushing's disease of the omentum"? Lancet. 1997;349:1210–3.
88. Pastucha D, Talafa V, Malincikova J, et al. Obesity, hypertension and insulin resistance in childhood–a pilot study. Biomed Pap Med Fac Univ Palacky Olomouc Czech Repub. 2010;154:77–81.
89. Bloomgarden ZT. Obesity, hypertension, and insulin resistance. Diabetes Care. 2002;25:2088–97.
90. Davy KP, Hall JE. Obesity and hypertension: two epidemics or one? Am J Physiol Regul Integr Comp Physiol. 2004;286:R803–13.
91. Anderson EA, Hoffman RP, Balon TW, Sinkey CA, Mark AL. Hyperinsulinemia produces both sympathetic neural activation and vasodilation in normal humans. J Clin Invest. 1991;87:2246–52.
92. Scherrer U, Owlya R, Trueb L. Sympathetic-nerve activity before and after resection of an insulinoma. N Engl J Med. 1996;335:1240–2.
93. Alvarez GE, Beske SD, Ballard TP, Davy KP. Sympathetic neural activation in visceral obesity. Circulation. 2002;106:2533–6.
94. De Vriese AS, Verbeuren TJ, Van de Voorde J, Lameire NH, Vanhoutte PM. Endothelial dysfunction in diabetes. Br J Pharmacol. 2000;130:963–74.
95. Hotta K, Funahashi T, Arita Y, et al. Plasma concentrations of a novel, adipose-specific protein, adiponectin, in type 2 diabetic patients. Arterioscler Thromb Vasc Biol. 2000;20:1595–9.
96. Iwashima Y, Katsuya T, Ishikawa K, et al. Hypoadiponectinemia is an independent risk factor for hypertension. Hypertension. 2004;43:1318–23.
97. Koch CA, Wofford M, Ayala AR, Pacak K. Overview of endocrine hypertension. Chapter 26 in Adrenal physiology and diseases (Chrousos GP, Section editor); 2009 http://www.endotext.org/adrenal/adrenal26/adrenalframe26.htm
98. Cardillo C, Kilcoyne CM, Cannon 3rd RO, Panza JA. Interactions between nitric oxide and endothelin in the regulation of vascular tone of human resistance vessels in vivo. Hypertension. 2000;35:1237–41.
99. Cardillo C, Kilcoyne CM, Cannon III RO, Panza JA. Increased activity of endogenous endothelin in patients with hypercholesterolemia. J Am Coll Cardiol. 2000;36:1483–8.
100. Cardillo C, Campia U, Iantorno M, Panza JA. Enhanced vascular activity of endogenous endothelin-1 in obese hypertensive patients. Hypertension. 2004;43:36–40.
101. Campia U, Cardillo C, Panza JA. Ethnic differences in the vasoconstrictor activity of endogenous endothelin-1 in hypertensive patients. Circulation. 2004;109:3191–5.
102. Jin JJ, Nakura J, Wu Z, et al. Association of endothelin-1 gene variant with hypertension. Hypertension. 2003;41:163–7.
103. Mather KJ, Lteif A, Steinberg HO, Baron AD. Interactions between endothelin and nitric oxide in the regulation of vascular tone in obesity and diabetes. Diabetes. 2004;53:2060–6.
104. Bloomfield GL, Sugerman HJ, Blocher CR, Gehr TW, Sica DA. Chronically increased intra-abdominal pressure produces systemic hypertension in dogs. Int J Obes Relat Metab Disord. 2000;24:819–24.
105. Sugerman H, Windsor A, Bessos M, Wolfe L. Intra-abdominal pressure, sagittal abdominal diameter and obesity comorbidity. J Intern Med. 1997;241:71–9.
106. Dwyer TM, Banks SA, Alonso-Galicia M, et al. Distribution of renal medullary hyaluronan in lean and obese rabbits. Kidney Int. 2000;58:721–9.

107. Kurukulasuriya LR, Stas S, Lastra G, Manrique C, Sowers JR. Hypertension in obesity. Endocrinol Metab Clin North Am. 2008;37:647–62; ix.
108. Hall JE, Brands MW, Henegar JR, Shek EW. Abnormal kidney function as a cause and a consequence of obesity hypertension. Clin Exp Pharmacol Physiol. 1998;25:58–64.
109. Kambham N, Markowitz GS, Valeri AM, Lin J, D'Agati VD. Obesity-related glomerulopathy: an emerging epidemic. Kidney Int. 2001;59:1498–509.
110. Redon J. Hypertension in obesity. Nutr Metab Cardiovasc Dis. 2001;11:344–53.
111. Bravo PE, Morse S, Borne DM, Aguilar EA, Reisin E. Leptin and hypertension in obesity. Vasc Health Risk Manag. 2006;2:163–9.
112. Hall JE, Crook ED, Jones DW, Wofford MR, Dubbert PM. Mechanisms of obesity-associated cardiovascular and renal disease. Am J Med Sci. 2002;324:127–37.
113. Stepniakowski KT, Goodfriend TL, Egan BM. Fatty acids enhance vascular alpha-adrenergic sensitivity. Hypertension. 1995;25:774–8.
114. Grekin RJ, Dumont CJ, Vollmer AP, Watts SW, Webb RC. Mechanisms in the pressor effects of hepatic portal venous fatty acid infusion. Am J Physiol. 1997;273:R324–30.
115. Steinberg HO, Tarshoby M, Monestel R, et al. Elevated circulating free fatty acid levels impair endothelium-dependent vasodilation. J Clin Invest. 1997;100:1230–9.
116. Steppan CM, Bailey ST, Bhat S, et al. The hormone resistin links obesity to diabetes. Nature. 2001;409:307–12.
117. Tan MS, Chang SY, Chang DM, Tsai JC, Lee YJ. Association of resistin gene 3′-untranslated region +62G–>A polymorphism with type 2 diabetes and hypertension in a Chinese population. J Clin Endocrinol Metab. 2003;88:1258–63.
118. Zhang J, Qin Y, Zheng X, et al. [The relationship between human serum resistin level and body fat content, plasma glucose as well as blood pressure]. Zhonghua Yi Xue Za Zhi. 2002;82:1609–12.
119. Nakao K, Ogawa Y, Suga S, Imura H. Molecular biology and biochemistry of the natriuretic peptide system. II: Natriuretic peptide receptors. J Hypertens. 1992;10:1111–4.
120. Nakao K, Ogawa Y, Suga S, Imura H. Molecular biology and biochemistry of the natriuretic peptide system. I: Natriuretic peptides. J Hypertens. 1992;10:907–12.
121. Ogawa Y, Nakao K, Nakagawa O, et al. Human C-type natriuretic peptide. Characterization of the gene and peptide. Hypertension. 1992;19:809–13.
122. Komatsu Y, Nakao K, Itoh H, Suga S, Ogawa Y, Imura H. Vascular natriuretic peptide. Lancet. 1992;340:622.
123. Melo LG, Veress AT, Chong CK, Pang SC, Flynn TG, Sonnenberg H. Salt-sensitive hypertension in ANP knockout mice: potential role of abnormal plasma renin activity. Am J Physiol. 1998;274:R255–61.
124. Melo LG, Pang SC, Ackermann U. Atrial natriuretic peptide: regulator of chronic arterial blood pressure. News Physiol Sci. 2000;15:143–9.
125. Melo LG, Steinhelper ME, Pang SC, Tse Y, Ackermann U. ANP in regulation of arterial pressure and fluid-electrolyte balance: lessons from genetic mouse models. Physiol Genomics. 2000;3:45–58.
126. Dessi-Fulgheri P, Sarzani R, Tamburrini P, et al. Plasma atrial natriuretic peptide and natriuretic peptide receptor gene expression in adipose tissue of normotensive and hypertensive obese patients. J Hypertens. 1997;15:1695–9.
127. Dessi-Fulgheri P, Sarzani R, Serenelli M, et al. Low calorie diet enhances renal, hemodynamic, and humoral effects of exogenous atrial natriuretic peptide in obese hypertensives. Hypertension. 1999;33:658–62.
128. Licata G, Volpe M, Scaglione R, Rubattu S. Salt-regulating hormones in young normotensive obese subjects. Effects of saline load. Hypertension. 1994;23:I20–4.
129. Sarzani R, Dessi-Fulgheri P, Salvi F, et al. A novel promoter variant of the natriuretic peptide clearance receptor gene is associated with lower atrial natriuretic peptide and higher blood pressure in obese hypertensives. J Hypertens. 1999;17:1301–5.
130. Abate NI, Mansour YH, Tuncel M, et al. Overweight and sympathetic overactivity in black Americans. Hypertension. 2001;38:379–83.

131. Berchtold P, Jorgens V, Finke C, Berger M. Epidemiology of obesity and hypertension. Int J Obes. 1981;5 Suppl 1:1–7.
132. Weyer C, Pratley RE, Snitker S, Spraul M, Ravussin E, Tataranni PA. Ethnic differences in insulinemia and sympathetic tone as links between obesity and blood pressure. Hypertension. 2000;36:531–7.
133. Castro JP, El-Atat FA, McFarlane SI, Aneja A, Sowers JR. Cardiometabolic syndrome: pathophysiology and treatment. Curr Hypertens Rep. 2003;5:393–401.
134. Good D, Morse SA, Ventura HO, Reisin E. Obesity, hypertension, and the heart. J Cardiometab Syndr. 2008;3:168–72.
135. Pilz B, Brasen JH, Schneider W, Luft FC. Obesity and hypertension-induced restrictive cardiomyopathy: a harbinger of things to come. Hypertension. 2004;43:911–7.
136. Kannel WB, Cobb J. Left ventricular hypertrophy and mortality–results from the Framingham Study. Cardiology. 1992;81:291–8.
137. Fox CS, Larson MG, Leip EP, Culleton B, Wilson PW, Levy D. Predictors of new-onset kidney disease in a community-based population. JAMA. 2004;291:844–50.
138. Palaniappan L, Carnethon M, Fortmann SP. Association between microalbuminuria and the metabolic syndrome: NHANES III. Am J Hypertens. 2003;16:952–8.
139. Chen J, Muntner P, Hamm LL, et al. The metabolic syndrome and chronic kidney disease in U.S. adults. Ann Intern Med. 2004;140:167–74.
140. Festa A, D'Agostino R, Howard G, Mykkanen L, Tracy RP, Haffner SM. Inflammation and microalbuminuria in nondiabetic and type 2 diabetic subjects: the Insulin Resistance Atherosclerosis Study. Kidney Int. 2000;58:1703–10.
141. Festa A, D'Agostino Jr R, Howard G, Mykkanen L, Tracy RP, Haffner SM. Chronic subclinical inflammation as part of the insulin resistance syndrome: the Insulin Resistance Atherosclerosis Study (IRAS). Circulation. 2000;102:42–7.
142. Das UN. Is obesity an inflammatory condition? Nutrition. 2001;17:953–66.
143. Rumore MM, Kim KS. Potential role of salicylates in type 2 diabetes. Ann Pharmacother. 2010;44:1207–21.
144. McCarty MF. Salsalate may have broad utility in the prevention and treatment of vascular disorders and the metabolic syndrome. Med Hypotheses. 2010;75:276–81.
145. Koska J, Ortega E, Bunt JC, et al. The effect of salsalate on insulin action and glucose tolerance in obese non-diabetic patients: results of a randomised double-blind placebo-controlled study. Diabetologia. 2009;52:385–93.
146. Fleischman A, Shoelson SE, Bernier R, Goldfine AB. Salsalate improves glycemia and inflammatory parameters in obese young adults. Diabetes Care. 2008;31:289–94.
147. Goldfine AB, Fonseca V, Jablonski KA, Pyle L, Staten MA, Shoelson SE. The effects of salsalate on glycemic control in patients with type 2 diabetes: a randomized trial. Ann Intern Med. 2010;152:346–57.
148. Konstantinides S, Schafer K, Loskutoff DJ. The prothrombotic effects of leptin possible implications for the risk of cardiovascular disease in obesity. Ann N Y Acad Sci. 2001;947:134–41; discussion 141–2.
149. Konstantinides S, Schafer K, Koschnick S, Loskutoff DJ. Leptin-dependent platelet aggregation and arterial thrombosis suggests a mechanism for atherothrombotic disease in obesity. J Clin Invest. 2001;108:1533–40.
150. Terzolo M, Reimondo G, Bovio S, Angeli A. Subclinical Cushing's syndrome. Pituitary. 2004;7:217–23.
151. Terzolo M, Bovio S, Pia A, et al. Subclinical Cushing's syndrome. Arq Bras Endocrinol Metabol. 2007;51:1272–9.
152. Mazzuco TL, Bourdeau I, Lacroix A. Adrenal incidentalomas and subclinical Cushing's syndrome: diagnosis and treatment. Curr Opin Endocrinol Diabetes Obes. 2009;16:203–10.
153. Gagliardi L, Torpy DJ. Subclinical Cushing's syndrome in adrenal incidentaloma: a common problem or an artefact of current diagnostic testing? Clin Endocrinol (Oxf). 2010; 72:277–8.

154. Terzolo M, Pia A, Ali A, et al. Adrenal incidentaloma: a new cause of the metabolic syndrome? J Clin Endocrinol Metab. 2002;87:998–1003.
155. Rossi R, Tauchmanova L, Luciano A, et al. Subclinical Cushing's syndrome in patients with adrenal incidentaloma: clinical and biochemical features. J Clin Endocrinol Metab. 2000;85:1440–8.
156. Baguet JP, Narkiewicz K, Mallion JM. Update on hypertension management: obstructive sleep apnea and hypertension. J Hypertens. 2006;24:205–8.
157. Tufik S, Santos-Silva R, Taddei JA, Bittencourt LR. Obstructive sleep apnea syndrome in the Sao Paulo Epidemiologic Sleep Study. Sleep Med. 2010;11:441–6.
158. Shah N, Roux F. The relationship of obesity and obstructive sleep apnea. Clin Chest Med. 2009;30:455–65; vii.
159. de Sousa AG, Cercato C, Mancini MC, Halpern A. Obesity and obstructive sleep apnea-hypopnea syndrome. Obes Rev. 2008;9:340–54.
160. Zhang XL. [Obstructive sleep apnea hypopnea and metabolic syndromes]. Zhonghua Jie He He Hu Xi Za Zhi. 2007;30:891–3.
161. Peppard PE, Young T, Palta M, Dempsey J, Skatrud J. Longitudinal study of moderate weight change and sleep-disordered breathing. JAMA. 2000;284:3015–21.
162. Peppard PE, Young T, Palta M, Skatrud J. Prospective study of the association between sleep-disordered breathing and hypertension. N Engl J Med. 2000;342:1378–84.
163. Morrell MJ, Finn L, Kim H, Peppard PE, Badr MS, Young T. Sleep fragmentation, awake blood pressure, and sleep-disordered breathing in a population-based study. Am J Respir Crit Care Med. 2000;162:2091–6.
164. Young T, Peppard P. Sleep-disordered breathing and cardiovascular disease: epidemiologic evidence for a relationship. Sleep. 2000;23 Suppl 4:S122–6.
165. Bausmer U, Gouveris H, Selivanova O, Goepel B, Mann W. Correlation of the Epworth Sleepiness Scale with respiratory sleep parameters in patients with sleep-related breathing disorders and upper airway pathology. Eur Arch Otorhinolaryngol. 2010;267:1645–8.
166. Jacobs CK, Coffey J. Clinical inquiries. Sleep apnea in adults: how accurate is clinical prediction? J Fam Pract. 2009;58:327–8.
167. Dimsdale JE, Coy T, Ziegler MG, Ancoli-Israel S, Clausen J. The effect of sleep apnea on plasma and urinary catecholamines. Sleep. 1995;18:377–81.
168. Narkiewicz K, Pesek CA, Kato M, Phillips BG, Davison DE, Somers VK. Baroreflex control of sympathetic nerve activity and heart rate in obstructive sleep apnea. Hypertension. 1998;32:1039–43.
169. Robinson GV, Stradling JR, Davies RJ. Sleep. 6: obstructive sleep apnoea/hypopnoea syndrome and hypertension. Thorax. 2004;59:1089–94.
170. Robinson GV, Pepperell JC, Segal HC, Davies RJ, Stradling JR. Circulating cardiovascular risk factors in obstructive sleep apnoea: data from randomised controlled trials. Thorax. 2004;59:777–82.
171. Lesske J, Fletcher EC, Bao G, Unger T. Hypertension caused by chronic intermittent hypoxia–influence of chemoreceptors and sympathetic nervous system. J Hypertens. 1997;15:1593–603.
172. Bao G, Metreveli N, Li R, Taylor A, Fletcher EC. Blood pressure response to chronic episodic hypoxia: role of the sympathetic nervous system. J Appl Physiol. 1997;83:95–101.
173. Bao G, Randhawa PM, Fletcher EC. Acute blood pressure elevation during repetitive hypocapnic and eucapnic hypoxia in rats. J Appl Physiol. 1997;82:1071–8.
174. Baguet JP, Erdine S, Mallion JM. European Society of Hypertension Scientific Newsletter: update on hypertension management: hypertension and dysrhythmias. J Hypertens. 2006;24:409–11.
175. Kato M, Roberts-Thomson P, Phillips BG, et al. Impairment of endothelium-dependent vasodilation of resistance vessels in patients with obstructive sleep apnea. Circulation. 2000;102:2607–10.

176. Duchna HW, Stoohs R, Guilleminault C, Christine Anspach M, Schultze-Werninghaus G, Orth M. Vascular endothelial dysfunction in patients with mild obstructive sleep apnea syndrome. Wien Med Wochenschr. 2006;156:596–604.
177. Duchna HW, Orth M, Schultze-Werninghaus G, Guilleminault C, Stoohs RA. Antihypertensive treatment and endothelium-dependent venodilation in sleep-disordered breathing. Sleep Breath. 2006;10:115–22.
178. Gjorup PH, Sadauskiene L, Wessels J, Nyvad O, Strunge B, Pedersen EB. Abnormally increased endothelin-1 in plasma during the night in obstructive sleep apnea: relation to blood pressure and severity of disease. Am J Hypertens. 2007;20:44–52.
179. Phillips BG, Narkiewicz K, Pesek CA, Haynes WG, Dyken ME, Somers VK. Effects of obstructive sleep apnea on endothelin-1 and blood pressure. J Hypertens. 1999;17:61–6.
180. Moller DS, Lind P, Strunge B, Pedersen EB. Abnormal vasoactive hormones and 24-hour blood pressure in obstructive sleep apnea. Am J Hypertens. 2003;16:274–80.
181. Pimenta E, Calhoun DA, Oparil S. Sleep apnea, aldosterone, and resistant hypertension. Prog Cardiovasc Dis. 2009;51:371–80.
182. Gonzaga CC, Calhoun DA. Resistant hypertension and hyperaldosteronism. Curr Hypertens Rep. 2008;10:496–503.
183. Calhoun DA, Nishizaka MK, Zaman MA, Harding SM. Aldosterone excretion among subjects with resistant hypertension and symptoms of sleep apnea. Chest. 2004;125:112–7.
184. Calhoun DA. Use of aldosterone antagonists in resistant hypertension. Prog Cardiovasc Dis. 2006;48:387–96.
185. Fletcher EC, Bao G, Li R. Renin activity and blood pressure in response to chronic episodic hypoxia. Hypertension. 1999;34:309–14.
186. Masserini B, Morpurgo PS, Donadio F, et al. Reduced levels of adiponectin in sleep apnea syndrome. J Endocrinol Invest. 2006;29:700–5.
187. Zhang XL, Yin KS, Wang H, Su S. Serum adiponectin levels in adult male patients with obstructive sleep apnea hypopnea syndrome. Respiration. 2006;73:73–7.
188. Makino S, Handa H, Suzukawa K, et al. Obstructive sleep apnoea syndrome, plasma adiponectin levels, and insulin resistance. Clin Endocrinol (Oxf). 2006;64:12–9.
189. Zhang XL, Yin KS, Li C, Jia EZ, Li YQ, Gao ZF. Effect of continuous positive airway pressure treatment on serum adiponectin level and mean arterial pressure in male patients with obstructive sleep apnea syndrome. Chin Med J (Engl). 2007;120:1477–81.
190. Wassertheil-Smoller S, Blaufox MD, Oberman AS, Langford HG, Davis BR, Wylie-Rosett J. The Trial of Antihypertensive Interventions and Management (TAIM) study. Adequate weight loss, alone and combined with drug therapy in the treatment of mild hypertension. Arch Intern Med. 1992;152:131–6.
191. Wofford MR, Smith G, Minor DS. The treatment of hypertension in obese patients. Curr Hypertens Rep. 2008;10:143–50.
192. Chobanian AV, Bakris GL, Black HR, et al. Seventh report of the Joint National Committee on Prevention, Detection, Evaluation, and Treatment of High Blood Pressure. Hypertension. 2003;42:1206–52.
193. Reisin E, Hutchinson HG. Obesity-hypertension:the effects on cardiovascular and renal systems–the therapeutic approach. In: Oparil S, Weber MA, editors. Hypertension. Philadelphia: W.B. Saunders; 1999. p. 206–10.
194. Battling Obesity & Hypertension. Does the DASH diet really reduce blood pressure? AWHONN Lifelines. 2002;6:21–3.
195. Appel LJ, Moore TJ, Obarzanek E, et al. A clinical trial of the effects of dietary patterns on blood pressure. DASH Collaborative Research Group. N Engl J Med. 1997;336:1117–24.
196. Reisin E, Abel R, Modan M, Silverberg DS, Eliahou HE, Modan B. Effect of weight loss without salt restriction on the reduction of blood pressure in overweight hypertensive patients. N Engl J Med. 1978;298:1–6.
197. Reisin E, Frohlich ED. Effects of weight reduction on arterial pressure. J Chronic Dis. 1982;35:887–91.

198. Kannel WB, Brand N, Skinner Jr JJ, Dawber TR, McNamara PM. The relation of adiposity to blood pressure and development of hypertension. The Framingham study. Ann Intern Med. 1967;67:48–59.
199. The effects of nonpharmacologic interventions on blood pressure of persons with high normal levels. Results of the Trials of Hypertension Prevention, Phase I. JAMA. 1992;267: 1213–20.
200. Whelton PK, Appel LJ, Espeland MA, et al. Sodium reduction and weight loss in the treatment of hypertension in older persons: a randomized controlled trial of nonpharmacologic interventions in the elderly (TONE). TONE Collaborative Research Group. JAMA. 1998;279:839–46.
201. Neter JE, Stam BE, Kok FJ, Grobbee DE, Geleijnse JM. Influence of weight reduction on blood pressure: a meta-analysis of randomized controlled trials. Hypertension. 2003;42:878–84.
202. Harsha DW, Bray GA. Weight loss and blood pressure control (Pro). Hypertension. 2008;51:1420–5; discussion 1425.
203. Sacks FM, Svetkey LP, Vollmer WM, et al. Effects on blood pressure of reduced dietary sodium and the Dietary Approaches to Stop Hypertension (DASH) diet. DASH-Sodium Collaborative Research Group. N Engl J Med. 2001;344:3–10.
204. Vollmer WM, Sacks FM, Svetkey LP. New insights into the effects on blood pressure of diets low in salt and high in fruits and vegetables and low-fat dairy products. Curr Control Trials Cardiovasc Med. 2001;2:71–4.
205. Vollmer WM, Sacks FM, Ard J, et al. Effects of diet and sodium intake on blood pressure: subgroup analysis of the DASH-sodium trial. Ann Intern Med. 2001;135:1019–28.
206. Weinberger MH. Salt sensitivity of blood pressure in humans. Hypertension. 1996;27: 481–90.
207. Hoffmann IS, Alfieri AB, Cubeddu LX. Salt-resistant and salt-sensitive phenotypes determine the sensitivity of blood pressure to weight loss in overweight/obese patients. J Clin Hypertens (Greenwich). 2008;10:355–61.
208. Gillum RF, Prineas RJ, Jeffery RW, et al. Nonpharmacologic therapy of hypertension: the independent effects of weight reduction and sodium restriction in overweight borderline hypertensive patients. Am Heart J. 1983;105:128–33.
209. Jeffery RW, Gillum R, Gerber WM, Jacobs D, Elmer PJ, Prineas RJ. Weight and sodium reduction for the prevention of hypertension: a comparison of group treatment and individual counseling. Am J Public Health. 1983;73:691–3.
210. Dunn AL, Marcus BH, Kampert JB, Garcia ME, Kohl III HW, Blair SN. Comparison of lifestyle and structured interventions to increase physical activity and cardiorespiratory fitness: a randomized trial. JAMA. 1999;281:327–34.
211. Andersen RE, Wadden TA, Bartlett SJ, Zemel B, Verde TJ, Franckowiak SC. Effects of lifestyle activity vs structured aerobic exercise in obese women: a randomized trial. JAMA. 1999;281:335–40.
212. Fagard R, Bielen E, Hespel P. Physical exercise in hypertension. In: Laralaragh J, Renner B, editors. Hypertension pathophysiology, diagnosis and management. New York: Raven Press; 1990. p. 1985–8.
213. Whelton SP, Chin A, Xin X, He J. Effect of aerobic exercise on blood pressure: a meta-analysis of randomized, controlled trials. Ann Intern Med. 2002;136:493–503.
214. Lichtenstein AH, Appel LJ, Brands M, et al. Summary of American Heart Association Diet and Lifestyle Recommendations revision 2006. Arterioscler Thromb Vasc Biol. 2006;26:2186–91.
215. Lichtenstein AH, Appel LJ, Brands M, et al. Diet and lifestyle recommendations revision 2006: a scientific statement from the American Heart Association Nutrition Committee. Circulation. 2006;114:82–96.
216. Trapp EG, Chisholm DJ, Freund J, Boutcher SH. The effects of high-intensity intermittent exercise training on fat loss and fasting insulin levels of young women. Int J Obes (Lond). 2008;32:684–91.

217. Institute of Medicine. Dietary reference intakes for energy, carbohydrates, fibre, fat, fatty acids, cholesterol and protein and amino acids. Washington DC: Food and Nutrition Board; 2002.
218. Reisin E, Jack AV. Obesity and hypertension: mechanisms, cardio-renal consequences, and therapeutic approaches. Med Clin North Am. 2009;93:733–51.
219. Fuchs FD. Vascular effects of alcoholic beverages: is it only alcohol that matters? Hypertension. 2005;45:851–2.
220. Gordon T, Kannel WB. Drinking habits and cardiovascular disease: the Framingham Study. Am Heart J. 1983;105:667–73.
221. Gordon T, Kannel WB. Drinking and its relation to smoking, BP, blood lipids, and uric acid. The Framingham study. Arch Intern Med. 1983;143:1366–74.
222. Klatsky AL, Friedman GD, Siegelaub AB, Gerard MJ. Alcohol consumption among white, black, or oriental men and women: Kaiser-Permanente multiphasic health examination data. Am J Epidemiol. 1977;105:311–23.
223. Klatsky AL, Friedman GD, Siegelaub AB, Gerard MJ. Alcohol consumption and blood pressure Kaiser-Permanente Multiphasic Health Examination data. N Engl J Med. 1977;296:1194–200.
224. Puddey IB, Parker M, Beilin LJ, Vandongen R, Masarei JR. Effects of alcohol and caloric restrictions on blood pressure and serum lipids in overweight men. Hypertension. 1992; 20:533–41.
225. Parker M, Puddey IB, Beilin LJ, Vandongen R. Two-way factorial study of alcohol and salt restriction in treated hypertensive men. Hypertension. 1990;16:398–406.
226. Klatsky AL, Gunderson E. Alcohol and hypertension: a review. J Am Soc Hypertens. 2008;2:307–17.
227. Boutelle KN, Kirschenbaum DS. Further support for consistent self-monitoring as a vital component of successful weight control. Obes Res. 1998;6:219–24.
228. Schouten R, Wiryasaputra DC, van Dielen FM, van Gemert WG, Greve JW. Long-term results of bariatric restrictive procedures: a prospective study. Obes Surg. 2010;20: 1617–26.
229. Abeles D, Shikora SA. Bariatric surgery: current concepts and future directions. Aesthet Surg J. 2008;28:79–84.
230. Sebastian JL. Bariatric surgery and work-up of the massive weight loss patient. Clin Plast Surg. 2008;35:11–26.
231. Grassi G, Seravalle G, Dell'Oro R, et al. Comparative effects of candesartan and hydrochlorothiazide on blood pressure, insulin sensitivity, and sympathetic drive in obese hypertensive individuals: results of the CROSS study. J Hypertens. 2003;21:1761–9.
232. Reisin E, Tuck ML. Obesity-associated hypertension: hypothesized link between etiology and selection of therapy. Blood Press Monit. 1999;4 Suppl 1:S23–6.
233. Richards RJ, Thakur V, Reisin E. Obesity-related hypertension: its physiological basis and pharmacological approaches to its treatment. J Hum Hypertens. 1996;10 Suppl 3:S59–64.
234. Masuo K, Mikami H, Ogihara T, Tuck ML. Weight reduction and pharmacologic treatment in obese hypertensives. Am J Hypertens. 2001;14:530–8.
235. Clasen R, Schupp M, Foryst-Ludwig A, et al. PPARgamma-activating angiotensin type-1 receptor blockers induce adiponectin. Hypertension. 2005;46:137–43.
236. Brenner BM, Cooper ME, de Zeeuw D, et al. Effects of losartan on renal and cardiovascular outcomes in patients with type 2 diabetes and nephropathy. N Engl J Med. 2001;345: 861–9.
237. Parving HH, Brenner BM, Cooper ME, et al. [Effect of losartan on renal and cardiovascular complications of patients with type 2 diabetes and nephropathy]. Ugeskr Laeger. 2001; 163:5514–9.
238. Lewis EJ, Hunsicker LG, Clarke WR, et al. Renoprotective effect of the angiotensin-receptor antagonist irbesartan in patients with nephropathy due to type 2 diabetes. N Engl J Med. 2001;345:851–60.

239. Julius S, Kjeldsen SE, Weber M, et al. Outcomes in hypertensive patients at high cardiovascular risk treated with regimens based on valsartan or amlodipine: the VALUE randomised trial. Lancet. 2004;363:2022–31.
240. Cohn JN, Julius S, Neutel J, et al. Clinical experience with perindopril in African-American hypertensive patients: a large United States community trial. Am J Hypertens. 2004;17:134–8.
241. Julius S, Cohn JN, Neutel J, et al. Antihypertensive utility of perindopril in a large, general practice-based clinical trial. J Clin Hypertens (Greenwich). 2004;6:10–7.
242. Dahlof B, Devereux RB, Kjeldsen SE, et al. Cardiovascular morbidity and mortality in the Losartan intervention for endpoint reduction in hypertension study (LIFE): a randomised trial against atenolol. Lancet. 2002;359:995–1003.
243. Effects of ramipril on cardiovascular and microvascular outcomes in people with diabetes mellitus: results of the HOPE study and MICRO-HOPE substudy. Heart Outcomes Prevention Evaluation Study Investigators. Lancet. 2000;355:253–9.
244. Wilson IM, Freis ED. Relationship between plasma and extracellular fluid volume depletion and the antihypertensive effect of chlorothiazide. Circulation. 1959;20:1028–36.
245. Weir MR, Reisin E, Falkner B, Hutchinson HG, Sha L, Tuck ML. Nocturnal reduction of blood pressure and the antihypertensive response to a diuretic or angiotensin converting enzyme inhibitor in obese hypertensive patients. TROPHY Study Group. Am J Hypertens. 1998;11:914–20.
246. Major outcomes in high-risk hypertensive patients randomized to angiotensin-converting enzyme inhibitor or calcium channel blocker vs diuretic: the antihypertensive and lipid-lowering treatment to prevent heart attack trial (ALLHAT). JAMA. 2002;288:2981–97.
247. Lithell H. Hypertension and hyperlipidemia. A review. Am J Hypertens. 1993;6:303S–8.
248. Gress TW, Nieto FJ, Shahar E, Wofford MR, Brancati FL. Hypertension and antihypertensive therapy as risk factors for type 2 diabetes mellitus. Atherosclerosis Risk in Communities Study. N Engl J Med. 2000;342:905–12.
249. Dahlof B, Sever PS, Poulter NR, et al. Prevention of cardiovascular events with an antihypertensive regimen of amlodipine adding perindopril as required versus atenolol adding bendroflumethiazide as required, in the Anglo-Scandinavian Cardiac Outcomes Trial-Blood Pressure Lowering Arm (ASCOT-BPLA): a multicentre randomised controlled trial. Lancet. 2005;366:895–906.
250. Lindholm LH, Carlberg B, Samuelsson O. Should beta blockers remain first choice in the treatment of primary hypertension? A meta-analysis. Lancet. 2005;366:1545–53.
251. Sowers JR, Bakris GL. Antihypertensive therapy and the risk of type 2 diabetes mellitus. N Engl J Med. 2000;342:969–70.
252. MacMahon SW, Macdonald GJ, Bernstein L, Andrews G, Blacket RB. Comparison of weight reduction with metoprolol in treatment of hypertension in young overweight patients. Lancet. 1985;1:1233–6.
253. MacMahon SW, Macdonald GJ, Bernstein L, Andrews G, Blacket RB. A randomized controlled trial of weight reduction and metoprolol in the treatment of hypertension in young overweight patients. Clin Exp Pharmacol Physiol. 1985;12:267–71.
254. Fagerberg B, Berglund A, Andersson OK, Berglund G, Wikstrand J. Cardiovascular effects of weight reduction versus antihypertensive drug treatment: a comparative, randomized, 1-year study of obese men with mild hypertension. J Hypertens. 1991;9:431–9.
255. Sarafidis PA, Bakris GL. Do the metabolic effects of beta blockers make them leading or supporting antihypertensive agents in the treatment of hypertension? J Clin Hypertens (Greenwich). 2006;8:351–6; quiz 357–8.
256. Sarafidis PA, Bakris GL. Are beta blockers passe for the treatment of hypertension? J Clin Hypertens (Greenwich). 2006;8:239–40.
257. Sarafidis PA, Bakris GL. Antihypertensive treatment with beta-blockers and the spectrum of glycaemic control. QJM. 2006;99:431–6.
258. Bakris GL, Fonseca V, Katholi RE, et al. Metabolic effects of carvedilol vs metoprolol in patients with type 2 diabetes mellitus and hypertension: a randomized controlled trial. JAMA. 2004;292:2227–36.

259. Hansson L, Zanchetti A, Carruthers SG, et al. Effects of intensive blood-pressure lowering and low-dose aspirin in patients with hypertension: principal results of the Hypertension Optimal Treatment (HOT) randomised trial. HOT Study Group. Lancet. 1998;351: 1755–62.
260. Staessen JA, Fagard R, Thijs L, et al. Randomised double-blind comparison of placebo and active treatment for older patients with isolated systolic hypertension. The Systolic Hypertension in Europe (Syst-Eur) Trial Investigators. Lancet. 1997;350:757–64.
261. Tuck ML, Bravo EL, Krakoff LR, Friedman CP. Endocrine and renal effects of nifedipine gastrointestinal therapeutic system in patients with essential hypertension. Results of a multicenter trial. The Modern Approach to the Treatment of Hypertension Study Group. Am J Hypertens. 1990;3:333S–41.
262. Krakoff LR, Bravo EL, Tuck ML, Friedman CP. Nifedipine gastrointestinal therapeutic system in the treatment of hypertension. Results of a multicenter trial. The Modern Approach to the Treatment of Hypertension (MATH) Study Group. Am J Hypertens. 1990;3:318S–25.
263. Bakris GL, Weir MR, Secic M, Campbell B, Weis-McNulty A. Differential effects of calcium antagonist subclasses on markers of nephropathy progression. Kidney Int. 2004;65: 1991–2002.
264. Major cardiovascular events in hypertensive patients randomized to doxazosin vs chlorthalidone: the antihypertensive and lipid-lowering treatment to prevent heart attack trial (ALLHAT). ALLHAT Collaborative Research Group. JAMA. 2000;283:1967–75.
265. Scheen AJ. Cardiovascular risk-benefit profile of sibutramine. Am J Cardiovasc Drugs. 2010;10:321–34.
266. Curfman GD, Morrissey S, Drazen JM. Sibutramine–another flawed diet pill. N Engl J Med. 2010;363:972–4.
267. James WP, Caterson ID, Coutinho W, et al. Effect of sibutramine on cardiovascular outcomes in overweight and obese subjects. N Engl J Med. 2010;363:905–17.
268. Gallhardo J, Davis N, Matthai S, Shield JP. European Medicines Agency withdrawal for sibutramine. Arch Dis Child. 2010;95:856.
269. Harrison-Woolrych M, Ashton J, Herbison P. Fatal and non-fatal cardiovascular events in a general population prescribed sibutramine in New Zealand: a prospective cohort study. Drug Saf. 2010;33:605–13.
270. Williams G. Withdrawal of sibutramine in Europe. BMJ. 2010;340:c824.
271. Aucott L, Poobalan A, Smith WC, Avenell A, Jung R, Broom J. Effects of weight loss in overweight/obese individuals and long-term hypertension outcomes: a systematic review. Hypertension. 2005;45:1035–41.
272. Avenell A, Broom J, Brown TJ, et al. Systematic review of the long-term effects and economic consequences of treatments for obesity and implications for health improvement. Health Technol Assess. 2004;8:iii–iv; 1–182.
273. Aucott L, Poobalan A, Smith WC, et al. Weight loss in obese diabetic and non-diabetic individuals and long-term diabetes outcomes–a systematic review. Diabetes Obes Metab. 2004;6:85–94.
274. Despres JP, Golay A, Sjostrom L. Effects of rimonabant on metabolic risk factors in overweight patients with dyslipidemia. N Engl J Med. 2005;353:2121–34.
275. Pi-Sunyer FX, Aronne LJ, Heshmati HM, Devin J, Rosenstock J. Effect of rimonabant, a cannabinoid-1 receptor blocker, on weight and cardiometabolic risk factors in overweight or obese patients: RIO-North America: a randomized controlled trial. JAMA. 2006;295:761–75.
276. Scheen AJ, Finer N, Hollander P, Jensen MD, Van Gaal LF. Efficacy and tolerability of rimonabant in overweight or obese patients with type 2 diabetes: a randomised controlled study. Lancet. 2006;368:1660–72.
277. Weaver TE, Chasens ER, Arora S. Modafinil improves functional outcomes in patients with residual excessive sleepiness associated with CPAP treatment. J Clin Sleep Med. 2009;5:499–505.
278. Bogan RK. Armodafinil in the treatment of excessive sleepiness. Expert Opin Pharmacother. 2010;11:993–1002.

279. Williams SC, Marshall NS, Kennerson M, Rogers NL, Liu PY, Grunstein RR. Modafinil effects during acute continuous positive airway pressure withdrawal: a randomized crossover double-blind placebo-controlled trial. Am J Respir Crit Care Med. 2010;181:825–31.
280. Ballard RD. Management of patients with obstructive sleep apnea. J Fam Pract. 2008; 57:S24–30.
281. Valentino RM, Foldvary-Schaefer N. Modafinil in the treatment of excessive daytime sleepiness. Cleve Clin J Med. 2007;74(561–6):568–71.
282. Abad VC, Guilleminault C. Pharmacological management of sleep apnoea. Expert Opin Pharmacother. 2006;7:11–23.
283. Boeve BF, Silber MH, Ferman TJ. Melatonin for treatment of REM sleep behavior disorder in neurologic disorders: results in 14 patients. Sleep Med. 2003;4:281–4.
284. Kryger M, Roth T, Wang-Weigand S, Zhang J. The effects of ramelteon on respiration during sleep in subjects with moderate to severe chronic obstructive pulmonary disease. Sleep Breath. 2009;13:79–84.
285. Nunes DM, Mota RM, Machado MO, Pereira ED, Bruin VM, Bruin PF. Effect of melatonin administration on subjective sleep quality in chronic obstructive pulmonary disease. Braz J Med Biol Res. 2008;41:926–31.
286. Tsaoussoglou M, Bixler EO, Calhoun S, Chrousos GP, Sauder K, Vgontzas AN. Sleep-disordered breathing in obese children is associated with prevalent excessive daytime sleepiness, inflammation, and metabolic abnormalities. J Clin Endocrinol Metab. 2010; 95(1):143–50.
287. Vgontzas AN, Liao D, Bixler EO, Chrousos GP, Vela-Bueno A. Insomnia with objective short sleep duration is associated with a high risk for hypertension. Sleep. 2009;32(4):491–7.
288. Vgontzas AN, Zoumakis E, Bixler EO, Lin HM, Collins B, Basta M, Peiovic S, Chrousos GP. Selective effects of CPAP on sleep apnoea-associated manifestations. Eur J Clin Invest. 2008;38(8):585–95.
289. Dorresteijn JA, Visseren FL, Spiering W. Mechanisms linking obesity to hypertension. Obes Rev. 2012;13:17–26.
290. Vasylyeva TL, Chennasamudram SP, Okogbo ME. Can we predict hypertension among pre-term children ? Clin Pediatr. 2011;50(10):936–42.
291. Humphreys MH. The brain splits obesity and hypertension. Nat Med. 2011;17(7):782–3.
292. Purkayastha S, Zhang G, Cai D. Uncoupling the mechanisms of obesity and hypertension by targeting hypothalamic IKK-beta and NF-kappaB. Nat Med. 2011;17(7):883–7.

Chapter 14
Central Mineralocorticoid Receptors and Cardiovascular Disease

Elise P. Gomez-Sanchez

Abstract This chapter briefly summarizes the history of the study of mineralocorticoid receptors (MR) in the CVO of the brain, hypothalamus, amygdala, and nucleus tractus solitarius, that modulate inflammatory response to injury and oxidative stress in the heart and vessels, as well as homeostatic control of the hemodynamic systems, including blood pressure, water and electrolyte balance, sodium appetite, and sympathetic drive to the heart and kidney. Unfortunately, much of our current knowledge is based on pathological functions. Though the currently available MR antagonists are valuable additions to the therapy for cardiovascular and renal disease, MR are expressed in specific neurons in other areas of the brain where they mediate diverse functions unrelated to the cardiovascular system, only some of which are well understood. The greatest expression of MR in the body is in the hippocampus where the receptors mediate trophic functions important to memory and cognition. Because of the crucial need to discover targets for the development of selective therapy for specific MR-mediated functions, the biology of the MR, transcriptional and non-transcriptional activity, and mechanisms conferring ligand specificity to aldosterone is also discussed.

Keywords Mineralocorticoid receptor • Brain • Hypertension • Inflammation • Aldosterone • Cardiovascular disease • Cortisol

E.P. Gomez-Sanchez (✉)
Research Service, G.V. (Sonny) Montgomery VA Medical Center, Jackson, MS, USA

Division of Endocrinology, Department of Medicine, The University of Mississippi Medical Center, Jackson, MS 39216, USA
e-mail: egomez-sanchez@umc.edu

C.A. Koch and G.P. Chrousos (eds.), *Endocrine Hypertension: Underlying Mechanisms and Therapy*, Contemporary Endocrinology, DOI 10.1007/978-1-60761-548-4_14,

Introduction

The term mineralocorticoid reflects the salient property of a class of adrenal corticosteroid hormones demonstrated at the time of the isolation of desoxycorticosterone (DOC) in the late 1930s: the regulated enhancement of vectorial transport of Na^+ and water in one direction, K^+ and H^+ in the other, across the epithelia of the renal tubule and amphibian urinary bladder [1]. It was also recognized very early that excessive mineralocorticoids raise the blood pressure [2–5] (reviewed in [6]). MR in non-epithelial cells, including those in neurons, cardiomyocytes, vascular smooth muscle, vascular endothelial cell, mediate diverse functions, only some of which are predicated on ion transport.

This chapter will address the MR in the brain, primarily neurons, that influence cardiovascular homeostasis and pathology, an area of study that increased dramatically in the 10 years since the clinical demonstration of the ameliorating effect of an MR antagonist in the RALES (Randomized ALdactone Evaluation Study) [7] trial. Interest in aldosterone has also been renewed by the recognition that primary aldosteronism is the most frequent cause of secondary hypertension [8] and that aldosterone levels within the high normal range predict the future development of hypertension in normotensive individuals [9, 10] and correlate with greater pathological myocardial remodeling in patients with essential hypertension [11, 12]. The crucial role of the inappropriate activation of MR within blood vessels, including cerebral vessels, in endothelial dysfunction and pathological remodeling will not be addressed [13]. Figure 14.1 illustrates brain areas that are important to mineralocorticoid hypertension.

History

A century after Addison described patients with adrenal cortical destruction as having "asthenic" hearts, deoxycorticosterone, DOC, the first mineralocorticoid to be isolated and synthesized, and deoxycorticosterone acetate (DOCA) were used to normalize fluid and electrolyte balance and strengthened cardiodynamics in patients with Addison's disease [14]. It was clear by then that overzealous replacement led to hypertension and renal damage in humans and experimental animals, particularly if paired with excess salt intake [2, 4, 5, 14]. Early studies demonstrated that subpressor doses of DOC augmented vascular responses to epinephrine and norepinephrine in healthy people on a normal salt diet, suggesting direct (vascular) and/or indirect (neural) effects on vascular tone led to the hypothesis that increased sympathetic drive was involved in essential hypertension [15].

Aldosterone, the primary endogenous mineralocorticoid, was isolated a few years later in 1952 [16–19], followed in 3 years by the description of the eponymous Conn's Syndrome, or Primary Aldosteronism, associated with hypertension and hypokalemia, and eventual heart and kidney failure [20]. Notwithstanding early evidence of direct cardiovascular and neural effects of mineralocorticoids [15, 21, 22]

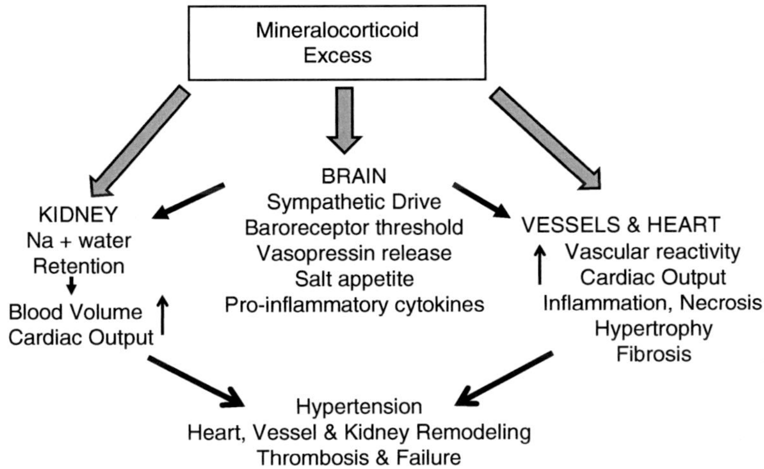

Fig. 14.1 Brain areas crucial to mineralocorticoid-salt and renovascular hypertension

and demonstration that DOCA produced hypertension in dialyzed animals after bilateral nephrectomy [23], retention of sodium and water by the kidneys became commonly accepted as primarily, if not exclusively, responsible for mineralocorticoid/salt excess hypertension, and the hypertension for pathological structural changes [2, 24, 25].

Mineralocorticoid Receptors in the Brain and Hypertension

Involvement of specific receptors for aldosterone in the neurohumoral control of cardiovascular and osmotic homeostasis was recognized by the 1960s [26, 27]. Autoradiographic studies demonstrated distinct receptors and binding characteristics for the two primary adrenal steroids, aldosterone and corticosterone, in the brain [28–30]. Among the areas of heaviest aldosterone binding are the hippocampus, circumventricular organ (CVO), some hypothalamic nuclei, and parts of the amygdala and brain stem. More recent immunohistochemical studies show that the MR is expressed in very specific neurons [31–34]. Ablation of specific hypothalamic and circumventricular areas, particularly an area anteroventral to the third ventricle, the AV3V area, prevented or attenuated the increase in blood pressure in renovascular and salt-sensitive forms of hypertension, including that of mineralocorticoid excess and some genetically hypertensive rat strains [35–41] (Fig. 14.1). Ablation of the AV3V area decreases sympathetic drive, baroreceptor sensitivity, and the systemic increases in vasopressin (VP) and serotonin produced by mineralocorticoid excess (reviewed in [42]). The AV3V area comprises the organum vasculosum of the lamina terminalis (OVLT), median preoptic nucleus, and afferents to the subfornical organ (SFO) and VP- and oxytocin-containing magnocellular neurons of the paraventricular nucleus (PVN). MR expression is dense in the OVLT,

SFO and in the area postrema (AP), all CVO outside the blood–brain barrier, where changes in osmotic pressure and concentrations of sodium and a large variety of circulating hormones and cytokines in the blood and cerebrospinal fluid are detected. Information from CVOs is relayed to the hypothalamus and other brain areas, including those regulating sympathetic drive to the heart, vessels, and kidneys [43–46]. While AV3V lesions prevent activation of the central sympathetic nervous system (SNS) in response to mineralocorticoids and centrally angiotensin II and attenuate the pressor response to systemic nitric oxide inhibition [45], they do not attenuate the vasoconstrictor actions of neural- or adrenal-derived catecholamines [43].

Selective infusions of mineralocorticoid receptor (MR) agonists and antagonists in various dog and rat models of hypertension confirmed and extended information from the ablation studies (reviewed in [47, 48]). Inappropriate activation of CVO MR mediates hypertension through an increase in sympathetic drive to the peripheral cardiovascular and renal systems, as well as through the release of VP and decreased baroreceptor sensitivity [42, 49–53] (see Fig. 14.2). Activation of MR of the amygdala increases sodium appetite [54–56].

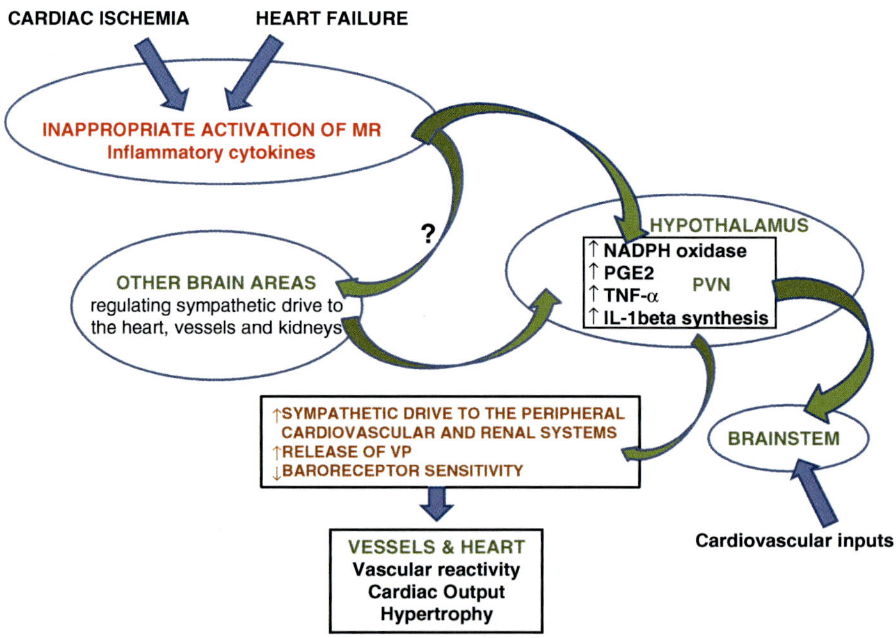

Fig. 14.2 Activation of MR in brain circumventricular organs during cardiac ischemia and heart failure paraventricular nucleus of hypothalamus (*PVN*), circumventricular organs (*CVO*), vasopressin (*VP*), see refs. [58, 60, 62] these are the primary and first to demonstrate the connection between heart damage, inflammation, the PVN and the SNS

Pivotal Role of the Central Sympathetic Nervous System

Patients with Primary Aldosteronism and renovascular hypertension have significantly greater sympathetic nerve activity than those with essential hypertension and non-hypertensive subjects and sympathetic nerve activity is normalized after surgical resolution of their disease [53, 57]. The persistent increase in sympathetic drive mediated by the activation of brain MR is responsible in part for the pathological structural remodeling and dysfunction following myocardial infarction in experimental animal models, even when circulating aldosterone levels are normal or low [58–63].

The central SNS is also activated by stress [64]. Cortisol, a major stress hormone, regulates the hypothalamic-pituitary-adrenal axis (HPA) through central glucocorticoid (GR) and mineralocorticoid receptors (MR). The activity of the HPA axis can be modulated by changes in function of the MR and GR [64–66].

MR, Inflammation, and Structural Changes in the Heart and Vessels

MR are involved and necessary in repair after tissue injury; however, prolonged and inappropriate activation leads to pathological remodeling and fibrosis. Inappropriate MR activation mediates the hypertrophy, inflammation, and fibrosis of the heart, vessels, and kidneys associated with Primary Aldosteronism [67–70], experimental mineralocorticoid/salt excess [6, 62, 71–75], and the hyperaldosteronism driven by elevated angiotensin II levels [72, 76–80]. These structural alterations and pathology can occur independently of significant hypertension [6, 48, 81, 82] and is preceded by inflammation in patients and animal models [6, 83–91]. The inappropriate activation of non-epithelial tissue MR also increases markers of oxidative stress, as well as diverse cellular mediators of inflammation in vitro and in vivo [92–97].

The progression of cardiac dysfunction to heart failure after experimental myocardial infarction is similar to that of mineralocorticoid excess and is mitigated by MR antagonists [58, 59, 98]. Inflammatory cytokines are involved in the communication between the injured heart and neurons in the PVN and AV3V area. Activation of MR in brain CVO during cardiac ischemia and heart failure leads to increased levels of neuronal activity, TNF-α and IL-1beta synthesis in the PVN, and TNF-α and IL-1beta levels in the blood and heart [59, 62, 99–104]. In addition, sympathetic afferent nerves from the injured heart signal to the brain to increase cytokine production [103] (Fig. 14.2).

Neurons of the AV3V area respond to IL-1beta, through a mechanism that includes the local synthesis of prostanoids, by exciting neurons of the medial preoptic area and PVN [105]. Circulating TNF-α and other proinflammatory cytokines induce cyclooxygenase (COX)-2 activity and synthesis of prostaglandin E2 by perivascular cells of vessels in the brain and thereby activate neurons in the PVN of hypothalamus, including corticotropin-releasing hormone (CRH) neurons. Treatment of a rat coronary ligation heart failure model with a MR antagonist significantly reduced cerebrospinal fluid prostaglandin E2, plasma norepinephrine, TNF-α, interleukin (IL)-1beta and IL-6, as well as hypothalamic COX-2 and CRH protein expression. The MR antagonist also decreased immunohistochemical staining in PVN neurons for TNF-α, interleukin (IL)-1beta, and CRH in the rat heart failure model. The effect of the MR antagonist was similar to that of etanercept and pentoxifylline, anti-cytokine drugs [106]. Along with amelioration of the inflammatory profile, left ventricular end-diastolic pressure and lower right ventricle/body weight and lung/body weight ratios were decreased; however, there was no improvement in left ventricular function of the MR antagonist-treated heart failure rats [103, 106]. These inflammatory responses are adaptive and necessary for the immediate response to injury and repair, presumably for the more common, less devastating insults to the myocardium [60]. Pretreatment and initiating MR antagonist treatment at the time of the coronary ligation decreased survival of the rats [60]. While the forebrain MR are crucial for repair and the short-term survival of cardiac ischemia induced by coronary ligation in the rat [60], their continued, excessive, and/or inappropriate activation exacerbates and accelerates the progression of heart failure due to inappropriate sympathetic nerve activity, volume retention, and inflammation that cannot be reversed with the systemic administration of antagonists of the renin-angiotensin system (RAS) [62].

Mineralocorticoid Receptor Biology

The MR is a member of the steroid nuclear receptor superfamily of ligand-activated transcription factors. Among these receptors, the MR shares the most homology with glucocorticoid receptors (GR). In addition to promoting gene transcription, MR also initiate rapid non-genomic effects through second messenger pathways [107–111] (reviewed by [109] and [112]). MR also appear to be activated in a steroid-independent fashion through transactivation by other signal transduction pathways, in particular that of angiotensin II [113].

The "Classical" genomic action of the MR is best understood (review [114]). Ligand-free MR is primarily located in the cytosol associated with chaperon and cell scaffolding proteins that alter the conformation of the molecule and anchor it in proximity to interacting proteins. Upon activation, MR are moved to the nucleus where they associate with the DNA as dimers [114–118]. MR form both homodimers and heterodimers with GR [119–121]. The effect of heterodimerization on transcriptional activity has not been completely elucidated, but is likely to have implications on glucocorticoid, as well as mineralocorticoid function [114, 122].

Like several other members of the steroid hormone transcription factor superfamily, notably the estrogen, androgen, and progesterone receptors, some MR are associated with the plasma membrane, probably in caveolae, and act through second messenger systems [109, 123–125]. Genomic or transcriptional effects mediated by

MR take several hours to occur; rapid non-genomic MR effects are initiated within minutes upon MR activation and may also result in the transcription of effector genes with a latency of 3 or more hours. Many, if not most, effects mediated by the MR, including the action of mineralocorticoids in the brain to increase salt appetite, as well as inflammation and repair, are mediated by both genomic and more rapid non-genomic actions [126–128].

Mineralocorticoid-mediated stimulation of the epithelial Na^+ channel and Na/K-ATPase pump were among the first MR-mediated intracellular effects studied, primarily in the nephron, colon, and toad bladder [129–131]. The increase in activity for both the ENaC and Na/K-ATPase are complex and multi-factorial, involving both genomic and non-genomic actions of MR leading to the net increase in channel activity and decrease in degradation [132–138]. Both ENaC and the Na/K-ATPase are instrumental in the central effects of aldosterone on blood pressure [139–142].

There is substantial evidence for an endogenous digitalis- or ouabain-like factor with an important role in the central control of the blood pressure [63, 142–148]. Endogenous ouabain is instrumental in the hypertension produced by the inappropriate activation of the MR during Na^+ repletion or excess in clinical and experimental conditions [142, 149–151]. Despite more than 30 years of concerted effort, the mechanism for its synthesis in a mammal has not been elucidated nor have intermediates been isolated [152, 153].

Mineralocorticoid Receptor Has Two Physiological Ligands

The MR are bound and, depending on the context, can be activated by two classes of steroid, the mineralocorticoids, principally aldosterone, and the glucocorticoids, cortisol, and corticosterone. The isolated or recombinant MR, which has also been called the "type I corticosteroid receptor," binds aldosterone, corticosterone, and cortisol with similar high affinity [154]. Circulating levels of aldosterone are regulated by Na^+, K^+, and angiotensin II in response to osmotic and hemodynamic need. Glucocorticoids are regulated by ACTH in a circadian manner and in response to energy needs and stress. As blood concentrations of glucocorticoids are normally 100–1,000 times greater than those of aldosterone, clearly circulating ligand concentrations are not the sole determinant of the extent of MR activation by aldosterone. MR splice variants so far described do not account for tissue-specific differences in MR ligand preference or activation specificity [155, 156]. MR specificity for aldosterone in epithelial mineralocorticoid target tissues is conferred extrinsically by the enzyme 11β-hydroxysteroid dehydrogenase type 2 (11β-HSD2) that converts cortisol and corticosterone to the inactive cortisone and 11-dehydrocorticosterone, allowing aldosterone access to the MR [157, 158]. 11β-HSD2 physically interacts with the MR within the endoplasmic reticulum membrane, thus the inactivation of cort and modulation of the relative levels of competing steroid occurs in very close proximity to the receptor [159–161]. Inactivating mutations of the 11β-HSD2 gene and pharmacological inhibition of the enzyme allow cortisol or corticosterone to activate renal tubular epithelial MR, producing Apparent Mineralocorticoid Excess characterized by Na^+ and water retention, K^+ and H^+ excretion, hypertension, and suppresses the renin-angiotensin-aldosterone system (RAAS) [162]. While the consequences of activation of the MR by aldosterone or cort are the same for some functions, including Na^+ retention in the kidney [163, 164], they are different for others, including many if not all of those in the CNS [165–171].

Another mechanism for 11β-HSD2 modulation of MR function has been proposed. MR in cells without 11β-HSD2 such as those in the hippocampus or heart are normally occupied by glucocorticoids and do not mediate inflammation or repair unless exposed to reactive oxygen species [89, 111, 172]. The hypothesis is that MR bound to glucocorticoids are inactive, including in cells that express 11β-HSD2. 11β-HSD2 requires NAD^+ as cofactor for dehydrogenase activity and generates NADH [159]. Inhibition of 11β-HSD2 allows the accumulation of the reactive oxygen species NAD^+, triggering the activation MR by glucocorticoids, for both specific functions normally attributed to aldosterone activation, as occurs in the renal tubule in AME, and inflammation and collagen formation, as occurs in the injured heart [173]. There are uncertainties about how 11β-HSD2 confers selectivity for aldosterone to the MR, yet it is clear that an understanding of the mechanisms that regulate glucocorticoid-activated MR activity is crucial to developing interventions into MR-mediated pathology, including the modulation of blood pressure and structural remodeling of the heart and vessels, by MR in the CNS, many of which do not appear to be associated with the 11β-HSD2 [174–176].

Autoradiography and functional tests demonstrate that MR in different parts of the brain have distinct preferences for either aldosterone or cort, with those in the hippocampus binding glucocorticoids and aldosterone in equal measure in adrenalectomized rats [29]. In vitro incubation of rat brain minces with tritiated precursors demonstrates the efficient conversion of corticosterone to the inactive steroid 11-dehydrocorticosterone [177, 178]. Moreover, intracerebroventricular infusions of three different 11beta-HSD inhibitors at doses too small to have an effect systemically produce hypertension. The central infusion of an MR antagonist abrogates the hypertension produced by the systemic administration of 11beta-HSD inhibitors, demonstrating a specific MR-driven response [47, 179, 180]. 11β-HSD2 mRNA was detected in the circumventricular nuclei by in situ hybridization [181] and both 11β-HSD2 and MR have been detected in the same neuron in select neurons of the NTS by immunohistochemistry [32–34].

As mentioned above, though some MR functions are initiated by either aldosterone or cort, others are ligand-specific [167, 171, 182]. The mechanisms for ligand-selectivity and functional specificity for MR in the brain are not adequately explained. In addition to the large differences between the circulating levels of aldosterone and glucocorticoids, there is the expression of the multiple drug resistance protein or p-glycoprotein that actively pumps specific compounds, including steroids out of cells, including those that form the blood brain barrier. p-glycoproteins are expressed in neurons, particularly those of the granular cell layer of the dentate gyrus, in addition to microvascular endothelial cells and astrocyte podocytes touching the microvessels of the brain [183]. In humans, transport by p-glycoprotein, i.e., exclusion from the brain, is significantly less for aldosterone than for cortisol, while corticosterone extrusion is minimal, suggesting that corticosterone, which circulates at 5–10% the level of cortisol in the human, is a significant ligand for the MR and GR in the human brain [184, 185]. Aldosterone concentrations in the rat brain are slightly lower than those in plasma, still 1–2 orders of magnitude levels of corticosterone, the major glucocorticoid in the rat [186]. Therefore for the Multiple Drug Resistant protein system to be a determinant of MR ligand specificity, it would have to function at the level of the individual neuron as it has been found in the hippocampus [183].

There is evidence for two other mechanisms that may increase local concentrations of aldosterone in or near aldosterone target cells: synthesis of aldosterone within the brain and the formation of an aldosterone derivative that is not a substrate for the p-gycoprotein and can activate the MR. Neurosteroids are those synthesized in the brain independently of the synthesis in the periphery [187, 188]. The requisite components for aldosterone synthesis, including StAR protein, required for cholesterol transport into the mitochondria, and the enzymes required for de novo aldosterone synthesis from cholesterol, including the aldo synthase enzyme unique to the formation of aldosterone, are expressed in rat and human brains [177, 178, 189–193]. Aldosterone synthase immunoreactivity is localized in neurons in several areas of the brain where MR expression is dense, including the cerebellum and hippocampus [194]. Aldosterone is produced *in vitro* from endogenous substrates, as well as tritiated deoxycorticosterone and corticosterone, by brain tissue from intact and adrenalectomized rats with similar efficiency [178, 190]. The aldosterone content of the brain reflects that of the plasma in adrenal-intact rats on diets of different salt content [193]. Extra-adrenal synthesis of aldosterone can only be appreciated by removal of the adrenals. In adrenalectomized rats the aldosterone content of the brain is very low, but consistently measurable and significantly higher than that of the plasma, which is usually below the limits of detection [193]. These data suggest that aldosterone synthesis does occur in the brain, but that normally most of the brain aldosterone is derived from the adrenal gland. Inappropriate aldosterone production within the brain appears to be involved in the pathogenesis of hypertension in the Dahl Salt Sensitive rat. Salt-induced hypertension in the Dahl SS is prevented by the central infusion of a MR antagonist, as well as AV3V ablation, implicating MR in the CVO in the hypertension, even though circulating aldosterone in these rats is suppressed by the high salt diet [195]. The salt-sensitive hypertension in the Dahl SS rat is also mitigated by the central infusion of inhibitors of steroidogenic enzymes, including one specific for aldosterone synthase, implicating aldosterone synthesis within the brain in this model [176, 177, 196]. Transgenic rats expressing the aldosterone synthase enzyme driven by the Synapsin 1 promoter which targets neurons have hypertension. Like the Dahl SS, circulating aldosterone levels are normal (unpublished data).

Aldosterone production by the adrenal is tightly regulated primarily by dietary sodium and angiotensin II; however, information about the regulation of the brain RAS, including the AT1 receptor, by sodium status in areas associated with hemodynamic homeostasis has been inconsistent [197–200]. However, inhibition of the central, but not systemic RAAS, decreases sympathetic drive and activation of the peripheral RAAS and increases tissue and circulating inflammatory cytokines produced by coronary ligation, suggesting that synthesis of aldosterone within the brain is regulated by the local RAAS [58, 59].

Aldosterone, cortisol, corticosterone, testosterone, and estradiol circulate as esters of fatty acids that are more hydrophobic than the parent compound, thus concentrate in tissues, particularly the brain and fat [201, 202], and regulation of the synthesis of esters may be a mechanism to control tissue concentration of these steroids [203, 204]. Both estrogen and aldosterone esters are potent activators of their respective receptors; some aldosterone esters have greater biological activity than aldosterone [205–209]. Aldosterone esters are hydrolysed to aldosterone very rapidly in blood, plasma, and serum and are not differentiated from aldosterone by common methods of measurement of aldosterone [209]. We confirmed studies done by the late Mary Lockett demonstrating the existence of significant amounts of an aldosterone ester in the heart and brain and found that aldosterone-18-monoacetate and -21-mono-oleate are more potent as hypertensinogens when infused intracerebroventricularly than the parent compound aldosterone [209]. As the enzymes responsible for steroid esterification are specific to the steroid [204], one could speculate that the local regulation of aldosterone ester formation may be a mechanism to exert aldosterone selectivity for the MR.

An area of study with great potential for finding mechanisms for MR ligand-selectivity and ligand functional specificity in different cells is that of the differential distribution of proteins which interact with steroid receptors [114]. Cell type-specific chaperone proteins may alter the conformation, thus binding affinity for aldosterone of the MR compared to the glucocorticoids in some tissues. Upon binding to a ligand, the MR sheds the chaperone proteins and dimerizes either as a homo or heterodimer with the GR in the nucleus, before or upon binding to hormone response elements in the promoter regions of specific genes, initiating the expression of these genes by recruiting requisite transcriptional machinery [120, 210–214]

Review [114]. MR and glucocorticoid receptors (GR) are co-expressed in many cells of the brain, including cerebellar purkinje and hippocampal pyramidal cells [215], where heterodimerization of MR and GR appears to be important in the transcriptional regulation of glucocorticoid-responsive genes in the brain [122] [216]. It is probable that GR and MR heterodimerization figures in the control of blood pressure and neurohumoral control of peripheral inflammation. Transcription efficiency is modulated by co-activators or co-repressors, proteins that bind activated receptors. To date, there are no cofactors or hormone response elements known to be specific for the MR; however, Steroid Receptor Co-activator protein family members have distinct anatomical distribution in the brain, with expression of SRC-1a mRNA prominent in the circumventricular areas of the brain associated with blood pressure homeostasis, as well as mineralocorticoid hypertension [114, 217–219].

In conclusion, mineralocorticoid receptors in specific neurons of the brain, primarily those of the CVO, hypothalamus, and amygdala mediate hemodynamic control, as well as modulate inflammation and repair in peripheral target organs.

However, most of what is known is about their role in pathological conditions; we know very little about the function of MR in the brains of healthy individuals. MR antagonists greatly ameliorate and slow the progress of heart and renal failure and their therapeutic use continues to increase, despite the fact that the preponderance of MR in the brain has functions unrelated to cardiovascular homeostasis or inflammation. More must be learned about the basic biology and function of the MR in the various areas of the brain to guide the development of targeted therapeutic agents.

Acknowledgments This work was supported by Merit Review Medical Research funds from the Department of Veterans Affairs and NIH grants HL27255, HL27737 and HL75321. We are grateful to Dr. Eugen Melcescu who helped with the illustrations.

There are no conflicts of interest.

References

1. Steiger M, Reichstein T. Desoxy-corticosterone (21-oxy-progesterone). Aus d-3-oxo-etiocholensäure. Helv Chim Acta. 1937;20:1164.
2. Kuhlman D, Ragan C, Ferrebee JW, Atchley DW, Loeb RF. Toxic effects of deoxycorticosterone esters in dogs. Science. 1939;90:496–7.
3. Rodbard S, Freed SC. The effect of desoxycorticosterone acetate on the blood pressure of the dog. Endocrinology. 1942;30:365–8.
4. Luft R, Sjogren B. The effect of desoxycorticosterone acetate and sodium chloride on blood pressure and renal function. Acta Endocrinol (Copenh). 1949;3(1):56–70.
5. Knowlton AI, Loeb EN, et al. Desoxycorticosterone acetate studies on the reversibility of its effect on blood pressure and renal damage in rats. Endocrinology. 1949;45(4): 435–45.
6. Gomez-Sanchez EP. Brain mineralocorticoid receptors: orchestrators of hypertension and end-organ disease. Curr Opin Nephrol Hypertens. 2004;13(2):191–6.
7. Pitt B, Zannad F, Cody R, Castaigne APA, Palensky J, Wittes J. The effect of spironolactone on mobidity and mortality in patients with severe heart failure. Randomized Aldactone evaluation study investigators. N Engl J Med. 1999;341:709–17.
8. Gomez-Sanchez CE, Rossi GP, Fallo F, Mannelli M. Progress in primary aldosteronism: present challenges and perspectives. Horm Metab Res. 2010;42(6):374–81.
9. Vasan RS, Evans JC, Larson MG, et al. Serum aldosterone and the incidence of hypertension in nonhypertensive persons. N Engl J Med. 2004;351(1):33–41.
10. Newton-Cheh C, Guo CY, Gona P, et al. Clinical and genetic correlates of aldosterone-to-renin ratio and relations to blood pressure in a community sample. Hypertension. 2007;49(4):846–56.
11. Vasan RS, Evans JC, Benjamin EJ, et al. Relations of serum aldosterone to cardiac structure: gender-related differences in the Framingham Heart Study. Hypertension. 2004;43(5):957–62.
12. Wang TJ, Gona P, Larson MG, et al. Multiple biomarkers and the risk of incident hypertension. Hypertension. 2007;49(3):432–8.
13. Osmond JM, Rigsby CS, Dorrance AM. Is the mineralocorticoid receptor a potential target for stroke prevention? Clin Sci (Lond). 2008;114(1):37–47.
14. Anderson E, Kinsell LW, et al. The treatment of Addison's disease by the intraoral administration of desoxycorticosterone acetate tablets. J Clin Endocrinol Metab. 1949;9(12):1324–32.
15. Raab W, Humphreys RJ, Lepeschkin E. Potentiation of pressor effects of nor-epinephrine and epinephrine in man by desoxycorticosterone acetate. J Clin Invest. 1950;29(10):1397–404.

16. Grundy HM, Simpson SA, Tait JF. Isolation of a highly active mineralocorticoid from beef adrenal extract. Nature. 1952;169(4306):795–6.
17. Simpson SA, Tait JF, Wettstein A, et al. Konstitution des aldosterons, des neuen mineralocorticoids. Experientia. 1953;10:132–3.
18. Tait JF, Tait SAS. A steroid memoir: a decade (or more) of electrocortin (aldosterone). Steroids. 1988;51:213–50.
19. Tait SA, Tait JF, Coghlan JP. The discovery, isolation and identification of aldosterone: reflections on emerging regulation and function. Mol Cell Endocrinol. 2004;217(1–2): 1–21.
20. Conn JW. Primary aldosteronism, a new clinical syndrome. J Lab Clin Med. 1955;45:3–7.
21. Vanatta JC, Cottle KE. Effect of desoxycorticosterone acetate on the peripheral vascular reactivity of dogs. Am J Physiol. 1955;151:119–22.
22. Jones AW, Hart RG. Altered ion transport in aortic smooth muscle during deoxycorticosterone acetate hypertension in rats. Circ Res. 1975;37:333–41.
23. Langford HG, Snavely JR. Effect of DCA on development of renoprival hypertension. Am J Physiol. 1959;196:449–50.
24. Coleman TG, Grange HJ, Guyton AC. Whole-body autoregulation and hypertension. Circ Res. 1971;28(29):11–76.
25. Guyton AC. Dominant role of the kidneys and accessory role of whole-body autoregulation in the pathogenesis of hypertension. Am J Hypertens. 1989;2:575–85.
26. Labadie P. [Osmo- and tenso-receptors; neuro-hormonal reflex arcs regulating fluid volume]. Rev Prat. 1964;14:1507–16.
27. Anderson ND, Fanestil DD. Corticoid receptors in rat brain: evidence for an aldosterone receptor. Endocrinology. 1976;98:676–84.
28. Stumpf WE, Sar M. Glucocorticosteroids and mineralocorticosteroid hormone target sites in the brain. Autoradiographic studies with corticosterone, aldosterone, deoxycorticosterone: in interaction within the brain-pituitary-adrenocortical system. In: Lones MT, Gillham B, Dallman MF, Chattopadhyay S, editors. Within the brain–pituitary–adrenocortical system. London: Academic; 1979. p. 137–47.
29. Birmingham MD, Stumpf WE, Sar M. Nuclear localization of aldosterone in rat brain cells assessed by autoradiography. Experientia. 1979;35:1240–1.
30. De Kloet ER. Brain corticosteroid receptor balance and homeostatic control. Front Neuroendocrinol. 1991;12:95–164.
31. Gomez-Sanchez CE, de Rodriguez AF, Romero DG, et al. Development of a panel of monoclonal antibodies against the mineralocorticoid receptor. Endocrinology. 2006;147(3): 1343–8.
32. Geerling JC, Engeland WC, Kawata M, Loewy AD. Aldosterone target neurons in the nucleus tractus solitarius drive sodium appetite. J Neurosci. 2006;26(2):411–7.
33. Geerling JC, Loewy AD. Aldosterone in the brain. Am J Physiol Renal Physiol. 2009; 297(3):F559–76.
34. Shekhtman E, Geerling JC, Loewy AD. Aldosterone-sensitive neurons of the nucleus of the solitary tract: multisynaptic pathway to the nucleus accumbens. J Comp Neurol. 2007;501(2):274–89.
35. Sanders BJ, Johnson AK. Lesions of the anteroventral third ventricle prevent salt-induced hypertension in the borderline hypertensive rat. Hypertension. 1989;14:619–22.
36. Tramposch AF, Lopes OU, Chernicky CL, Ferrario CM. Alternative mechanism for attenuated pressor responses in AV3V-lesioned dogs. Am J Physiol. 1989;257:R431–8.
37. Brody MJ, Fink GD, Buggy J, Haywood JR, Gordon FJ, Johnson AK. The role of the anteroventral third ventrical (AV3V) region in experimental hypertension. Circ Res. 1978;43:2–13.
38. Buggy J, Fink GD, Haywood JR, Johnson AK, Brody MJ. Interruption of the maintenance phase of established hypertension by ablation of the anteroventral third ventricle (AV3V) in rats. Clin Exp Hypertens. 1978;1(3):337–53.
39. Brody MJ, Haywood JR, Touw KB. Neural mechanisms in hypertension. Annu Rev Physiol. 1978;42:441–53.

40. Songu-Mize E, Bealer SL, Caldwell RW. Effect of AV3V lesions on development of DOCA-salt hypertension and vascular Na+-pump activity. Hypertension. 1982;4(5):575–80.
41. Moreira TS, Takakura AC, Colombari E, Menani JV. Antihypertensive effects of central ablations in spontaneously hypertensive rats. Am J Physiol Regul Integr Comp Physiol. 2009;296(6):R1797–806.
42. Brody MJ, Varner KJ, Vasquez EC, Lewis SJ. Central nervous system and the pathogenesis of hypertension. Sites and mechanisms. Hypertension. 1991;18(5 Suppl):III7–12.
43. Whalen EJ, Beltz TG, Lewis SJ, Johnson AK. AV3V lesions attenuate the cardiovascular responses produced by blood-borne excitatory amino acid analogs. Am J Physiol. 1999;276(5 Pt 2):H1409–15.
44. Whalen EJ, Schoorlemmer GH, Beltz TG, Johnson AK, Lewis SJ. Effects of chronic lesions of the anteroventral region of the third ventricle on cardiac beta-adrenoceptor function in conscious rats. Brain Res. 2001;913(1):82–5.
45. Lewis SJ, Whalen EJ, Beltz TG, Johnson AK. Role of the anterior region of the third ventricle in the cardiovascular responses produced by systemic injection of a nitric oxide synthase inhibitor. Brain Res. 1999;830(1):191–4.
46. Brooks VL, Haywood JR, Johnson AK. Translation of salt retention to central activation of the sympathetic nervous system in hypertension. Clin Exp Pharmacol Physiol. 2005; 32(5–6):426–32.
47. Gomez-Sanchez EP. Central hypertensive effects of aldosterone. Front Neuroendocrinol. 1997;18:440–62.
48. Gomez-Sanchez EP, Gomez-Sanchez CE. Central regulation of blood pressure by the mineralocorticoid receptor. Mol Cell Endocrinol. 2012;350(2):289–98.
49. Janiak P, Brody MJ. Central interactions between aldosterone and vasopressin on cardiovascular system. Am J Physiol. 1988;255(1 Pt 2):R166–73.
50. Janiak PC, Lewis SJ, Brody MJ. Role of central mineralocorticoid binding sites in development of hypertension. Am J Physiol. 1990;259(5 Pt 2):R1025–34.
51. Bealer SL. Anteroventral third ventricle periventricular tissue contributes to cardiac baroreflex responses. Clin Exp Pharmacol Physiol. 2000;27(5–6):460–4.
52. Wei SG, Felder RB. Forebrain renin-angiotensin system has a tonic excitatory influence on renal sympathetic nerve activity. Am J Physiol Heart Circ Physiol. 2002;282(3):H890–5.
53. Kontak AC, Wang Z, Arbique D, et al. Reversible sympathetic overactivity in hypertensive patients with primary aldosteronism. J Clin Endocrinol Metab. 2010;95(10):4756–61.
54. Sakai RR, Nicolaidis S, Epstein AN. Salt appetite is suppressed by interference with angiotensin II and aldosterone. Am J Physiol. 1986;251:R762–8.
55. Sakai RR, Ma LY, Zhang DM, McEwen BS, Fluharty SJ. Intracerebral administration of mineralocorticoid receptor antisense oligonucleotides attenuate adrenal steroid-induced salt appetite in rats. Neuroendocrinology. 1996;64:425–9.
56. Sakai RR, McEwen BS, Fluharty SJ, Ma LY. The amygdala: site of genomic and nongenomic arousal of aldosterone-induced sodium intake. Kidney Int. 2000;57:1337–45.
57. Miyajima E, Yamada Y, Yoshida Y, et al. Muscle sympathetic nerve activity in renovascular hypertension and primary aldosteronism. Hypertension. 1991;17(6 Pt 2):1057–62.
58. Felder RB, Francis J, Weiss RM, Zhang ZH, Wei SG, Johnson AK. Neurohumoral regulation in ischemia-induced heart failure. Role of the forebrain. Ann N Y Acad Sci. 2001;940:444–53.
59. Francis J, Weiss RM, Wei SG, et al. Central mineralocorticoid receptor blockade improves volume regulation and reduces sympathetic drive in heart failure. Am J Physiol Heart Circ Physiol. 2001;281(5):H2241–51.
60. Francis J, Wei SG, Weiss RM, Beltz T, Johnson AK, Felder RB. Forebrain-mediated adaptations to myocardial infarction in the rat. Am J Physiol Heart Circ Physiol. 2002;282(5): H1898–906.
61. Zhang ZH, Francis J, Weiss RM, Felder RB. The renin-angiotensin-aldosterone system excites hypothalamic paraventricular nucleus neurons in heart failure. Am J Physiol Heart Circ Physiol. 2002;283(1):H423–33.

62. Felder RB, Francis J, Zhang ZH, Wei SG, Weiss RM, Johnson AK. Heart failure and the brain: new perspectives. Am J Physiol Regul Integr Comp Physiol. 2003;284(2): R259–76.
63. Huang BS, Leenen FH. The brain renin-angiotensin-aldosterone system: a major mechanism for sympathetic hyperactivity and left ventricular remodeling and dysfunction after myocardial infarction. Curr Heart Fail Rep. 2009;6(2):81–8.
64. Chrousos GP. Stress and disorders of the stress system. Nat Rev Endocrinol. 2009;5(7):374–81.
65. DeRijk RH, de Kloet ER. Corticosteroid receptor polymorphisms: determinants of vulnerability and resilience. Eur J Pharmacol. 2008;583(2–3):303–11.
66. Klok MD, Vreeburg SA, Penninx BWJH, Zitman FG, de Kloet ER, DeRijk RH. Common functional mineralocorticoid receptor polymorphisms modulate the cortisol awakening response: interactions with SSRIs. Psychoneuroendocrinology. 2011;36:484–94.
67. Tarazi RC, Ibrahim MM, Bravo EL, Dustan HP. Hemodynamic characteristics of primary aldosteronism. N Engl J Med. 1973;289(25):1330–5.
68. Tanabe A, Naruse M, Naruse K, et al. Left ventricular hypertrophy is more prominent in patients with primary aldosteronism than in patients with other types of secondary hypertension. Hypertens Res. 1997;20:85–90.
69. Rossi GP, Di Bello V, Ganzaroli C, et al. Excess aldosterone is associated with alterations of myocardial texture in primary aldosteronism. Hypertension. 2002;40(1):23–7.
70. Luft FC. Workshop: mechanisms and cardiovascular damage in hypertension. Hypertension. 2001;37(2 Pt 2):594–8.
71. Brilla CG, Murphy RL, Smits JF, Struijker Boudier HA. The concept of cardioreparation: part 1. Pathophysiology of remodelling. J Cardiovasc Risk. 1996;3:281–5.
72. Brilla CG, Rupp H, Funck R, Maisch B. The renin-angiotensin-aldosterone system and myocardial collagen matrix remodelling in congestive heart failure. Eur Heart J. 1995; 16(Suppl O):107–9.
73. Gerling IC, Sun Y, Ahokas RA, et al. Aldosteronism: an immunostimulatory state precedes proinflammatory/fibrogenic cardiac phenotype. Am J Physiol Heart Circ Physiol. 2003;285(2): H813–21.
74. Ahokas RA, Warrington KJ, Gerling IC, et al. Aldosteronism and peripheral blood mononuclear cell activation: a neuroendocrine-immune interface. Circ Res. 2003;93(10):e124–35.
75. Weber KT. Aldosteronism revisited: perspectives on less well-recognized actions of aldosterone. J Lab Clin Med. 2003;142(2):71–82.
76. Chander PN, Rocha R, Ranaudo J, Singh G, Zuckerman A, Stier Jr CT. Aldosterone plays a pivotal role in the pathogenesis of thrombotic microangiopathy in SHRSP. J Am Soc Nephrol. 2003;14(8):1990–7.
77. Brilla CG. The cardiac structure-function relationship and the renin-angiotensin-aldosterone system in hypertension and heart failure. Curr Opin Cardiol. 1994;9 Suppl 1:2–10.
78. Brilla CG, Reams GP, Maisch B, Weber KT. Renin-angiotensin system and myocardial fibrosis in hypertension: regulation of the myocardial collagen matrix. Eur Heart J. 1993;14(Suppl J):57–61.
79. Brilla CG, Matsubara LS, Weber KT. Anti-aldosterone treatment and the prevention of myocardial fibrosis in primary and secondary hyperaldosteronism. J Mol Cell Card. 1993;25:563–75.
80. Yu Y, Wei SG, Zhang ZH, Gomez-Sanchez E, Weiss RM, Felder RB. Does aldosterone upregulate the brain renin-angiotensin system in rats with heart failure? Hypertension. 2008;51(3):727–33.
81. Rocha R, Funder JW. The pathophysiology of aldosterone in the cardiovascular system. Ann N Y Acad Sci. 2002;970:89–100.
82. Young MJ. Mechanisms of mineralocorticoid receptor-mediated cardiac fibrosis and vascular inflammation. Curr Opin Nephrol Hypertens. 2008;17(2):174–80.
83. Rocha R, Stier CT, Kifor I, et al. Aldosterone: a mediator of myocardial necrosis and renal arteriopathy. Endocrinology. 2000;141:3871–8.

84. Rocha R, Rudolph AE, Frierdich GE, et al. Aldosterone induces a vascular inflammatory phenotype in the rat heart. Am J Physiol Heart Circ Physiol. 2002;283(5):H1802–10.
85. Blasi ER, Rocha R, Rudolph AE, Blomme EA, Polly ML, McMahon EG. Aldosterone/salt induces renal inflammation and fibrosis in hypertensive rats. Kidney Int. 2003;63(5): 1791–800.
86. Weber KT. The proinflammatory heart failure phenotype: a case of integrative physiology. Am J Med Sci. 2005;330(5):219–26.
87. Quinkler M, Zehnder D, Eardley KS, et al. Increased expression of mineralocorticoid effector mechanisms in kidney biopsies of patients with heavy proteinuria. Circulation. 2005;112(10): 1435–43.
88. Joffe HV, Adler GK. Effect of aldosterone and mineralocorticoid receptor blockade on vascular inflammation. Heart Fail Rev. 2005;10(1):31–7.
89. Funder JW. RALES, EPHESUS and redox. J Steroid Biochem Mol Biol. 2005;93(2–5):121–5.
90. Godfrey V, Farquharson CA, Macdonald JE, Yee KM, Struthers AD. Effect of spironolactone on C-reactive protein levels in patients with heart disease. Int J Cardiol. 2007;117(2):282–4.
91. Fiebeler A, Nussberger J, Shagdarsuren E, et al. Aldosterone synthase inhibitor ameliorates angiotensin II-induced organ damage. Circulation. 2005;111(23):3087–94.
92. Brown NJ. Aldosterone and end-organ damage. Curr Opin Nephrol Hypertens. 2005;14(3): 235–41.
93. Gilbert KC, Brown NJ. Aldosterone and inflammation. Curr Opin Endocrinol Diabetes Obes. 2010;17(3):199–204.
94. Brown NJ. Aldosterone and vascular inflammation. Hypertension. 2008;51(2):161–7.
95. Marney AM, Brown NJ. Aldosterone and end-organ damage. Clin Sci (Lond). 2007;113(6): 267–78.
96. Luther JM, Gainer JV, Murphey LJ, et al. Angiotensin II induces interleukin-6 in humans through a mineralocorticoid receptor-dependent mechanism. Hypertension. 2006;48(6):1050–7.
97. Kraus D, Jager J, Meier B, Fasshauer M, Klein J. Aldosterone inhibits uncoupling protein-1, induces insulin resistance, and stimulates proinflammatory adipokines in adipocytes. Horm Metab Res. 2005;37(7):455–9.
98. Francis J, Weiss RM, Wei SG, Johnson AK, Felder RB. Progression of heart failure after myocardial infarction in the rat. Am J Physiol Regul Integr Comp Physiol. 2001;281(5):R1734–45.
99. Francis GS. Aldosterone inhibition and heart failure: too good to be true? Am Heart J. 2001;141(1):1–2.
100. Zhang ZH, Wei SG, Francis J, Felder RB. Cardiovascular and renal sympathetic activation by blood-borne TNF-alpha in rat: the role of central prostaglandins. Am J Physiol Regul Integr Comp Physiol. 2003;284(4):R916–27.
101. Francis J, Beltz T, Johnson AK, Felder RB. Mineralocorticoids act centrally to regulate blood-borne tumor necrosis factor-alpha in normal rats. Am J Physiol Regul Integr Comp Physiol. 2003;285(6):R1402–9.
102. Francis J, Weiss RM, Johnson AK, Felder RB. Central mineralocorticoid receptor blockade decreases plasma TNF-alpha after coronary artery ligation in rats. Am J Physiol Regul Integr Comp Physiol. 2003;284(2):R328–35.
103. Francis J, Zhang ZH, Weiss RM, Felder RB. Neural regulation of the proinflammatory cytokine response to acute myocardial infarction. Am J Physiol Heart Circ Physiol. 2004;287(2):H791–7.
104. Francis J, Chu Y, Johnson AK, Weiss RM, Felder RB. Acute myocardial infarction induces hypothalamic cytokine synthesis. Am J Physiol Heart Circ Physiol. 2004;286(6):H2264–71.
105. Ota K, Katafuchi T, Takaki A, Hori T. AV3V neurons that send axons to hypothalamic nuclei respond to the systemic injection of IL-1beta. Am J Physiol. 1997;272(2 Pt 2):R532–40.
106. Kang YM, Zhang ZH, Johnson RF, et al. Novel effect of mineralocorticoid receptor antagonism to reduce proinflammatory cytokines and hypothalamic activation in rats with ischemia-induced heart failure. Circ Res. 2006;99(7):758–66.
107. Fuller PJ, Young MJ. Mechanisms of mineralocorticoid action. Hypertension. 2005;46(6): 1227–35.

108. Funder JW. The nongenomic actions of aldosterone. Endocr Rev. 2005;26(3):313–21.
109. Grossmann C, Benesic A, Krug AW, et al. Human mineralocorticoid receptor expression renders cells responsive for nongenotropic aldosterone actions. Mol Endocrinol. 2005;19(7):1697–710.
110. Karst H, Berger S, Turiault M, Tronche F, Schutz G, Joels M. Mineralocorticoid receptors are indispensable for nongenomic modulation of hippocampal glutamate transmission by corticosterone. Proc Natl Acad Sci U S A. 2005;102(52):19204–7.
111. Mihailidou AS, Funder JW. Nongenomic effects of mineralocorticoid receptor activation in the cardiovascular system. Steroids. 2005;70(5–7):347–51.
112. Connell JM, Davies E. The new biology of aldosterone. J Endocrinol. 2005;186(1):1–20.
113. Jaffe IZ, Mendelsohn ME. Angiotensin II and aldosterone regulate gene transcription via functional mineralocortocoid receptors in human coronary artery smooth muscle cells. Circ Res. 2005;96(6):643–50.
114. Viengchareun S, Le Menuet D, Martinerie L, Munier M, Pascual-Le Tallec L, Lombes M. The mineralocorticoid receptor: insights into its molecular and (patho)physiological biology. Nucl Recept Signal. 2007;5:e012.
115. Hellal-Levy C, Fagart J, Souque A, Rafestin-Oblin ME. Mechanistic aspects of mineralocorticoid receptor activation. Kidney Int. 2000;57:1250–5.
116. Pearce D, Verrey F, Chen SY, et al. Role of SGK in mineralocorticoid-regulated sodium transport. Kidney Int. 2000;57:1283–9.
117. Bratton MR, Gomez-Sanchez EP, Gomez-Sanchez CE, Subauste JS. The myosin binding protein is a novel mineralocorticoid receptor binding partner. Mol Cell Endocrinol. 2004;217(1–2):221–7.
118. Echeverria PC, Mazaira G, Erlejman A, Gomez-Sanchez C, Pilipuk GP, Galigniana MD. Nuclear import of the glucocorticoid receptor-hsp90 complex through the nuclear pore complex is mediated by its interaction with Nup62 and importin beta. Mol Cell Biol. 2009;29(17):4788–97.
119. Savory JG, Prefontaine GG, Lamprecht C, et al. Glucocorticoid receptor homodimers and glucocorticoid-mineralocorticoid receptor heterodimers form in the cytoplasm through alternative dimerization interfaces. Mol Cell Biol. 2001;21(3):781–93.
120. Nishi M, Tanaka M, Matsuda K, Sunaguchi M, Kawata M. Visualization of glucocorticoid receptor and mineralocorticoid receptor interactions in living cells with GFP-based fluorescence resonance energy transfer. J Neurosci. 2004;24(21):4918–27.
121. Tsugita M, Iwasaki Y, Nishiyama M, et al. Glucocorticoid receptor plays an indispensable role in mineralocorticoid receptor-dependent transcription in GR-deficient BE(2)C and T84 cells *in vitro*. Mol Cell Endocrinol. 2009;302(1):18–25.
122. Trapp T, Rupprecht R, Castren M, Reul JM, Holsboer F. Heterodimerization between mineralocorticoid and glucocorticoid receptor: a new principle of glucocorticoid action in the CNS. Neuron. 1994;13:1457–62.
123. Rossol-Haseroth K, Zhou Q, Braun S, et al. Mineralocorticoid receptor antagonists do not block rapid ERK activation by aldosterone. Biochem Biophys Res Commun. 2004;318(1):281–8.
124. Haseroth K, Gerdes D, Berger S, et al. Rapid nongenomic effects of aldosterone in mineralo corticoid-receptor-knockout mice. Biochem Biophys Res Commun. 1999;266(1): 257–61.
125. Pedram A, Razandi M, Sainson RC, Kim JK, Hughes CC, Levin ER. A conserved mechanism for steroid receptor translocation to the plasma membrane. J Biol Chem. 2007; 282(31):22278–88.
126. Pietranera L, Saravia FE, McEwen BS, Lucas LL, Johnson AK, De Nicola AF. Changes in Fos expression in various brain regions during deoxycorticosterone acetate treatment: relation to salt appetite, vasopressin mRNA and the mineralocorticoid receptor. Neuroendocrinology. 2001;74(6):396–406.
127. Grossmann C, Gekle M. Nongenotropic aldosterone effects and the EGFR: interaction and biological relevance. Steroids. 2008;73(9–10):973–8.

128. Grossmann C, Gekle M. New aspects of rapid aldosterone signaling. Mol Cell Endocrinol. 2009;308(1–2):53–62.
129. Petty KJ, Kokko JP, Marver D. Secondary effect of aldosterone on Na-KATPase activity in the rabbit cortical collecting tubule. J Clin Invest. 1981;68(6):1514–21.
130. Marver D. Models of aldosterone action on sodium transport: emerging concepts. Adv Exp Med Biol. 1986;196:153–71.
131. Horisberger J-D, Canessa C, Rossier BC. The epithelial sodium channel: recent developments. Cell Physiol Biochem. 1993;3:283–94.
132. Zhang W, Xia X, Reisenauer MR, et al. Aldosterone-induced Sgk1 relieves Dot1a-Af9-mediated transcriptional repression of epithelial Na+ channel alpha. J Clin Invest. 2007;117(3): 773–83.
133. Pearce D, Kleyman TR. Salt, sodium channels, and SGK1. J Clin Invest. 2007;117(3):592–5.
134. Michlig S, Mercier A, Doucet A, et al. ERK1/2 controls Na, K-ATPase activity and transepithelial sodium transport in the principal cell of the cortical collecting duct of the mouse kidney. J Biol Chem. 2004;279(49):51002–12.
135. Mihailidou AS, Mardini M, Funder JW. Rapid, nongenomic effects of aldosterone in the heart mediated by epsilon protein kinase C. Endocrinology. 2004;145(2):773–80.
136. Summa V, Camargo SM, Bauch C, Zecevic M, Verrey F. Isoform specificity of human Na(+), K(+)-ATPase localization and aldosterone regulation in mouse kidney cells. J Physiol. 2004;555(Pt 2):355–64.
137. Nielsen J, Kwon TH, Frokiaer J, Knepper MA, Nielsen S. Maintained ENaC trafficking in aldosterone-infused rats during mineralocorticoid and glucocorticoid receptor blockade. Am J Physiol Renal Physiol. 2007;292(1):F382–94.
138. Musch MW, Lucioni A, Chang EB. Aldosterone regulation of intestinal Na absorption involves SGK-mediated changes in NHE3 and Na+ pump activity. Am J Physiol Gastrointest Liver Physiol. 2008;295(5):G909–19.
139. Gomez-Sanchez EP, Gomez-Sanchez CE. Effect of central amiloride infusion on mineralocorticoid hypertension. Am J Physiol. 1994,267:E754–8.
140. Gomez-Sanchez EP, Gomez-Sanchez CE. The effect of the central infusion of benzamil on Dahl S rat hypertension. Am J Physiol. 1995;269:H1044–7.
141. Gomez-Sanchez EP, Foecking MF, Sellers D, Blankenship MS, Gomez-Sanchez CE. Is the circulating ouabain-like compound ouabain? Am J Hypertens. 1994;7:647–50.
142. Gomez-Sanchez EP, Gomez-Sanchez CE, Fort C. Immunization of Dahl SS/jr rats with a ouabain conjugate mitigates salt-induced hypertension. Am J Hypertens. 1994;7:591–6.
143. Lichtstein D, Samuelov S. Endogenous digitalis-like activity in rat brain. Biochem Biophys Res Commun. 1980;96:1518–23.
144. Takahashi H, Matsuzawa M, Okabayashi H, et al. Evidence for a digitalis-like substance in the hypothalamopituitary axis in rats: implications in the central cardiovascular regulation associated with an excess intake of sodium. Jap Circ J. 1987;51:1199–207.
145. Buckalew VM, Haddy FJ. The role of digitalis-like factor in the pathophysiology of hypertension. In: Laragh JH, Brenner BM, editors. Endocrine mechanism in hypertension. 2nd ed. New York: Raven; 1989. p. 307–34.
146. Hamlyn JM, Manunta P. Ouabain, digitalis-like factors and hypertension. J Hypertens. 1992;10:S99–111.
147. Lichtstein D, Samuelov S. Endogenous ouabain like activity in rat brain. Biochem Biophys Res Commn. 1991;96:1518–23.
148. Wang H, Huang BS, Leenen FH. Brain sodium channels and ouabainlike compounds mediate central aldosterone-induced hypertension. Am J Physiol Heart Circ Physiol. 2003;285(6): H2516–23.
149. Blaustein MP, Hamlyn JM. Pathogenesis of essential hypertension. A link between dietary salt and high blood pressure. Hypertension. 1991;18:III184–95.
150. Blaustein MP, Hamlyn JM. Signaling mechanisms that link salt retention to hypertension: endogenous ouabain, the Na(+) pump, the Na(+)/Ca(2+) exchanger and TRPC proteins. Biochim Biophys Acta. 2010;1802(12):1219–29.

151. Manunta P, Hamlyn JM, Simonini M, et al. Endogenous ouabain and the renin-angiotensin-aldosterone system: distinct effects on Na handling and blood pressure in human hypertension. J Hypertens. 2011;29(2):349–56.
152. Hamlyn JM, Laredo J, Shah JR, Lu ZR, Hamilton BP. 11-Hydroxylation in the biosynthesis of endogenous ouabain: multiple implications. Ann N Y Acad Sci. 2003;986:685–93.
153. Tripodi G, Citterio L, Kouznetsova T, et al. Steroid biosynthesis and renal excretion in human essential hypertension: association with blood pressure and endogenous ouabain. Am J Hypertens. 2009;22(4):357–63.
154. Arriza JW, Weinberger C, Cerelli G, et al. Cloning of human mineralocorticoid receptor complementary DNA: structural and functional kinship with the glucocorticoid receptor. Science. 1987;237:268–75.
155. Zennaro MC, Farman N, Bonvalet JP, Lombes M. Tissue-specific expression of alpha and beta messenger ribonucleic acid isoforms of the human mineralocorticoid receptor in normal and pathological states. J Clin Endocrinol Metab. 1997;82:1345–52.
156. Zhou M-Y, Gomez-Sanchez CE, Gomez-Sanchez EP. An alternatively spliced mineralocorticoid receptor mRNA causing truncation of the steroid binding domain. Mol Cell Endocrinol. 2000;159:125–31.
157. Stewart PM, Corrie JET, Shackleton CHL, Edwards CRW. Syndrome of apparent mineralocorticoid excess. A defect in the cortisol-cortisone shuttle. J Clin Invest. 1988;82:340–9.
158. Funder JW, Pearce PT, Smith R, Smith AI. Mineralocorticoid action: target tissue specificity is enzyme, not receptor, mediated. Science. 1988;242:583–5.
159. Naray-Fejes-Toth A, Fejes-Toth G. Subcellular localization of the type 2 11beta-hydroxysteroid dehydrogenase. A green fluorescent protein study. J Biol Chem. 1996;271: 15436–42.
160. Naray-Fejes-Toth A, Fejes-Toth G. Extranuclear localization of endogenous 11beta-hydroxysteroid dehydrogenase-2 in aldosterone target cells. Endocrinology. 1998;139:2955–9.
161. Odermatt A, Arnold P, Frey FJ. The intracellular localization of the mineralocorticoid receptor is regulated by 11beta-hydroxysteroid dehydrogenase type 2. J Biol Chem. 2001;276(30): 28484–92.
162. White PC. 11beta-Hydroxysteroid dehydrogenase and its role in the syndrome of apparent mineralocorticoid excess. Am J Med Sci. 2001;322(6):308–15.
163. Ulick S, Levine LS, Gunczler P. A syndrome of apparent mineralocorticoid excess associated with defects in the peripheral metabolism of cortisol. J Clin Endocrinol Metab. 1979;49:757–64.
164. Funder JW, Pearce PT, Myles K, Roy LP. Apparent mineralocorticoid excess, pseudohypoaldosteronism, and urinary electrolyte excretion: toward a redefinition of mineralocorticoid action. FASEB J. 1990;4:3234–8.
165. De Kloet ER, Versteeg DHG, Kovacs GL. Aldosterone blocks the response to corticosterone in the raphe-hippocampal serotonin system. Brain Res. 1983;264:323–7.
166. Reul JMHM, van den Bosch FR, De Kloet ER. Relative occupation of type-I and type-II corticosteroid receptors in rat brain following stress and dexamethasone treatment: functional implications. J Endocrinol. 1987;115:459–67.
167. Gomez-Sanchez EP, Venkataraman MT, Thwaites D. ICV infusion of Corticosterone antagonizes ICV-aldosterone hypertension. Am J Physiol. 1990;258:E649–53.
168. van den Berg DTWM, De Kloet ER, van Dijken HH, de Jong W. Differential central effects of mineralocorticoid and glucocorticoid agonists and antagonists on blood pressure. Endocrinology. 1990;126:118–24.
169. Oitzl MS, van Haarst AD, Sutanto W, De Kloet ER. Corticosterone, brain mineralocorticoid receptors (MRs) and the activity of the hypothalamic-pituitary-adrenal (HPA) axis: the Lewis rat as an example of increased central MR capacity and a hyporesponsive HPA axis. Psychoneuroendocrinology. 1995;20:655–75.
170. van Acker SA, Oitzl MS, Fluttert MF, de Kloet ER. Centrally regulated blood pressure response to vasoactive peptides is modulated by corticosterone. J Neuroendocrinol. 2002;14(1):56–63.

171. Wilson P, Morgan J, Funder JW, Fuller PJ, Young MJ. Mediators of mineralocorticoid receptor-induced profibrotic inflammatory responses in the heart. Clin Sci (Lond). 2009;116(9): 731–9.
172. Funder JW. Mineralocorticoid receptors: distribution and activation. Heart Fail Rev. 2005;10(1):15–22.
173. Funder JW. Mineralocorticoid receptor activation and oxidative stress. Hypertension. 2007; 50(5):840–1.
174. Frey FJ, Odermatt A, Frey BM. Glucocorticoid-mediated mineralocorticoid receptor activation and hypertension. Curr Opin Nephrol Hypertens. 2004;13(4):451–8.
175. Mihailidou AS, Le Loan TY, Mardini M, Funder JW. Glucocorticoids activate cardiac mineralocorticoid receptors during experimental myocardial infarction. Hypertension. 2009;54(6): 1306–12.
176. Gomez-Sanchez EP. The mammalian mineralocorticoid receptor: tying down a promiscuous receptor. Exp Physiol. 2010;95(1):13–8.
177. Gomez-Sanchez CE, Zhou MY, Cozza EN, Morita H, Eddleman FC, Gomez-Sanchez EP. Corticosteroid synthesis in the central nervous system. Endocr Res. 1996;22:463–70.
178. Gomez-Sanchez CE, Zhou MY, Cozza EN, Morita H, Foecking MF, Gomez-Sanchez EP. Aldosterone biosynthesis in the rat brain. Endocrinology. 1997;138:3369–73.
179. Gomez-Sanchez EP, Gomez-Sanchez CE. Central hypertensinogenic effects of glycyrrhizic acid and carbenoxolone. Am J Physiol. 1992;263:E1125–30.
180. Gomez-Sanchez EP, Gomez-Sanchez CE. Maternal hypertension and progeny blood pressure: role of aldosterone and 11β-HSD. Hypertension. 1999;33:1369–73.
181. Roland BL, Li KX, Funder JW. Hybridization histochemical localization of 11 beta-hydroxysteroid dehydrogenase type 2 in rat brain. Endocrinology. 1995;136(10):4697–700.
182. De Kloet ER, Van Acker SA, Sibug RM, et al. Brain mineralocorticoid receptors and centrally regulated functions. Kidney Int. 2000;57:1329–36.
183. Karssen AM, Meijer O, Pons D, De Kloet ER. Localization of mRNA expression of P-glycoprotein at the blood-brain barrier and in the hippocampus. Ann N Y Acad Sci. 2004;1032:308–11.
184. Karssen AM, Meijer OC, van der Sandt IC, et al. Multidrug resistance P-glycoprotein hampers the access of cortisol but not of corticosterone to mouse and human brain. Endocrinology. 2001;142(6):2686–94.
185. Karssen AM, Meijer OC, van der Sandt IC, De Boer AG, De Lange EC, De Kloet ER. The role of the efflux transporter P-glycoprotein in brain penetration of prednisolone. J Endocrinol. 2002;175(1):251–60.
186. Gomez-Sanchez EP, Gomez-Sanchez CE. Is aldosterone synthesized in the CNS regulated and functional? Trends Endocrinol Metab. 2003;14(10):444–6.
187. Selye H. The anesthetic effect of steroid hormones. Proc Soc Exp Biol Med. 1941;46:116–21.
188. Le Goascogne C, Robel P, Gouézou M, Sananes N, Baulieu E, Waterman M. Neurosteroids: cytochrome P-450scc in Rat Brain. Science. 1987;237:1212–5.
189. Mellon SH, Deschepper CF. Neurosteroid biosynthesis: genes for adrenal steroidogenic enzymes are expressed in the brain. Brain Res. 1993;629:283–92.
190. MacKenzie SM, Clark CJ, Ingram MC, et al. Corticosteroid production by fetal rat hippocampal neurons. Endocr Res. 2000;26(4):531–5.
191. Yu L, Romero DG, Gomez-Sanchez CE, Gomez-Sanchez EP. Steroidogenic enzyme gene expression in the human brain. Mol Cell Endocrinol. 2002;190(1–2):9–17.
192. King SR, Manna PR, Ishii T, et al. An essential component in steroid synthesis, the steroidogenic acute regulatory protein, is expressed in discrete regions of the brain. J Neurosci. 2002;22(24):10613–20.
193. Gomez-Sanchez EP, Ahmad N, Romero DG, Gomez-Sanchez CE. Is aldosterone synthesized within the rat brain? Am J Physiol Endocrinol Metab. 2005;288(2):E342–6.
194. MacKenzie SM, Clark CJ, Fraser R, Gomez-Sanchez CE, Connell JMC, Davies E. Expression of 11b-hydroxylase and aldosterone synthase genes in rat brain. J Mol Endocrinol. 2000;24:321–8.

195. Gomez-Sanchez EP, Fort C, Thwaites D. Central mineralocorticoid receptor antagonism blocks hypertension in Dahl S/JR rats. Am J Physiol. 1992;262:E96–9.
196. Gomez-Sanchez EP, Samuel J, Vergara G, Ahmad N. Effect of 3{beta}-hydroxysteroid dehydrogenase inhibition by trilostane on blood pressure in the Dahl salt-sensitive rat. Am J Physiol Regul Integr Comp Physiol. 2005;288(2):R389–93.
197. Sandberg K, Ji H, Catt KJ. Regulation of angiotensin II receptors in rat brain during dietary sodium changes. Hypertension. 1994;23:I137–41.
198. Jo H, Yang EK, Lee WJ, Park KY, Kim HJ, Park JS. Gene expression of central and peripheral renin-angiotensin system components upon dietary sodium intake in rats. Regul Pept. 1996;67:115–21.
199. Ye P, Kenyon CJ, MacKenzie SM, et al. Regulation of aldosterone synthase gene expression in the rat adrenal gland and central nervous system by sodium and angiotensin II. Endocrinology. 2003;144(8):3321–8.
200. Huang BS, White RA, Jeng AY, Leenen FH. Role of central nervous system aldosterone synthase and mineralocorticoid receptors in salt-induced hypertension in Dahl salt-sensitive rats. Am J Physiol Regul Integr Comp Physiol. 2009;296(4):R994–1000.
201. Hochberg RB, Pahuja SL, Zielinski JE, Larner JM. Steroidal fatty acid esters. J Steroid Biochem Mol Biol. 1991;40:577–85.
202. Borg W, Shackleton CH, Pahuja SL, Hochberg RB. Long-lived testosterone esters in the rat. Proc Natl Acad Sci U S A. 1995;92(5):1545–9.
203. Hochberg RB. Biological esterification of steroids. Endocr Rev. 1998;19(3):331–48.
204. Pahuja SL, Zielinski JE, Giordano G, McMurray WJ, Hochberg RB. The biosynthesis of d-ring fatty acid esters of estriol. J Biol Chem. 1991;266(12):7410–6.
205. Petrazzuoli M, Pahuja SL, Larner JM, Hochberg RB. Biological activity of the fatty acid ester metabolites of corticoids. Endocrinology. 1990;127:555–9.
206. Lockett MF, Retallack RW. The influence of heart rate on the secretion of a substance closely resembling the 18-monoacetate of D-aldosterone by the hearts of cats under chloralose anaesthesia. J Physiol. 1970;208:21–32.
207. Lockett MF. Changes in the flow and composition of the urine induced by the 18 monoacetate of D-aldosterone, in cats. J Physiol. 1969;202:671–82.
208. Lockett MF. Hormonal actions of the heart and of lungs on the isolated kidney. J Physiol. 1967;193:661–79.
209. Gomez-Sanchez CE, Foecking MF, Gomez-Sanchez EP. Aldosterone esters and the heart. Am J Hypertens. 2001;14:200S–5.
210. Pearce D, Naray-Fejes-Toth A, Fejes-Toth G. Determinants of subnuclear organization of mineralocorticoid receptor characterized through analysis of wild type and mutant receptors. J Biol Chem. 2002;277(2):1451–6.
211. Lombes M, Farman N, Oblin ME. Immunohistochemical localization of renal mineralocorticoid receptor by using an anti-idiotypic antibody that is an internal image of aldosterone. Proc Natl Acad Sci. 1990;87:1086–8.
212. Couette B, Fagart J, Jalaguier S, Lombes M, Souque A, Rafestin-Oblin ME. Ligand-induced conformational change in the human mineralocorticoid receptor occurs within its hetero-oligomeric structure. Biochem J. 1996;315:421–7.
213. Fejes-Toth G, Pearce D, Naray-Fejes-Toth A. Subcellular localization of mineralocorticoid receptors in living cells: effects of receptor agonists and antagonists. Proc Natl Acad Sci USA. 1998;95:2973–8.
214. Pilipuk GP, Vinson GP, Gomez-Sanchez CE, Galigniana MD. Evidence for NL1-independent nuclear translocation of the mineralocorticoid receptor. Biochemistry. 2007;46(5):1389–97.
215. Trapp T, Holsboer F. Ligand-induced conformational changes in the mineralocorticoid receptor analyzed by protease mapping. Biochem Biophys Res Commun. 1995;215:286–91.
216. Rupprecht R, Arriza J, Spengler D, et al. Transactivation and synergistic properties of the mineralocorticoid receptor: relationship to the glucocorticoid receptor. Mol Endocrinol. 1993;7:597–603.

217. Meijer OC, Steenbergen PJ, De Kloet ER. Differential expression and regional distribution of steroid receptor coactivators SRC-1 and SRC-2 in brain and pituitary. Endocrinology. 2000;141(6):2192–9.
218. Pascual-Le Tallec L, Lombes M. The mineralocorticoid receptor: a journey exploring its diversity and specificity of action. Mol Endocrinol. 2005;19(9):2211–21.
219. Stanisic V, Lonard DM, O'Malley BW. Modulation of steroid hormone receptor activity. Prog Brain Res. 2010;181:153–76.

Index

C.A. Koch and G.P. Chrousos (eds.), *Endocrine Hypertension: Underlying Mechanisms and Therapy*, Contemporary Endocrinology, DOI 10.1007/978-1-60761-548-4,

Made in the USA
Las Vegas, NV
16 September 2026

ad3440e3-2abb-426b-83c4-586804c1cc2cR04